MEDICINAL CHEMISTRY: AN INTRODUCTION

Edited by
Levitah Castil Mapatac

Delve Publishing

Medicinal Chemistry: An Introduction

Edited by Levitah Castil Mapatac

Edition 2018

Delve Publishing

Published by

Delve Publishing LLC

708 3rd Avenue, 6th Floor

New York

NY 10801

United States of America

www.delvepublishing.com

ISBN: 978-1-68095-725-9 (Hardback)

Printed in United States of America

Library of Congress Control Number: 2016920405

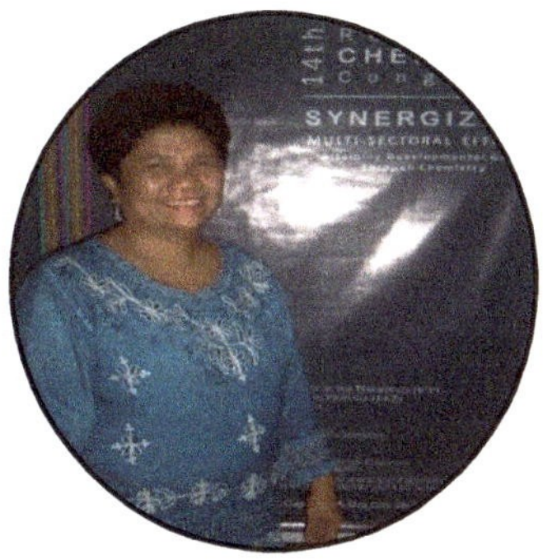

About the Editor

Levitah Castil Mapatac

Levitah C. Mapatac is an Associate Professor, researcher, writer and a PhD holder from the University in Science and Technology of Southern Philippines. Her interest varies from different chemistry concepts and applications and currently doing research in traditional medicines, water waste pollution and environmental chemistry in the aspect of contamination pathways, profilling and rehabilatation of mining waste.

Table of Contents

3 PROCESS OF DRUG DISCOVERY

4 PERSONALIZED MEDICINE

5 DRUG DESIGN

6 TARGETED DRUG DELIVERY: METHODS AND APPLICATIONS

7 MECHANISM AND MODE OF ACTION

8 DRUG CLASS

9 PHARMACODYNAMICS AND PHARMACOKINETICS

10 PHARMACOLOGY

11 ENZYME INHIBITOR AND LIGAND EFFICIENCY

List of Abbreviations

ANDA	Abbreviated New Drug Application
ARMD	Age Related Macular Degeneration
ACE	Angiotensin Converting Enzyme
BEI	Binding Efficiency Index
CCB	Calcium Channel Blockers
CNS	Central Nervous System
CDS	Chemical Delivery Systems
CMC	Chemistry, Manufacturing, and Control
CML	Chronic Myeloid Leukemia
DAT	Dopamine Transporter
DLS	Dynamic Light Scattering
FDA	Food and Drug Administration
FBLD	Fragment Based Lead Discovery
GAD	Generalized Anxiety Disorder
GIVE	Generic Initiative for Value and Efficiency
GINA	Genetic Information Nondiscrimination Act
GWAS	Genome Wide Association Study
GLP	Good Laboratory Practices
HTS	High Throughput Screening
ITC	Isothermal Titration Calorimetry
LE	Ligand Efficiency
MOA	Mechanism of Action
MST	Microscale Thermophoresis

MOA	Mode of Action
MCPD	Multicellular Pharmacodynamics
NDA	New Drug Application
NME	New Molecular Entity
NOAC	Novel Oral Anticoagulants
NMR	Nuclear Magnetic Resonance
OCD	Obsessive Compulsive Disorder
OCFS	Open Cell Free Synthesis
PBP	Penicillin Binding Proteins
PAE	Post Antibiotic Effect
RES	Reticuloendothelial System
SNRI	Serotonin Norepinephrine Reuptake Inhibitor
SAR	Structural Activity Relationship
SPR	Surface Plasmon Resonance
SEI	Surface Binding Efficiency Index
SIADH	Syndrome of Inappropriate Antidiuretic Hormone
SILENT	Syndrome of Irreversible Lithium Effected Neurotoxicity
TCM	Traditional Chinese Medicine
VS	Virtual screening

Preface

Medicinal chemistry is the application of biology and chemistry to the design of new drugs for treating disease. It is the chemistry discipline concerned with the design, development and synthesis of pharmaceutical drugs. The discipline combines expertise from chemistry and pharmacology to identify, develop and synthesize chemical agents that have a therapeutic use and to evaluate the properties of existing drugs. Medicinal chemists apply their chemistry training to the process of synthesizing new pharmaceuticals. They also improve the processes by which existing pharmaceuticals are made. Medicinal chemists are focused on drug discovery and development and are concerned with the isolation of medicinal agents found in plants, as well as the creation of new synthetic drug compounds. Most chemists work with a team of scientists from different disciplines, including biologists, toxicologists, pharmacologists, theoretical chemists, microbiologists, and biopharmacists. Medicinal chemistry is a stimulating field as it links many scientific disciplines and allows for collaboration with other scientists in researching and developing new drugs. In particular, medicinal chemistry in its most common practice —focusing on small organic molecules—encompasses synthetic organic chemistry and aspects of natural products and computational chemistry in close combination with chemical biology, enzymology and structural biology, together aiming at the discovery and development of new therapeutic agents. Practically speaking, it involves chemical aspects of identification, and then systematic, thorough synthetic alteration of new chemical entities to make them suitable for therapeutic use. It includes synthetic and computational aspects of the study of existing drugs and agents in development in relation to their bioactivities, i.e., understanding their structure-activity relationships. Pharmaceutical chemistry is focused on quality aspects of medicines and aims to assure fitness for purpose of medicinal products. This book provides an introduction to medicinal chemistry. It covers basic principles and background, and describes the general tactics and strategies involved in effective drug design and development.

Content Coverage

Chapter One is intended to provide an overview of medicinal chemistry and its applications in the path of drug discovery.

Chapters Two provides the features of chemogenomics, an emerging discipline that combines the latest tools of genomics and chemistry and applies them to target and drug discovery.

Chapters Three and *Four* discuss about the process of drug discovery and personalized medicine procedures that separates patients into different groups—with medical decisions, practices, interventions and/or products being tailored to the individual patient based on their predicted response or risk of disease, respectively.

Chapter Five and *Six* present the approaches of drug design and smart drug delivery system. The drug delivery system is highly integrated and requires various disciplines, such as chemists, biologist and engineers, to join forces to optimize this system.

Chapters Seven is mechanism and mode of action that describes the process by which a molecule, such as a drug, functions to produce a pharmacological effect. A drug's mechanism of action may refer to its effects on a biological readout such as cell growth, or its interaction and modulation of its direct biomolecular target.

Chapter Eight and *Nine* discusses about drug class and the study of the biochemical and physiologic effects of drugs, separately.

Chapter Ten and *Eleven* provides the knowledge of drug action on biological systems and enzyme inhibitors molecules, correspondingly. Many drug molecules are enzyme inhibitors, so their discovery and improvement is an active area of knowledge in pharmacology.

CHAPTER 1

Introduction to Medicinal Chemistry

Chapter Contents

Medicinal chemistry involves the application of a number of specialized disciplinary approaches all focused on the ultimate goal of drug discovery. Drug target identification and validation, rational (target-based) drug design, structural biology, computational-based drug design, methods development (chemical, biochemical, and computational), and "Hit-to-lead" development are all aspects of medicinal chemistry. The techniques and approaches of chemical biology, synthetic organic chemistry, combinatorial (bio)chemistry, mechanistic enzymology, computational chemistry, chemical genomics, and high-throughput screening process are all applied and used by medicinal chemists towards drug discovery.

INTRODUCTION

Medicinal chemistry and pharmaceutical chemistry are disciplines at the intersection of chemistry, especially synthetic organic chemistry, and pharmacology and various other biological specialties, where they are involved with design, chemical synthesis and development for market of pharmaceutical agents, or bio-active molecules (drugs).

Compounds used as medicines are most often organic compounds, which are often divided into the broad classes of small organic molecules (e.g., atorvastatin, fluticasone, clopidogrel) and "biologics" (infliximab, erythropoietin, insulin glargine), the latter of which are most often medicinal preparations of proteins (natural and recombinant antibodies, hormones, etc.). Inorganic and organometallic compounds are also useful as drugs (e.g., lithium and platinum-based agents such as lithium carbonate and cis-platin as well as gallium).

In particular, medicinal chemistry in its most common practice —focusing on small organic molecules—encompasses synthetic organic chemistry and aspects of natural products and computational chemistry in close combination with chemical biology, enzymology and structural biology, together aiming at the discovery and development of new therapeutic agents. Practically speaking, it involves chemical aspects of identification, and then systematic, thorough synthetic alteration of new chemical entities to make them suitable for therapeutic use. It includes synthetic and computational aspects of the study of existing drugs and agents in development in relation to their bioactivities (biological activities and properties), i.e., understanding their structure-activity relationships (SAR). Pharmaceutical chemistry is focused on quality aspects of medicines and aims to assure fitness for purpose of medicinal products.

At the biological interface, medicinal chemistry combines to form a set of highly interdisciplinary sciences, setting its organic, physical, and computational emphasis alongside biological areas such as biochemistry, molecular biology, pharmacognosy and pharmacology, toxicology and veterinary and human medicine along with project management, statistics, and pharmaceutical business practices, systematically oversee altering identified chemical agents such that after pharmaceutical formulation, they are safe and efficacious, and therefore suitable for use in treatment of disease.

MEDICINAL CHEMISTRY IN THE PATH OF DRUG DISCOVERY

Discovery

Discovery is the identification of novel active chemical compounds, often called "hits" which are typically found by assay of compounds for a desired biological activity. Initial hits can come from repurposing existing agents toward a new pathologic processes, and from observations of biologic effects of new or existing natural products from bacteria, fungi, plants, etc. In addition, hits also routinely originate from structural observations of small molecule "fragments" bound to therapeutic (enzymes, receptors, etc.) where the fragments serve as starting points to develop more chemically complex forms by synthesis. Finally, hits also regularly originate from *en-masse* testing of chemical compounds against biological targets, where the compounds may be from novel synthetic chemical libraries known to have particular properties (kinase inhibitory activity, diversity or drug-likeness, etc.) or from historic chemical compound collections or libraries created through combinatorial chemistry. While a number of approaches toward the identification and development of hits exist, the most successful techniques are based on chemical and biological intuition developed in team environments through years of rigorous practice aimed solely at discovering new therapeutic agents.

Hit to Lead and lead Optimization

Further chemistry and analysis is necessary, first to identify the "triage" compounds that do not provide series displaying suitable SAR and chemical characteristics associated with long-term potential for development, then to improve remaining hit series with regard to the desired primary activity, as well as secondary activities and physiochemical properties such that the agent will be useful when administered in real patients. In this regard, chemical modifications can improve the recognition and binding geometries (pharmacophores) of the candidate compounds, and so their affinities for their targets, as well as improving the physicochemical properties of the molecule that underlie necessary pharmacokinetic/pharmacodynamic (PK/PD), and toxicologic profiles (stability toward metabolic degradation, lack of geno-, hepatic, and cardiac toxicities, etc.) such that the chemical compound or biologic is suitable for introduction into animal and human studies.

Process Chemistry and Development

The final synthetic chemistry stages involves the production of a lead compound in suitable quantity and quality to allow large scale animal testing, and then human clinical trials. This involves the optimization of the synthetic route for bulk industrial production, and discovery of the most suitable drug formulation. The former of these is still the bailiwick of medicinal chemistry, the latter brings in the specialization of formulation science (with its components of physical and polymer chemistry and materials science). The synthetic chemistry specialization in medicinal chemistry aimed in the adaptation and optimization of the synthetic route for industrial scale syntheses by hundreds of kilograms or more is termed process synthesis, and involves thorough knowledge of acceptable synthetic practice in the context of large scale reactions (reaction thermodynamics, economics, safety, etc.). Critical at this stage is the transition to more stringent GMP requirements for material sourcing, handling, and chemistry.

TRAINING IN MEDICINAL CHEMISTRY

Medicinal chemistry is by nature an interdisciplinary science, and practitioners have a strong background in organic chemistry, which must eventually be coupled with a broad understanding of biological concepts related to cellular drug targets. Scientists in the field of medicinal chemistry can be classified as industrial scientist and can work together in an interdisciplinary team applying his/her expertize in chemistry ability, synthetic ability using chemistry principles inorder to design effective therapeutic agents. The length of training is intense with practitioners often required to attain a 4-year bachelor's followed by a 4-6 year Ph.D. in organic chemistry. Most training regimens include a postdoctoral fellowship period of 2 or more years after receiving a Ph.D. in chemistry making the length of training ranging from *10-12* years of college education. However, employment opportunities at the Master's graduate can be employed in pharmaceutical industries while the Ph.D. graduates will have a better opportunities in the academe either in the private and government sector. Many medicinal chemists, particularly in academia and research, also earn a Pharm.D (doctor of pharmacy). Some of these PharmD/PhD researchers are RPh's (Registered Pharmacists).

Graduate level programs in medicinal chemistry can be found in traditional medicinal chemistry or pharmaceutical sciences departments, departments associated with the schools of pharmarcy and chemistry divisions. However, the majority of working medicinal chemists have graduate degrees (MS, but especially Ph.D.) in organic chemistry, rather than medicinal chemistry, and the preponderance of positions are in discovery where the net is necessarily cast the widest and most broadest synthetic activity occurs.

In the discovery of small molecule therapeutics wherein an emphasis was given on the trainings and breadth of experience of an individual in the application of synthetic and natural products in the doctoral and post doctoral positions. (e.g., for individuals with pure synthetic organic and natural products synthesis in Ph.D. and post-doctoral positions, ibid.). In the medicinal chemistry specialty areas associated with the design and synthesis of chemical libraries or the execution of process chemistry aimed at viable commercial syntheses (areas generally with fewer opportunities), training paths are often much more varied (e.g., including focused training in physical organic chemistry, library-related syntheses, etc.). Most entry level workers in medicinal chemistry especially in U.S. has no formal trainings in medicinal chemistry but had received the necessary background of employment in medicinal and pharmacologic chemistry applications. formal training in medicinal chemistry but receive the necessary medicinal chemistry and pharmacologic background after employment—at entry into their work in a pharmaceutical company, where the company provides its particular understanding or model of "medichem" training through active involvement in practical synthesis on therapeutic projects. (The same is somewhat true of computational medicinal chemistry specialties, but not to the same degree as in synthetic areas.)

REFERENCES

1. Hughes, Jp; Rees, S; Kalindjian, Sb; Philpott, Kl (2011-03-01). "Principles of early drug discovery". British Journal of Pharmacology. 162 (6): 1239–1249. doi:10.1111/j.1476-5381.2010.01127.x. ISSN 1476-5381. PMC 3058157Freely accessible. PMID 21091654.
2. Johnston, Kelly L.; Ford, Louise; Umareddy, Indira; Townson, Simon; Specht, Sabine; Pfarr, Kenneth; Hoerauf, Achim; Altmeyer, Ralf; Taylor, Mark J. (2014-12-01). "Repurposing of approved drugs from the human pharmacopoeia to target Wolbachia endosymbionts of onchocerciasis and lymphatic filariasis". International Journal for Parasitology: Drugs and Drug Resistance. Includes articles from two meetings: "Anthelmintics: From Discovery to Resistance", pp. 218--315, and "Global Challenges for New Drug Discovery Against Tropical Parasitic Diseases", pp. 316--357. 4 (3): 278–286. doi:10.1016/j.ijpddr.2014.09.001. PMC 4266796Freely accessible. PMID 25516838.
3. Harvey, Alan L. (2008-10-01). "Natural products in drug discovery". Drug Discovery Today. 13 (19–20): 894–901. doi:10.1016/j.drudis.2008.07.004.
4. Cragg, Gordon M.; Newman, David J. (2013-06-01). "Natural products: A continuing source of novel drug leads". Biochimica et Biophysica Acta (BBA) - General Subjects. 1830 (6): 3670–3695. doi:10.1016/j.bbagen.2013.02.008. PMC 3672862Freely accessible. PMID 23428572.

CHAPTER 2

Chemogenomics: Strategy and Applications

Chapter Contents

- **Introduction**
- **Medicinal Chemistry in the Path of Drug Discovery**
- **Training in Medicinal Chemistry**

Chemogenomics is an emerging discipline that combines the latest tools of genomics and chemistry and applies them to target and drug discovery. Its strength lies in eliminating the bottleneck that currently occurs in target identification by measuring the broad, conditional effects of chemical libraries on whole biological systems or by screening large chemical libraries quickly and efficiently against selected targets. The hope in chemogenomics will shed light in the identification and validation of therapeutic targets that can detect drug candidates that will rapidly and effectively generate new treatments and other applications for many human diseases.

INTRODUCTION

Chemogenomics, or chemical genomics, is the systematic screening of targeted chemical libraries of small molecules against individual drug target families (e.g., GPCRs, nuclear receptors, kinases, proteases, etc.) with the ultimate goal of identification of novel drugs and drug targets. Typically some members of a target library have been well characterized where both the functions has been determined and compounds that modulate the function of those targets (ligands in the case of receptors, inhibitors of enzymes, or blockers of ion channels) have been identified. Other members of the target family may have unknown functions with no known ligands can be classified as orphan receptors. By identifying screening hits that modulate the activity of the less well characterized members of the target family, the function of these novel targets can be elucidated. Furthermore, the hits for these targets can be used as a starting point for drug discovery. The completion of the human genome project has provided an abundant potential targets for therapeutic interventions. Chemogenomics strives to study the intersection of all possible in all the aspect of the potential targets.

A common method to construct a targeted chemical library is to include known ligands of at least one and preferably several members of the target family. Since a portion of ligands that were designed and synthesized to bind to one family member will also bind to additional family members, the compounds contained in a targeted chemical library should collectively bind to a high percentage of the target family.

STRATEGY

Chemogenomics integrates target and drug discovery by using active compounds, which function as ligands, as probes to characterize proteome functions. The interaction between a small compound and a protein induces a phenotype. Once the phenotype is characterized , this could be associated to a protein molecular events. Compared with genetics, chemogenomics techniques are able to modify the function of a protein rather than the gene. Also, chemogenomics is able to observe the interaction as well as reversibility in real-time. For example, the modification of a phenotype can be observed only after addition of a specific compound and can be interrupted after its withdrawal from the medium.

Currently, there are two experimental chemogenomic approaches: forward (classical) chemogenomics and reverse chemogenomics. Forward chemogenomics attempts to identify drug targets by searching for molecules which give a certain phenotype on cells or animals, while reverse chemogenomics aims to validate phenotypes by searching for molecules that interact specifically with a given protein. Both of these approaches requires a suitable collection of compounds and an appropriate model system for screening the compounds and looking for the parallel identification of biological targets and biologically active compounds. The biologically active compounds that are discovered through forward or reverse chemogenomics approaches are known as "modulators" because they bind to and modulate specific molecular targets thus, they could be used as "targeted therapeutics".

Forward Chemogenomics

In forward chemogenomics, which is also known as classical chemogenomics, a particular phenotype is studied and small compound interacting with this function are identified. The molecular basis of this desired phenotype is unknown. Once the modulators have been identified, they will be used as tools to look for the protein responsible for the phenotype. For example, a loss-of-function phenotype could be an arrest of tumor growth. Once a compound that lead to a target phenotype have been identified, identifying the gene and protein targets should be the next step. The main challenge of forward chemogenomics strategy lies in designing phenotypic assays that lead immediately from screening to target identification.

Reverse Chemogenomics

In reverse chemogenomics, small compounds that perturb the function of an enzyme in the context of an in vitro enzymatic test will be identified. Once the modulators have been identified, the phenotype induced by the molecule is analyzed in a test on cells or on whole organisms. This method will identify or confirm the role of the enzyme in the biological response. Reverse chemogenomics used to be virtually identical to the target-base approaches that have been applied in drug discovery and molecular pharmacology over the past decades. This strategy is now enhanced by parallel screening and by the ability to perform lead optimization on many targets that belong to one target family.

Applications

Determining Mode of Action

Chemogenomics has been used to identify mode of action (MOA) for traditional Chinese medicine (TCM) and Ayurveda. Compounds contained in traditional medicines are usually more soluble than synthetic compounds, have "privileged structures" (chemical structures that are more frequently found to bind in different living organisms), and have more comprehensively known safety and tolerance factors. Therefore, this makes them especially attractive as a resource for lead structures in when developing new molecular entities. Databases containing chemical structures of compounds used in alternative medicine along with their phenotypic effects, in silico analysis may be of use to assist in determining MOA for example, by predicting ligand targets that were relevant to known phenotypes for traditional medicines. In a case study for TCM, the therapeutic class of 'toning and replenishing medicine" was evaluated. Therapeutic actions (or phenotypes) for that class include anti-inflammatory, antioxidant, neuroprotective, hypoglycemic activity, immunomodulatory, antimetastatic, and hypotensive. Sodium-glucose transport proteins and PTP1B (an insulin signaling regulator) were identified as targets which link to the hypoglycemic phenotype suggested. The case study for Ayurveda involved anti-cancer formulations. In this case, the target prediction program enriched for targets directly connected to cancer progression such as steroid-5-alpha-reductase and synergistic targets like the efflux pump P-gp. These target-phenotype links can help identify novel MOAs.

Beyond TCM and Ayurveda, chemogenomics can be applied early in drug discovery to determine a compound's mechanism of action and take advantage of genomic biomarkers of toxicity and efficacy for application to Phase I and II clinical trials.

Identifying New Drug Targets

Chemogenomics profiling can be used to identify totally new therapeutic targets, for example new antibacterial agents. The study capitalized on the availability of an existing ligand library for an enzyme called murD that is used in the peptidoglycan synthesis pathway. Relying on the chemogenomics similarity principle, the researchers mapped the murD ligand library to other members of the mur ligase family (murC, murE, murF, murA, and murG) to identify new targets for the known ligands. Ligands identified would be expected to be broad-spectrum Gram-negative inhibitors in experimental assays since peptidoglycan synthesis is exclusive to bacteria. Structural and molecular docking studies revealed candidate ligands for murC and murE ligases.

Identifying Genes in Biological Pathway

Thirty years after the post translationally modified histidine derivative diphthamide was determined, chemogenomics was used to discover the enzyme responsible for the final step in its synthesis. Dipthamide is a post translationally modified histidine residue found on the translation elongation factor 2 (eEF-2). The first two steps of the biosynthesis pathway leading to dipthine have been known, but the enzyme responsible for the amidation of dipthine to diphthamide remained a mystery. The researchers capitalized on Saccharomyces cerevisiae cofitness data. Cofitness data is data representing the similarity of growth fitness under various conditions between any two different deletion strains. Under the assumption that strains lacking the diphthamide synthetase gene should have high cofitness with strain lacking other diphthamide biosynthesis genes, they identified ylr143w as the strain with the highest cofitness to the all other strains lacking known diphthamide biosynthesis genes. Subsequent experimental assays confirmed that YLR143W was required for diphthamide synthesis and was the missing diphthamide synthetase.

CHEMICAL GENETICS

Chemical genetics is the investigation of the function of proteins and signal transduction pathways in cells by the screening of chemical libraries of small molecules. Chemical genetics is analogous to classical genetic screen where random mutations are introduced in organisms, the phenotype of these mutants is observed, and finally the specific gene mutation (genotype) that produced that phenotype is identified. In chemical genetics, the phenotype is disturbed not by introduction of mutations, but by exposure to small molecule tool compounds. Phenotypic screening of chemical libraries is used to identify drug targets (forward genetics) or to validate those targets in experimental models of disease (reverse genetics). Recent applications of this topic have been implicated in signal transduction, which may play a role in discovering new cancer treatments. Chemical genetics can serves as a unifying study between chemistry and biology.

Method

Chemical genetic screens are preformed using libraries of small molecules that have known activities or simply diverse chemical structures. These screens can be done in a high-throughput mode, using 96 well-plates, where each well contains cells treated with a unique compound. In addition to cells, *Xenopus* or zebrafish embryos can also be screened in 96 well format where compounds are dissolved in the media in which embryos grow. Embryos are let developed until the stage of interest and then the phenotype can be analyzed. Several concentrations can be tested in order to determine the toxic and the optimal concentrations.

Applications

Adding compounds to developing embryos allow comprehension of mechanism of action of drugs, their toxicity and developmental processes involving their targets. Chemical screens have been mostly performed on either wild type or transgenic *Xenopus* and zebrafish organisms as they produce a large amount of synchronized, fast-to-develop and transparent eggs easy to visually score. The use of chemicals in developmental biology offers two main advantages. Firstly, it is easy to perform high-throughput screen using wide spectrum or specific target compounds and reveal important genes or pathways involved in developmental processes. Secondly, it allows narrowing the time of action of a particular gene. It can also be used as a tool in drug development to test toxicity in whole organism. Procedures such as FETAX (Frog Embryo Teratogenesis Assay – Xenopus) are being developed to implement chemical screenings to test toxicity.Zebrafish and *Xenopus* embryos have also been used to identify new drugs targeting a particular gene of interest.

HIGH-THROUGHPUT SCREENING

High-throughput screening (HTS) is a method for scientific experimentation especially used in drug discovery and relevant to the fields of biology and chemistry. Using robotics, data processing and control software, liquid handling devices, and sensitive detectors, high-throughput screening allows a researcher to quickly conduct millions of chemical, genetic, or pharmacological tests. Through this process one can rapidly identify active compounds, antibodies, or genes that modulate a particular biomolecular pathway. The results of these experiments provide a starting points for drug design and for understanding the interaction or role of a particular biochemical process in biology.

Assay Plate Preparation

The key labware or testing vessel of HTS is the microtiter plate: a small container, usually disposable and made of plastic, that features a grid of small, open divots called *wells*. In general, modern (circa 2013) microplates for HTS have either 384, 1536, or 3456 wells. These are all multiples of 96, reflecting the original 96-well microplate with spaced wells of 8 x 12 9 mm . Most of the wells contain test items, depending on the nature of the experiment. These could be different chemical compounds dissolved e.g. in an aqueous solution of dimethyl sulfoxide (DMSO). The wells could also contain cells or enzymes of some type. (The other wells may be empty or contain pure solvent or untreated samples, intended for use as experimental controls.)

A screening facility typically holds a library of *stock plates*, whose contents are carefully catalogued, and each of which may have been created by the lab or obtained from a commercial source. These stock plates themselves are not directly used in experiments instead a separate *assay plates* are created as needed. An assay plate is simply a copy of a stock plate, created by pipetting a small amount of liquid (often measured in nanoliters) from the wells of a stock plate to the corresponding wells of a completely empty plate.

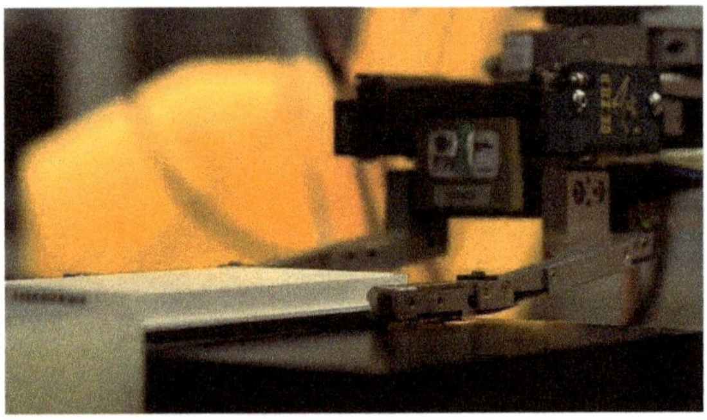

A robot arm handles an assay plate

Reaction Observation

To prepare for an assay, the researcher fills each well of the plate with some biological entity that they wish to conduct the experiment upon, such as a protein, cells, or an animal embryo. After some incubation time has passed to allow the biological matter to absorb, bind to, or otherwise react (or fail to react) with the compounds in the wells, measurements are taken across all the plate's wells, either manually or by a machine. Manual measurements are often necessary when the researcher is using microscopy to (for example) seek changes or defects in embryonic development caused by the well's compounds, looking for effects that a computer could not easily determine by itself. Otherwise, a specialized automated analysis machine can run a number of experiments on the wells (such as shining polarized light on them and measuring reflectivity, which can be an indication of protein binding). In this case, the machine outputs the result of each experiment as a grid of numeric values, with each number mapping to the value obtained from a single well. A high-capacity analysis machine can measure dozens of plates in the space of a few minutes like this, generating thousands of experimental data points at a high speed..

Depending on the results of this first assay, the researcher can perform follow up assays within the same screen by "cherrypicking" liquid from the source wells that gave interesting results (known as "hits") into new assay plates, and then re-running the experiment to collect further data on this narrowed set, confirming and refining observations.

Automation systems

Automation is an important element in HTS's usefulness. Typically, an integrated robot system consisting of one or more robots transports assay-microplates from station to station for sample and reagent addition, mixing, incubation, and finally readout or detection.

An HTS system can usually prepare, incubate, and analyze many plates simultaneously, further speeding the data-collection process. HTS robots that can test up to 100,000 compounds per day currently exist. Automatic colony pickers pick thousands of microbial colonies for high throughput genetic screening. The term uHTS or *ultra-high-throughput screening* refers (circa 2008) to screening in excess of 100,000 compounds per day.

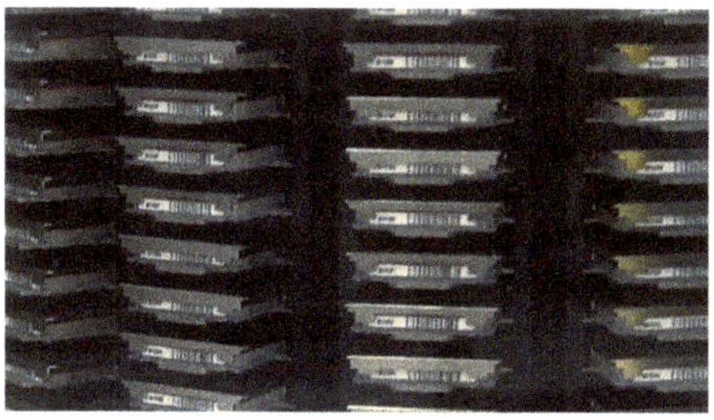

A carousel system to store assay plates for high storage capacity and high speed access

Experimental Design and Data Analysis

With the ability of rapid screening of diverse compounds (such as small molecules or siRNAs) to identify active compounds, HTS has led to an explosion in the rate of data generated in recent years. Consequently, one of the most fundamental challenges in HTS experiments is to glean biochemical significance from mounds of data, which relies on the development and adoption of appropriate experimental designs and analytic methods for both quality control and hit selection. HTS research is one of the fields that have a feature described by John Blume, Chief Science Officer for Applied Proteomics, Inc. Soon, if a scientist does not understand some statistics or rudimentary data-handling technologies, he or she may not be considered to be a true molecular biologist and, thus, will simply become "a dinosaur."

Quality Control

High-quality HTS assays are critical in HTS experiments. The development of high-quality HTS assays requires the integration of both experimental and computational approaches for quality control (QC). Three important means of QC are (i) good plate design, (ii) the selection of effective positive and negative chemical/biological controls, and (iii) the development of effective QC metrics to measure the degree of differentiation so that assays with inferior data quality can be identified. A good plate design helps to identify systematic errors (especially those linked with well position) and determine what normalization should be used to remove/reduce the impact of systematic errors on both QC and hit selection.

Effective analytic QC methods serve as a gatekeeper for excellent quality assays. In a typical HTS experiment, a clear distinction between a positive control and a negative reference such as a negative control is an index for good quality. Many quality-assessment measures have been proposed to measure the degree of differentiation between a positive control and a negative reference. Signal-to-background ratio, signal-to-noise ratio, signal window, assay variability ratio, and Z-factor have been adopted to evaluate data quality. Strictly standardized mean difference (SSMD) has recently been proposed for assessing data quality in HTS assays.

Hit Selection

A compound with a desired size of effects in an HTS is called a "hit". The process of selecting hits is called hit selection. The analytic methods for hit selection in screens without replicates (usually in primary screens) differ from those with replicates (usually in confirmatory screens). For example, the z-score method is suitable for screens without replicates whereas the t-test is suitable for screens with replicates. The calculation of SSMD for screens without replicates also differs from that for screens with replicates .

For hit selection in primary screens without replicates, the easily interpretable ones are average fold change, mean difference, percent inhibition, and percent activity. However, they do not capture data variability effectively. The z-score method or SSMD, which can capture data variability based on an assumption that every compound has the same variability as a negative reference in the screens. However, outliers are common in HTS experiments, and methods such as z-score are sensitive to outliers and can be problematic. As a consequence, robust methods such as the z*-score method, SSMD*, B-score method, and quantile-based method have been proposed and adopted for hit selection.

In a screen with replicates, we can directly estimate variability for each compound; as a consequence, we should use SSMD or t-test that does not rely on the strong assumption that the z-score and z*-score rely on. One issue with the use of t-test and associated p-values is that they are affected by both sample size and effect size. They come from testing for no mean difference, and thus are not designed to measure the size of compound effects. For hit selection, the major interest is the size of effect in a tested compound. SSMD directly assesses the size of effects. SSMD has also been shown to be better than other commonly used effect sizes. The population value of SSMD is comparable across experiments and, thus, we can use the same cutoff for the population value of SSMD to measure the size of compound effects .

Techniques for Increased Throughput and Efficiency

Unique distributions of compounds across one or many plates can be employed either to increase the number of assays per plate or to reduce the variance of assay results, or both. The simplifying assumption made in this approach is that any N compounds in the same well will not typically interact with each other, or the assay target, in a manner that fundamentally changes the ability of the assay to detect true hits.

For example, imagine a plate wherein compound A is in wells 1-2-3, compound B is in wells 2-3-4, and compound C is in wells 3-4-5. In an assay of this plate against a given target, a hit in wells 2, 3, and 4 would indicate that compound B is the most likely agent, while also providing three measurements of compound B's efficacy against the specified target. Commercial applications of this approach involve combinations in which no two compounds ever share more than one well, to reduce the (second-order) possibility of interference between pairs of compounds being screened.

Recent Advances

In March 2010, research was published demonstrating an HTS process allowing 1,000 times faster screening (100 million reactions in 10 hours) at 1-millionth the cost (using 10^{-7} times the reagent volume) than conventional techniques using drop-based microfluidics. Drops of fluid separated by oil replace microplate wells and allow analysis and hit sorting while reagents are flowing through channels.

In 2010, researchers developed a silicon sheet of lenses that can be placed over microfluidic arrays to allow the fluorescence measurement of 64 different output channels simultaneously with a single camera. This process can analyze 200,000 drops per second.

Whereby traditional HTS drug discovery uses purified proteins or intact cells, very interesting recent development of the technology is associated with the use of intact living organisms, like the nematode *Caenorhabditis elegans* and zebrafish (*Danio rerio*).

Increasing Utilization of HTS in Academia for Biomedical Research

HTS is a relatively recent innovation, made feasible largely through modern advances in robotics and high-speed computer technology. It still takes a highly specialized and expensive screening lab to run an HTS operation, so in many cases a small- to moderate-size research institution will use the services of an existing HTS facility rather than set up one for itself.

There is a trend in academia for universities to have their own drug discovery enterprise. These facilities, which normally are found only in industry, are now increasingly found at universities as well. UCLA, for example, features an open access HTS laboratory Molecular Screening Shared Resources (MSSR, UCLA), which can screen more than 100,000 compounds a day on a routine basis. The open access policy ensures that researchers from all over the world can take advantage of this facility without lengthy intellectual property negotiations. With a compound library of over 200,000 small molecules, the MSSR has one of the largest compound deck of all universities on the west coast. Also, the MSSR features full functional genomics capabilities (genome wide siRNA, shRNA, cDNA and CRISPR) which are complementary to molecule efforts. Thus, functional genomics leverages HTS capabilities to execute genome wide screens which examine the function of each gene in the context of interest by either knocking each gene out or overexpressing it. Parallel access to high-throughput small molecule screen and a genome wide screen enables researcher to perform target identification and validation for given disease or the mode of action determination on a small molecule. The most accurate results can be obtained by use of "arrayed" functional genomics libraries, i.e. each library contains a single construct such as a single siRNA or cDNA. Functional genomics is typically paired with high content screening using e.g. epifluorescent miscroscopy or laser scanning cytometry. The University of Illinois also has a facility for HTS, as does the University of Minnesota. The Life Sciences Institute at the University of Michigan houses the HTS facility in the Center for Chemical Genomics. The Rockefeller University has an open-access HTS Resource Center HTSRC (The Rockefeller University, HTSRC), which offers a library of over 165,000 compounds. Northwestern University's High Throughput Analysis Laboratory supports target identification, validation, assay development, and compound screening. The non-profit Sanford Burnham Prebys Medical Discovery Institute also has a long-standing HTS facility in the Conrad Prebys Center for Chemical Genomics which was part of the MLPCN.

In the United States, the National Institutes of Health or NIH has created a nationwide consortium of small-molecule screening centers to produce innovative chemical tools for use in biological research. The Molecular Libraries Probe Production Centers Network, or MLPCN, performs HTS on assays provided by the research community, against a large library of small molecules maintained in a central molecule repository.

Virtual Screening

Virtual screening (VS) is a computational technique used in drug discovery to search libraries of small molecules in order to identify those structures which are most likely to bind to a drug target, typically a protein receptor or enzyme.

Virtual screening has been defined as the "automatically evaluating very large libraries of compounds" using computer programs. As this definition suggests, VS has largely been a numbers game focusing on how the enormous chemical space of over 10^{60} conceivable compounds can be filtered to a manageable number that can be synthesized, purchased, and tested. Although searching the entire chemical universe may be a theoretically interesting problem, more practical VS scenarios focus on designing and optimizing targeted combinatorial libraries and enriching libraries of available compounds from in-house compound repositories or vendor offerings. As the accuracy of the method has increased, virtual screening has become an integral part of the drug discovery process.

Methods

There are two broad categories of screening techniques: ligand-based and structure-based.

Ligand-Based

Given a set of structurally diverse ligands that binds to a receptor, a model of the receptors that can built up by exploiting the collective information contained in such set of ligands. These are known as pharmacophore models. A candidate ligand can then be compared to the pharmacophore model to determine whether it is compatible with it and therefore likely to bind.

Another approach to ligand-based virtual screening is to use 2D chemical similarity analysis methods to scan a database of molecules against one or more active ligand structure.

A popular approach to ligand-based virtual screening is based on searching molecules with shape similar to that of known actives, as such molecules will fit the target's binding site and hence will be likely to bind the target. There are a number of prospective applications of this class of techniques in the literature. Pharmacophoric extensions of these 3D methods are also freely-available as webservers.

Structure-Based

Structure-based virtual screening involves docking of candidate ligands into a protein target followed by applying a scoring function to estimate the likelihood that the ligand will bind to the protein with high affinity. Webservers oriented to prospective virtual screening are available to all.

Computing Infrastructure

The computation of pair-wise interactions between atoms, which is a prerequisite for the operation of many virtual screening programs, is of $O(N^2)$ computational complexity, where N is the number of atoms in the system. Because of the quadratic scaling with respect to the number of atoms, the computing infrastructure may vary from a laptop computer for a ligand-based method to a mainframe for a structure-based method.

Ligand-Based

Ligand-based methods typically require a fraction of a second for a single structure comparison operation. A single CPU is enough to perform a large screening within hours. However, several comparisons can be made in parallel in order to expedite the processing of a large database of compounds.

Structure-Based

The size of the task requires a parallel computing infrastructure, such as a cluster of Linux systems, running a batch queue processor to handle the work, such as Sun Grid Engine or Torque PBS.

A means of handling the input from large compound libraries is needed. This requires a form of compound database that can be queried by the parallel cluster, delivering compounds in parallel to the various compute nodes. Commercial database engines may be too ponderous, and a high speed indexing engine, such as Berkeley DB, may be a better choice. Furthermore, it may not be efficient to run one comparison per job, because the ramp up time of the cluster nodes could easily outstrip the amount of useful work. To work around this, it is necessary to process batches of compounds in each cluster job, aggregating the results into some kind of log file. A secondary process, to mine the log files and extract high scoring candidates, can then be run after the whole experiment has been run.

Accuracy

The aim of virtual screening is to identify molecules of novel chemical structure that binds to the macromolecular target of interest. Thus, success of a virtual screen is defined in terms of finding interesting new scaffolds rather than the total number of hits. Interpretations of virtual screening accuracy should therefore be considered with caution. Low hit rates of interesting scaffolds are clearly preferable over high hit rates of already known scaffolds.

Most tests of virtual screening studies in the literature are retrospective. In these studies, the performance of a VS technique is measured by its ability to retrieve a small set of previously known molecules with affinity to the target of interest (active molecules or just actives) from a library containing a much higher proportion of assumed inactives or decoys. By contrast, in prospective applications of virtual screening, the resulting hits are subjected to experimental confirmation (e.g., IC_{50}measurements). There is consensus that retrospective benchmarks are not good predictors of prospective performance and consequently only prospective studies constitute conclusive proof of the suitability of a technique for a particular target.

REFERENCES

1. Bredel M, Jacoby E (Apr 2004). "Chemogenomics: an emerging strategy for rapid target and drug discovery". Nature Reviews. Genetics. 5 (4): 262–75. doi:10.1038/nrg1317. PMID 15131650.
2. Namchuk M (2002). "Finding the molecules to fuel chemogenomics". Targets. 1 (4): 125–129. doi:10.1016/S1477-3627(02)02206-7.
3. Caron PR, Mullican MD, Mashal RD, Wilson KP, Su MS, Murcko MA (Aug 2001). "Chemogenomic approaches to drug discovery". Current Opinion in Chemical Biology. 5 (4): 464–70. doi:10.1016/S1367-5931(00)00229-5. PMID 11470611.
4. Ambroise Y. "Chemogenomic techniques". Retrieved 28 July 2013.
5. Wuster A, Madan Babu M (May 2008). "Chemogenomics and biotechnology". Trends in Biotechnology. 26 (5): 252–8. doi:10.1016/j.tibtech.2008.01.004. PMID 18346803.
6. Mohd Fauzi F, Koutsoukas A, Lowe R, Joshi K, Fan TP, Glen RC, Bender A (Mar 2013). "Chemogenomics approaches to rationalizing the mode-of-action of traditional Chinese and Ayurvedic medicines". Journal of Chemical Information and Modeling. 53 (3): 661–73. doi:10.1021/ci3005513. PMID 23351136.
7. Engelberg A (Sep 2004). "Iconix Pharmaceuticals, Inc.--removing barriers to efficient drug discovery through chemogenomics". Pharmacogenomics. 5 (6): 741–4. doi:10.1517/14622416.5.6.741. PMID 15335294.
8. Bhattacharjee B, Simon RM, Gangadharaiah C, Karunakar P (Jun 2013). "Chemogenomics profiling of drug targets of peptidoglycan biosynthesis pathway in Leptospira interrogans by virtual screening approaches". Journal of Microbiology and Biotechnology. 23 (6): 779–84. doi:10.4014/jmb.1206.06050. PMID 23676922.
9. Cheung-Ong K, Song KT, Ma Z, Shabtai D, Lee AY, Gallo D, Heisler LE, Brown GW, Bierbach U, Giaever G, Nislow C (Nov 2012). "Comparative chemogenomics to examine the mechanism of action of dna-targeted platinum-acridine anticancer agents". ACS Chemical Biology. 7 (11): 1892–901. doi:10.1021/cb300320d. PMID 22928710.

10. Kubinyi H (2006). "Chemogenomics in drug discovery". In Weinmann H, Jaroch S. Chemical genomics small molecule probes to study cellular function. Berlin: Springer. ISBN 3-540-27865-6.

11. Russel K, Michne WF (2004). "The value of chemical genetics in drug discovery". In Folkers G, Kubinyi H, Müller G, Mannhold R. Chemogenomics in drug discovery: a medicinal chemistry perspective. Weinheim: Wiley-VCH. pp. 69–96. ISBN 3-527-30987-X.

12. Carlson SM, White FM (May 2012). "Expanding applications of chemical genetics in signal transduction". Cell Cycle. 11 (10): 1903–9. doi:10.4161/cc.19956. PMID 22544320.

13. O'Connor CJ, Laraia L, Spring DR (Aug 2011). "Chemical genetics". Chemical Society Reviews. 40 (8): 4332–45. doi:10.1039/C1CS15053G. PMID 21562678.

14. Branca M (Feb 2003). "Conquering Infinity with Chemical Genetics". Bio IT World.

15. Tomlinson ML, Rejzek M, Fidock M, Field RA, Wheeler GN (Apr 2009). "Chemical genomics identifies compounds affecting Xenopus laevis pigment cell development". Molecular bioSystems. 5 (4): 376–84. doi:10.1039/B818695B. PMID 19396374.

16. Kälin RE, Bänziger-Tobler NE, Detmar M, Brändli AW (Jul 2009). "An in vivo chemical library screen in Xenopus tadpoles reveals novel pathways involved in angiogenesis and lymphangiogenesis". Blood. 114 (5): 1110–22. doi:10.1182/blood-2009-03-211771. PMC 2721788Freely accessible. PMID 19478043.

17. Taylor KL, Grant NJ, Temperley ND, Patton EE (2010-06-12). "Small molecule screening in zebrafish: an in vivo approach to identifying new chemical tools and drug leads". Cell Communication and Signaling. 8 (1): 11. doi:10.1186/1478-811x-8-11. PMC 2912314Freely accessible. PMID 20540792.

18. Ny A, Autiero M, Carmeliet P (Mar 2006). "Zebrafish and Xenopus tadpoles: small animal models to study angiogenesis and lymphangiogenesis". Experimental Cell Research. Special Issue on Angiogenesis. 312 (5): 684–93. doi:10.1016/j.yexcr.2005.10.018. PMID 16309670.

19. Tomlinson ML, Guan P, Morris RJ, Fidock MD, Rejzek M, Garcia-Morales C, Field RA, Wheeler GN (Jan 2009). "A chemical genomic approach identifies matrix metalloproteinases as playing an essential and specific role in Xenopus melanophore migration". Chemistry & Biology. 16 (1): 93–104. doi:10.1016/j.chembiol.2008.12.005. PMID 19171309.

20. Hu L, Zhu J, Rotchell JM, Wu L, Gao J, Shi H (Mar 2015). "Use of the enhanced frog embryo teratogenesis assay-Xenopus (FETAX) to determine chemically-induced phenotypic effects". The Science of the Total Environment. 508: 258–65. doi:10.1016/j.scitotenv.2014.11.086. PMID 25481254.

21. Molina G, Vogt A, Bakan A, Dai W, Queiroz de Oliveira P, Znosko W, Smithgall TE, Bahar I, Lazo JS, Day BW, Tsang M (Sep 2009). "Zebrafish chemical screening reveals an inhibitor of Dusp6 that expands cardiac cell lineages". Nature Chemical Biology. 5 (9): 680–7. doi:10.1038/nchembio.190. PMC 2771339Freely

accessible. PMID 19578332.

22. Rester U (July 2008). "From virtuality to reality - Virtual screening in lead discovery and lead optimization: a medicinal chemistry perspective". Current Opinion in Drug Discovery & Development. 11 (4): 559–68. PMID 18600572.
23. Rollinger JM, Stuppner H, Langer T (2008). "Virtual screening for the discovery of bioactive natural products". Progress in Drug Research. Progress in Drug Research. 65 (211): 211, 213–49. doi:10.1007/978-3-7643-8117-2_6. ISBN 978-3-7643-8098-4. PMID 18084917.
24. Walters WP, Stahl MT, Murcko MA (1998). "Virtual screening – an overview". Drug Discov. Today. 3 (4): 160–178. doi:10.1016/S1359-6446(97)01163-X.
25. Bohacek RS, McMartin C, Guida WC (1996). "The art and practice of structure-based drug design: a molecular modeling perspective". Med. Res. Rev. 16: 3–50. doi:10.1002/(SICI)1098-1128(199601)16:1<3::AID-MED1>3.0.CO;2-6.
26. McGregor, Malcolm J; Luo, Zhaowen; Jiang, Xuliang (June 11, 2007). "Chapter 3: Virtual screening in drug discovery". In Huang, Ziwei. Drug Discovery Research. New Frontiers in the Post-Genomic Era. Wiley-VCH: Weinheim, Germany. pp. 63–88. ISBN 978-0-471-67200-5.
27. McInnes C (October 2007). "Virtual screening strategies in drug discovery". Current Opinion in Chemical Biology. 11 (5): 494–502. doi:10.1016/j.cbpa.2007.08.033. PMID 17936059.
28. Sun H (2008). "Pharmacophore-based virtual screening". Current Medicinal Chemistry. 15 (10): 1018–24. doi:10.2174/092986708784049630. PMID 18393859.
29. Willet P, Barnard JM, Downs GM (1998). "Chemical similarity searching". J Chem Inf Comput Sci. 38 (6): 983–996. doi:10.1021/ci9800211.
30. Rush TS, Grant JA, Mosyak L, Nicholls A (March 2005). "A shape-based 3-D scaffold hopping method and its application to a bacterial protein-protein interaction". Journal of Medicinal Chemistry. 48 (5): 1489–95. doi:10.1021/jm040163o. PMID 15743191.
31. Ballester PJ, Westwood I, Laurieri N, Sim E, Richards WG (February 2010). "Prospective virtual screening with Ultrafast Shape Recognition: the identification of novel inhibitors of arylamine N-acetyltransferases". Journal of the Royal Society, Interface / the Royal Society. 7 (43): 335–42. doi:10.1098/rsif.2009.0170. PMC 2842611Freely accessible. PMID 19586957.
32. Li H, Leung KS, Wong MH, Ballester PJ (July 2016). "USR-VS: a web server for large-scale prospective virtual screening using ultrafast shape recognition techniques". Nucleic Acids Research. 44 (W1): W436–41. doi:10.1093/nar/gkw320. PMID 27106057.
33. Sperandio O, Petitjean M, Tuffery P (July 2009). "wwLigCSRre: a 3D ligand-based server for hit identification and optimization". Nucleic Acids Research. 37 (Web Server issue): W504–9. doi:10.1093/nar/gkp324. PMC 2703967Freely accessible. PMID 19429687.
34. Kroemer RT (August 2007). "Structure-based drug design: docking

and scoring". Current Protein & Peptide Science. 8 (4): 312–28. doi:10.2174/138920307781369382. PMID 17696866.

35. Cavasotto CN, Orry AJ (2007). "Ligand docking and structure-based virtual screening in drug discovery". Current Topics in Medicinal Chemistry. 7 (10): 1006–14. doi:10.2174/156802607780906753. PMID 17508934.
36. Kooistra AJ, Vischer HF, McNaught-Flores D, Leurs R, de Esch IJ, de Graaf C (2016). "Function-specific virtual screening for GPCR ligands using a combined scoring method". Scientific Reports. 6: 28288. doi:10.1038/srep28288. PMID 27339552.
37. Irwin JJ, Shoichet BK, Mysinger MM, Huang N, Colizzi F, Wassam P, Cao Y (September 2009). "Automated docking screens: a feasibility study". Journal of Medicinal Chemistry. 52 (18): 5712–20. doi:10.1021/jm9006966. PMC 2745826Freely accessible. PMID 19719084.
38. Li H, Leung KS, Ballester PJ, Wong MH (2014-01-24). "istar: a web platform for large-scale protein-ligand docking". PloS One. 9 (1): e85678. doi:10.1371/journal.pone.0085678. PMC 3901662Freely accessible. PMID 24475049.
39. Irwin JJ (2008). "Community benchmarks for virtual screening". Journal of Computer-Aided Molecular Design. 22 (3-4): 193–9. doi:10.1007/s10822-008-9189-4. PMID 18273555.
40. Good AC, Oprea TI (2008). "Optimization of CAMD techniques 3. Virtual screening enrichment studies: a help or hindrance in tool selection?". Journal of Computer-Aided Molecular Design. 22 (3-4): 169–78. doi:10.1007/s10822-007-9167-2. PMID 18188508.
41. Schneider G (April 2010). "Virtual screening: an endless staircase?". Nature Reviews. Drug Discovery. 9 (4): 273–6. doi:10.1038/nrd3139. PMID 20357802.
42. Ballester PJ (January 2011). "Ultrafast shape recognition: method and applications". Future Medicinal Chemistry. 3 (1): 65–78. doi:10.4155/fmc.10.280. PMID 21428826.

CHAPTER 3

Process of Drug Discovery

Chapter Contents

- **Introduction**
- **Historical Background**
- **Drug Targets**
- **Drug Metabolism**
- **Fragment-Based Lead Discovery**

Drug discovery is the process through which potential new medicines are identified. It involves a wide range of scientific disciplines, including biology, chemistry and pharmacology. In the fields of medicine, biotechnology and pharmacology despite advances in technology and ever-greater understanding of biological systems, the drug discovery process can too often be a lengthy, expensive, difficult, and inefficient process. Once a compound has shown its value in testing it will begin the process of drug development prior to clinical trials.

Drug discovery and design requires the identification of candidates, synthesis, characterization, screening, and assays for therapeutic efficacy.

INTRODUCTION

In the fields of medicine, biotechnology and pharmacology, drug discovery is the process by which new candidate medications are discovered. Historically, drugs were discovered through identifying the active ingredient from traditional remedies or by serendipitous discovery. Later chemical libraries of synthetic small molecules, natural products or extracts were screened in intact cells or whole organisms to identify substances that have a desirable therapeutic effect in a process known as classical pharmacology. Since sequencing of the human genome which allowed rapid cloning and synthesis of large quantities of purified proteins, it has become common practice to use high throughput screening of large compounds libraries against isolated biological targets which are hypothesized to be disease modifying in a process known as reverse pharmacology. Hits from these screens are then tested in cells and then in animals for efficacy.

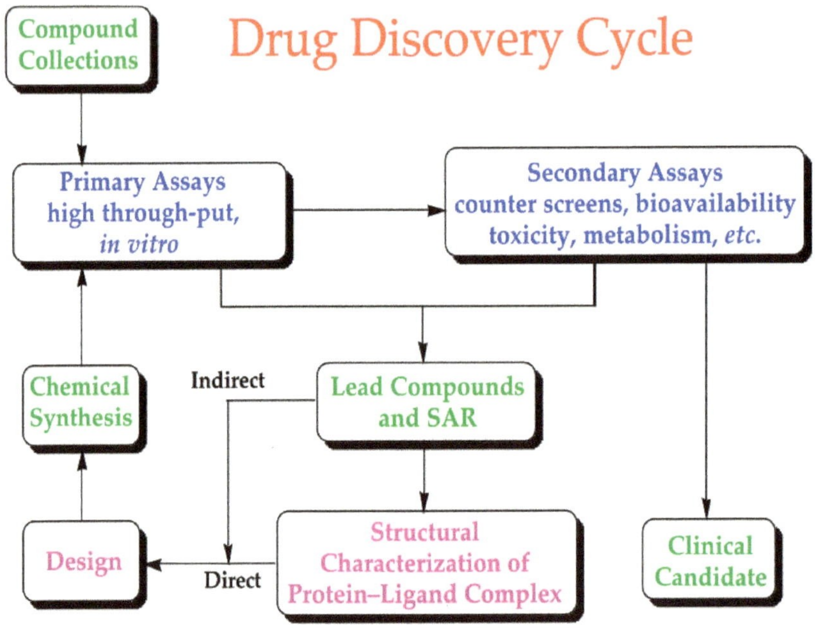

Modern drug discovery involves the identification of screening hits, medicinal chemistry and optimization of those hits to increase the affinity, selectivity (to reduce the potential of side effects), efficacy/potency, metabolicstability (to increase the half-life), and oral bioavailability. Once a compound that fulfills all of these requirements has been identified, it will begin the process of drug development prior to clinical trials. One or more of these steps may not necessarily involved in the computer aided drug design. Modern drug discovery is thus usually a capital-intensive process that involves large investments by pharmaceutical industry corporations as well as national governments (who provide grants and loan guarantees). Despite advances in technology and understanding of biological systems, drug discovery is still a lengthy, "expensive, difficult, and inefficient process" with low rate of new therapeutic discovery. In 2010, the research and development cost of each new molecular entity (NME) was approximately US$1.8 billion. Drug discovery is done by pharmaceutical companies, with research assistance from universities. The "final product" of drug discovery is a patent on the potential drug. The drug requires very expensive Phase I, II and III clinical trials, and most of them fail. Small companies have a critical role, often then selling the rights to larger companies that have the resources to run the clinical trials.

Discovering drugs that may be a commercial success, or a public health success, involves a complex interaction between investors, industry, academia, patent laws, regulatory exclusivity, marketing and the need to balance secrecy with communication. Meanwhile, for disorders whose rarity means that no large commercial success or public health effect can be expected, the orphan drug funding process ensures that people who experience those disorders can have some hope of pharmacotherapeutic advances.

HISTORICAL BACKGROUND

The idea that the effect of a drug in the human body is mediated by specific interactions of the drug molecule with biological macromolecules, (proteins or nucleic acids in most cases) led scientists to the conclusion that individual chemicals are required for the biological activity of the drug. This made for the beginning of the modern era in pharmacology, as pure chemicals, instead of crude extracts, became the standard drugs. Examples of drug compounds isolated from crude preparations are morphine, the active agent in opium, and digoxin, a heart stimulant originating from Digitalis lanata. Organic chemistry also led to the synthesis of many of the natural products isolated from biological sources.

Historically substances, whether crude extracts or purified chemicals were screened for biological activity without knowledge of the biological target. Only after an active substance was identified was an effort made to identify the target. This approach is known as classical pharmacology, forward pharmacology, or phenotypic drug discovery.

Later, small molecules were synthesized to specifically target a known physiological/ pathological pathways rather than adopting the mass screening of banks of stored compounds. This led to great success, such as the work of Gertrude Elion and George H. Hitchings on purine metabolism, the work of James Black on beta blockers and cimetidine, and the discovery of statins by Akira Endo. Another champion of the approach of developing chemical analogues of known active substances was Sir David Jack at Allen and Hanbury's, later Glaxo, who pioneered the first inhaled selective beta2-adrenergic agonist for asthma, the first inhaled steroid for asthma, ranitidine as a successor to cimetidine, and supported the development of the triptans.

Gertrude Elion, working mostly with a group of fewer than 50 people in purine analogues contributed to the discovery of the following; the first anti viral medicine, the first drug to induce remission of childhood leukemia, pivotal anti-cancer treatments, an anti-malarial, an anti-bacterial and medicine for the treatment of gout.

Cloning of human proteins made possible by screening of large libraries of compounds against specific targets thought to be linked to specific diseases. This approach is known as reverse pharmacology and is the most frequently used approach today.

DRUG TARGETS

The definition of "target" itself is something argued within the pharmaceutical industry. Generally, the "target" is the naturally existing cellular or molecular structure involved in line with the interest of pathology especially in drug development. However, the distinction between a "new" and "established" target can be made without a full understanding of just what a "targets" is. This distinction is typically made by pharmaceutical companies engaged in discovery and development of therapeutics. In 2011, there was an estimated 435 genome products discovered and identified as a therapeutic drug targets as approved by the FDA.

"Established targets" are those for which there is a good scientific understanding, supported by a lengthy publication history, of both how the target functions in normal physiology and how it is involved in human pathology. This does not imply that the mechanism of action of drugs that are thought to act through a particular established target is fully understood. Rather, "established" relates directly to the amount of background information available on a target, in particular functional information. The more such information is available, the less investment is (generally) required to develop a therapeutic directed against the target. The process of gathering such functional information is called "target validation" in pharmaceutical industry parlance. Established targets also include those that the pharmaceutical industry has had experience mounting drug discovery campaigns against in the past, such a history provides information on the chemical feasibility of developing a small molecular therapeutic against the target and can provide licensing opportunities and freedom-to-operate indicators with respect to small-molecule therapeutic candidates.

In general, "new targets" are all those targets that are not "established targets" but this had been subjected to drug discovery campaigns. These typically include newly discovered proteins whose function has now become clear as a result of basic scientific research.

The majority of targets currently selected for drug discovery efforts are proteins. Two classes predominate: G-protein-coupled receptors (or GPCRs) and protein kinases.

Screening and Design

The process of finding a new drug against a chosen target for a particular disease usually involves high-throughput screening (HTS), wherein large libraries of chemicals are tested for their ability to modify the target. For example, if the target is a novel GPCR, compounds will be screened for their ability to inhibit or stimulate that receptor (see antagonist and agonist) and if the target kinase, the chemicals will be tested for their ability to inhibit that kinase.

Another important function of HTS is to show how selective the compounds are for the chosen target. The ideal is to find a molecule which will interfere with the chosen target and not the other targets. To this end, other screening runs will be made to see whether the "hits" against the chosen target will interfere with other related targets – this is the process of cross-screening. Cross-screening is important, because the more unrelated targets a compound hits, the more likely that off-target toxicity will occur with that compound once it reaches the clinic.

It is very unlikely that a perfect drug candidate will emerge from these early screening runs. It is more often observed that several compounds are found to have some degree of activity, and if these compounds share common chemical features, one or more pharmacophores can then be developed. At this point, medicinal chemists will attempt to use structure-activity relationships (SAR) to improve certain features of the lead compound:

- increase activity against the chosen target;
- reduce activity against unrelated targets and
- improve the druglikeness or ADME properties of the molecule.

This process will require several iterative screening runs which hopes that the properties of properties of the new molecular entities will improve, and allow the favoured compounds to go forward to in vitro and in vivo testing for activity in the disease model of choice.

Amongst the physico-chemical properties associated with drug absorption include ionization (pKa), and solubility; permeability can be determined by PAMPA and Caco-2. PAMPA is attractive as an early screen due to the low consumption of drug and the low cost compared to tests such as Caco-2, gastrointestinal tract (GIT) and Blood–brain barrier (BBB) with which there is a high correlation.

A range of parameters can be used to assess the quality of compounds or series of compounds as proposed in the Lipinski's Rule of Five. Such parameters include calculated properties such as cLogP to estimate lipophilicity, molecular weight, polar surface area and measured properties, such as potency, in-vitro measurement of enzymatic clearance etc. Some descriptors such as ligand efficiency (LE) and lipophilic efficiency (LiPE) combine such parameters to assess druglikeness.

While HTS is a commonly used method for novel drug discovery, this is not the only method. It is often possible to start from a molecule which already has some of the desired properties. Such a molecule might be extracted from a natural product or even be a drug on the market which could be improved upon (so-called "me too" drugs). Other methods, such as virtual high throughput screening, where screening is done using computer-generated models and attempting to "dock" virtual libraries to a target, are also often used.

Another important method for drug discovery is *de novo* drug design, in which a prediction is made of the sorts of chemicals that might (e.g.) fit into an active site of the target enzyme. For example, virtual screening and computer-aided drug design are often used to identify new chemical moieties that may interact with a target protein. Molecular modelling and molecular dynamics simulations can be used as a guide to improve the potency and properties of new drug leads.

There is also a paradigm shift in the drug discovery community to shift away from HTS, which is expensive and may only cover limited chemical space, to the screening of smaller libraries (maximum a few thousand compounds). These include fragment-based lead discovery (FBDD) and protein-directed dynamic combinatorial chemistry. The ligands in these approaches are usually much smaller, and they bind to the target protein with weaker binding affinity than those hits that are identified from HTS. Further modified through organic synthesis into lead compounds are often required. Such modifications are often guided by protein X-ray crystallography of the protein-fragment complex. The advantages of these approaches are that they allow more efficient screening and the compound library, although small, typically covers a large chemical space when compared to HTS.

Once a lead compound series has been established with sufficient target potency and selectivity and favourable drug-like properties, one or two compounds will then be proposed for drug development. The best of these is generally called the lead compound, while the other will be designated as the "backup".

Nature as Source of Drugs

Traditionally many drugs and other chemicals with biological activity have been discovered by studying allelopathy – chemicals that organisms create that affect the activity of other organisms in the fight for survival.

Despite the rise of combinatorial chemistry as an integral part of lead discovery process, natural products still play a major role as starting material for drug discovery. A 2007 report found that of the 974 small molecule new chemical entities developed between 1981 and 2006, 63% were natural derived or semisynthetic derivatives of natural products. For certain therapy areas, such as antimicrobials, antineoplastics, antihypertensive and anti-inflammatory drugs, the numbers were higher. In many cases, these products have been used traditionally for many years.

Natural products may be useful as a source of novel chemical structures for modern techniques of development of antibacterial therapies.

Despite the implied potential, only a fraction of Earth's living species has been tested for bioactivity.

Plant-Derived

Prior to Paracelsus, the vast majority of traditionally used crude drugs in Western medicine were plant-derived extracts. This has resulted in a pool of information about the potential of plant species as an important source of starting material for drug discovery. A different set of metabolites is sometimes produced in the different anatomical parts of the plant (e.g. root, leaves and flower), and botanical knowledge is crucial also for the correct identification of bioactive plant materials.

Microbial Metabolites

Microbes compete for living space and nutrients. To survive in these conditions, many microbes have developed abilities to prevent competing species from proliferating. Microbes are the main source of antimicrobial drugs. *Streptomyces* species have been a valuable source of antibiotics. The classical example of an antibiotic discovered as a defense mechanism against another microbe is the discovery of penicillin in bacterial cultures contaminated by *Penicillium* fungi in 1928.

Marine Invertebrates

Marine environments are potential sources for new bioactive agents. Arabinose nucleosides discovered from marine invertebrates in 1950's demonstrating for the first time that sugar moieties other than ribose and deoxyribose can yield bioactive nucleoside structures. However, it was 2004 when the first marine-derived drug was approved. The cone snail toxin ziconotide, also known as Prialt, was approved by the Food and Drug Administration to treat severe neuropathic pain. Several other marine-derived agents are now in clinical trials for indications such as cancer, anti-inflammatory use and pain. One class of these agents are bryostatin-like compounds, under investigation as anti-cancer therapy.

Chemical Diversity of Natural Products

As above mentioned, combinatorial chemistry was a key technology enabling the efficient generation of large screening libraries for the needs of high-throughput screening. However, now, after two decades of combinatorial chemistry, it has been pointed out that despite the increased efficiency in chemical synthesis, no increase in lead or drug candidates has been reached. This has led to analysis of chemical characteristics of combinatorial chemistry products, compared to existing drugs or natural products. The chemoinformatics concepts in chemical diversity as dipected in the distribution of of compounds in the chemical space based on their physicochemical characteristics, is often used to describe the difference between the combinatorial chemistry libraries and natural products. The synthetic, combinatorial library compounds seem to cover only a limited and quite uniform chemical space, whereas existing drugs and particularly natural products, exhibit much greater chemical diversity, distributing more evenly to the chemical space. The most prominent differences between natural products and compounds in combinatorial chemistry libraries is the number of chiral centers (much higher in natural compounds), structure rigidity (higher in natural compounds) and number of aromatic moieties (higher in combinatorial chemistry libraries). Other chemical differences between these two groups include the nature of heteroatoms (O and N enriched in natural products, and S and halogen atoms more often present in synthetic compounds), as well as level of non-aromatic unsaturation (higher in natural products). As both structure rigidity and chirality are both well-established factors in medicinal chemistry known to enhance compounds specificity and efficacy as a drug. It has been suggested that natural products compare favorable to today's combinatorial chemistry libraries as potential lead molecules.

Natural Product

Screening

Two main approaches exist for the findings of new bioactive chemical entities from natural sources.

The first is sometimes referred to as random collection and screening of material, but in fact the collection is often far from random in that biological (often botanical) knowledge is used about which families show promise, based on a number of factors, including past screening. This approach is based on the fact that only a small part of earth's biodiversity has ever been tested for pharmaceutical activity. It is also based on the fact that organisms living in a species-rich environment need to evolve defensive and competitive mechanisms to survive, mechanisms which might usefully be exploited in the development of drugs that can cure diseases affecting humans. A collection of plant, animal and microbial samples from rich ecosystems can potentially give rise to novel biological activities worth exploiting in the drug development process. One example of a successful use of this strategy is the screening for antitumour agents by the National Cancer Institute, started in the 1960's. Paclitaxel was identified from Pacific yew tree *Taxus brevifolia*. Paclitaxel showed anti-tumour activity by a previously undescribed mechanism (stabilization of microtubules) and is now approved for clinical use for the treatment of lung, breast and ovarian cancer, as well as for Kaposi's sarcoma. Early in the 21st century, Cabazitaxel (made by Sanofi, a French firm), another relative of taxol has been shown effective against prostate cancer, also because it works by preventing the formation of microtubules, which pull the chromosomes apart in dividing cells (such as cancer cells). Other examples are: 1. Camptotheca (Camptothecin Topotecan Irinotecan Rubitecan Belotecan); 2. Podophyllum (Etoposide Teniposide); 3a. Anthracyclines (Aclarubicin · Daunorubicin Doxorubicin Epirubicin Idarubicin Amrubicin Pirarubicin Valrubicin · Zorubicin); 3b. Anthracenediones (Mitoxantrone Pixantrone).

The second main approach involves ethnobotany, the study of the general use of plants in society, and ethnopharmacology, an area inside ethnobotany, which is focused specifically on medicinal uses.

Both of these two main approaches can be used in selecting starting materials for future drugs. Artemisinin, an antimalarial agent from sweet wormtree *Artemisia annua*, used in Chinese medicine since 200BC is one drug used as part of combination therapy for multiresistant *Plasmodium falciparum*.

Structural Elucidation

The elucidation of the chemical structure is critical to avoid the re-discovery of a chemical agent that is already known for its structure and chemical activity. Mass spectrometry is a method in which individual compounds are identified based on their mass/charge ratio, after ionization. Chemical compounds exist in nature as mixtures, so the combination of liquid chromatography and mass spectrometry (LC-MS) is often used to separate the individual chemicals. Databases of mass spectras for known compounds are available, and can be used to assign a structure to an unknown mass spectrum. Nuclear magnetic resonance spectroscopy is the primary technique for determining chemical structures of natural products. NMR yields information about individual hydrogen and carbon atoms in the structure, allowing detailed reconstruction of the molecule's architecture.

DRUG METABOLISM

Drug metabolism is the metabolic breakdown of drugs by living organisms, usually through specialized enzymatic systems. More generally, xenobiotic metabolism (from the Greek xenos "stranger" and biotic "related to living beings") is the set of metabolic pathways that modify the chemical structure of xenobiotics, which are compounds foreign to an organism's normal biochemistry, such any drug or poison. These pathways are being formed by biotransformation present in all major groups of organisms, and are considered to be of ancient origin. These reactions often act to detoxify poisonous compounds (although in some cases the intermediates in xenobiotic metabolism can themselves cause toxic effects). The study of drug metabolism is called pharmacokinetics.

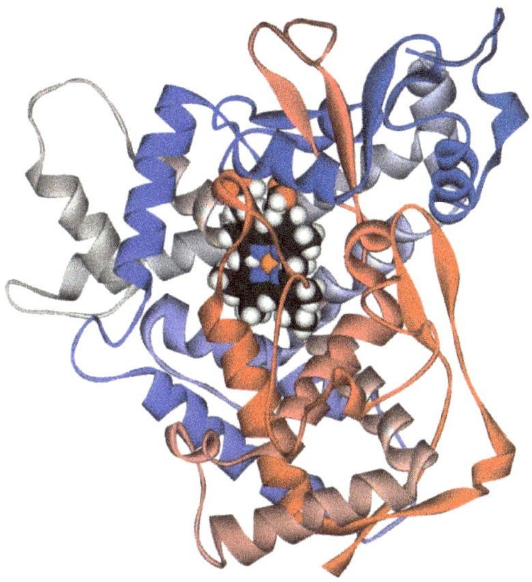

Cytochrome P450 oxidases are important enzymes in xenobiotic metabolism.

The metabolism of pharmaceutical drugs is an important aspect of pharmacology and medicine. For example, the rate of metabolism determines the duration and intensity of a drug's pharmacologic action. Drug metabolism also affects multidrug resistance in infectious diseases and in chemotherapy for cancer, and the actions of some drugs as substrates or inhibitors of enzymes involved in xenobiotic metabolism are a common reason for hazardous drug interactions. These pathways are also important in environmental science, with the xenobiotic metabolism of microorganisms determining whether a pollutant will be broken down during bioremediation, or persist in the environment. The enzymes of xenobiotic metabolism, particularly the glutathione S-transferases are also important in agriculture, since they may produce resistance to pesticides and herbicides.

Drug metabolism is divided into three phases. In phase I, enzymes such as cytochrome P450 oxidases introduce reactive or polar groups into xenobiotics. These modified compounds are then conjugated to polar compounds in phase II reactions. These reactions are catalyzed by transferase enzymes such as glutathione S-transferases. Finally, in phase III, the conjugated xenobiotics may be further processed, before being recognized by efflux transporters and pumped out of cells. Drug metabolism often converts lipophilic compounds into hydrophilic products that are more readily excreted.

Permeability Barriers and Detoxification

The exact compounds an organism is exposed to will be largely unpredictable, and may differ widely overtime these are major characteristics of xenobiotic toxic stress. The major challenge faced by xenobiotic detoxification systems is that they must be able to remove the almost-limitless number of xenobiotic compounds from the complex mixture of chemicals involved in normal metabolism. The solution that has evolved to address this problem is an elegant combination of physical barriers and low-specificity enzymatic systems.

All organisms use cell membranes as hydrophobic permeability barriers to control access to their internal environment. Polar compounds cannot diffuse across these cell membranes, and the uptake of useful molecules is mediated through transport proteins that specifically select substrates from the extracellular mixture. This selective uptake means that most hydrophilic molecules cannot enter cells, since they are not recognized by any specific transporters. In contrast, the diffusion of hydrophobic compounds across these barriers cannot be controlled and organisms therefore, cannot exclude lipid-soluble xenobiotics using membrane barriers.

However, the existence of a permeability barrier means that organisms were able to evolve detoxification systems that exploit the hydrophobicity common to membrane-permeable xenobiotics. These systems therefore solve the specificity problem by possessing such broad substrate specificities that they metabolize almost any non-polar compound. Useful metabolites are excluded since they are polar, and in general contain one or more charged groups.

The detoxification of the reactive by-products of normal metabolism cannot be achieved by the systems outlined above, because these species are derived from normal cellular constituents and usually share their polar characteristics. However, since these compounds are few in number, specific enzymes can recognize and remove them. Examples of these specific detoxification systems are the glyoxalase system, which removes the reactive aldehyde methylglyoxal, and the various antioxidant systems that eliminate reactive oxygen species.

Phases of Detoxification

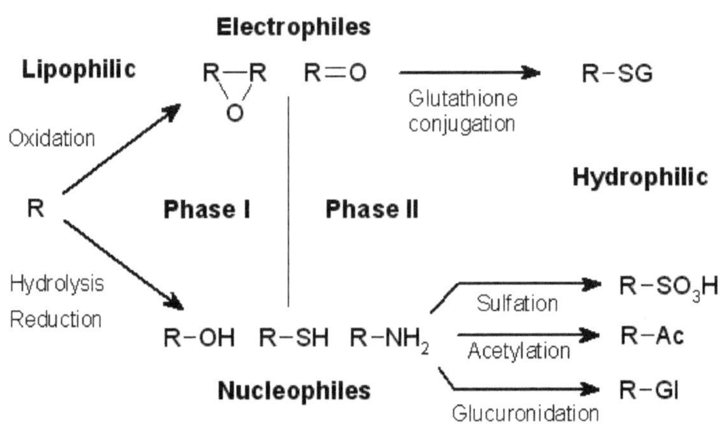

Phases I and II of the metabolism of a lipophilic xenobiotic.

The metabolism of xenobiotics is often divided into three phases: modification, conjugation and excretion. These reactions act in concert to detoxify xenobiotics and remove them from cells.

Phase I – Modification

In phase I, a variety of enzymes act to introduce reactive and polar groups into their substrates. One of the most common modifications is hydroxylation catalyzed by the cytochrome P-450-dependent mixed-function oxidase system. These enzyme complexes act to incorporate an atom of oxygen into nonactivated hydrocarbons, which can result in either the introduction of hydroxyl groups or N-, O- and S-dealkylation of substrates. The reaction mechanism of the P-450 oxidases proceeds through the reduction of cytochrome-bound oxygen and the generation of a highly-reactive oxyferryl species, according to the following scheme:

$$O_2 + NADPH + H^+ + RH \rightarrow NADP^+ + H_2O + ROH$$

Phase I reactions (also termed nonsynthetic reactions) may occur by oxidation, reduction, hydrolysis, cyclization, decyclization, and addition of oxygen or removal of hydrogen and being carried out by mixed function of oxidases which is found in the liver. These oxidative reactions typically involve a cytochrome P450 monooxygenase (often abbreviated CYP), NADPH and oxygen. The classes of pharmaceutical drugs that utilize this method for their metabolism include phenothiazines, paracetamol, and steroids. If the metabolites of phase I reactions are sufficiently polar, they may be readily excreted at this point. However, many phase I products are not eliminated rapidly and undergo a subsequent reaction in which an endogenous substrate combines with the newly incorporated functional group to form a highly polar conjugate.

A common Phase I oxidation involves conversion of a C-H bond to a C-OH. This reaction sometimes converts a pharmacologically inactive compound (a prodrug) to a pharmacologically active one. By the same token, Phase I can turn a nontoxic molecule into a poisonous one (toxification). Simple hydrolysis in the stomach is normally an innocuous reaction, however there are exceptions. For example, phase I metabolism converts acetonitrile to $HOCH_2CN$, which rapidly dissociates into formaldehyde and hydrogen cyanide, both of which are toxic.

Phase I metabolism of drug candidates can be simulated in the laboratory using non-enzyme catalysts. This example of a biomimetic reaction tends to give products that often contains the Phase I metabolites. As an example, the major metabolite of the pharmaceutical trimebutine, desmethyltrimebutine (nor-trimebutine), can be efficiently produced by in vitro oxidation of the commercially available drug. Hydroxylation of an N-methyl group leads to expulsion of a molecule of formaldehyde, while oxidation of the O-methyl groups takes place to a lesser extent.

Oxidation

- Cytochrome P450 monooxygenase system;
- Flavin-containing monooxygenase system;

- Alcohol dehydrogenase and aldehyde dehydrogenase;
- Monoamine oxidase;
- Co-oxidation by peroxidases;

Reduction

- NADPH-cytochrome P450 reductase

Cytochrome P450 reductase, also known as NADPH:ferrihemoprotein oxidoreductase, NADPH:hemoprotein oxidoreductase, NADPH:P450 oxidoreductase, P450 reductase, POR, CPR, CYPOR, is a membrane-bound enzyme required for electron transfer to cytochrome P450 in the microsome of the eukaryotic cell from a FAD- and FMN-containing enzyme NADPH:cytochrome P450 reductase The general scheme of electron flow in the POR/ P450 system is: NADPH → FAD → FMN → P450 → O_2

- Reduced (ferrous) cytochrome P450

During reduction reactions, a chemical can enter *futile cycling*, in which it gains a free-radical electron, then promptly loses it to oxygen (to form a superoxide anion).

Hydrolysis

- Esterases and amidase and
- Epoxide hydrolase.

Phase II – Conjugation

In subsequent phase II reactions, these activated xenobiotic metabolites are conjugated with charged species such as glutathione (GSH), sulfate, glycine, or glucuronic acid. Sites on drugs where conjugation reactions occur include carboxyl (-COOH), hydroxyl (-OH), amino (NH_2), and sulfhydryl (-SH) groups. Products of conjugation reactions have increased molecular weight and tend to be less active than their substrates, unlike Phase I reactions which often produce active metabolites. The addition of large anionic groups (such as GSH) detoxifies reactive electrophiles and produces more polar metabolites that cannot diffuse across membranes, and may, therefore, be actively transported.

These reactions are catalyzed by a large group of broad-specificity transferases, which in combination can metabolise almost any hydrophobic compound that contains nucleophilic or electrophilic groups. One of the most important classes of this group is that of the glutathione S-transferases (GSTs).

Mechanism	Involved enzyme	Co-factor	Location
methylation	methyltransferase	S-adenosyl-L-methionine	liver, kidney, lung, CNS
sulphation	sulfotransferases	3'-phosphoadenosine-5'-phosphosulfate	liver, kidney, intestine

acetylation	• N-acetyltransferases • bile acid-CoA:amino acid N-acyltransferases	acetyl coenzyme A	liver, lung, spleen, gastric mucosa, RBCs, lymphocytes
glucuronidation	UDP-glucuronosyltransferases	UDP-glucuronic acid	liver, kidney, intestine, lung, skin, prostate, brain
glutathione conjugation	glutathione S-transferases	glutathione	liver, kidney
glycine conjugation	acetyl Co-enzyme As	glycine	liver, kidney

Phase III – Further Modification and Excretion

After phase II reactions, the xenobiotic conjugates may be further metabolised. A common example is the processing of glutathione conjugates to acetylcysteine (mercapturic acid) conjugates. Here, the γ-glutamate and glycine residues in the glutathione molecule are removed by Gamma-glutamyl transpeptidase and dipeptidases. In the final step, the cystine residue in the conjugate is acetylated.

Conjugates and their metabolites can be excreted from cells in phase III of their metabolism, with the anionic groups acting as affinity tags for a variety of membrane transporters of the multidrug resistance protein (MRP) family. These proteins are members of the family of ATP-binding cassette transporters and can catalyse the ATP-dependent transport of a huge variety of hydrophobic anions, and thus act to remove phase II products to the extracellular medium, where they may be further metabolized or excreted.

Endogenous Toxins

The detoxification of endogenous reactive metabolites such as peroxides and reactive aldehydes often cannot be achieved by the system described above. This is the result of these specie's being derived from normal cellular constituents and usually sharing their polar characteristics. However, since these compounds are few in number, it is possible for enzymatic systems to utilize specific molecular recognition to recognize and remove them. The similarity of these molecules to useful metabolites therefore means that different detoxification enzymes are usually required for the metabolism of each group of endogenous toxins. Examples of these specific detoxification systems are the glyoxalase system, which acts to dispose of the reactive aldehyde methylglyoxal, and the various antioxidant systems that remove reactive oxygen species.

Sites

Quantitatively, the smooth endoplasmic reticulum of the liver cell is the principal organ of drug metabolism, although every biological tissue has some ability to metabolize drugs. Factors responsible for the liver's contribution to drug metabolism include that it is a large organ, that it is the first organ perfused by chemicals absorbed in the gut, and that there are very high concentrations of most drug-metabolizing enzyme systems relative to other organs. If a drug is taken into the GI tract, where it enters hepatic circulation through the portal vein, it becomes well-metabolized and is said to show the *first pass effect*.

Other sites of drug metabolism include epithelial cells of the gastrointestinal tract, lungs, kidneys, and the skin. These sites are usually responsible for localized toxicity reactions.

Factors that Affect Drug Metabolism

The duration and intensity of pharmacological action of most lipophilic drugs are determined by the rate they are metabolized to inactive products. The Cytochrome P450 monooxygenase system is the most important pathway in this regard. In general, anything that *increases* the rate of metabolism (*e.g.*, enzyme induction) of a pharmacologically active metabolite will *decrease* the duration and intensity of the drug action. The opposite is also true (*e.g.*, enzyme inhibition). However, in cases where an enzyme is responsible for metabolizing a pro-drug into a drug, enzyme induction can speed up this conversion and increase drug levels, potentially causing toxicity.

Various *physiological* and *pathological* factors can also affect drug metabolism. Physiological factors that can influence drug metabolism ncludes; age, individual variation (*e.g.*, pharmacogenetics), enterohepatic circulation, nutrition, intestinal flora, or sex differences.

In general, drugs are metabolized more slowly in fetal, neonatal and elderly humans and animals than in adults.

Genetic variation (polymorphism) accounts for some of the variability in the effect of drugs. With N-acetyltransferases (involved in *Phase II* reactions), individual variation creates a group of people who acetylate slowly (*slow acetylators*) and those who acetylate quickly, split roughly 50:50 in the population of Canada. This variation may have dramatic consequences, as the slow acetylators are more prone to dose-dependent toxicity.

Cytochrome P450 monooxygenase system enzymes can also vary across individuals, with deficiencies occurring in 1 – 30% of people, depending on their ethnic background.

Pathological factors can also influence drug metabolism, including liver, kidney, or heart diseases.

In silico modelling and simulation methods allow drug metabolism to be predicted in virtual patient populations prior to performing clinical studies in human subjects. This can be used to identify individuals most at risk from adverse reaction.

FRAGMENT-BASED LEAD DISCOVERY

Fragment-based lead discovery (FBLD) also known as fragment-based drug discovery (FBDD) is a method used for finding lead compounds as part of the drug discovery process. It is based on identifying small chemical fragments, which may bind only weakly to the biological target, and then growing them or combining them to produce a lead with a higher affinity. FBLD can be compared with high-throughput screening (HTS).

In HTS, libraries with up to millions of compounds, with molecular weights of around 500 Da, are screened, and nanomolar binding affinities are sought. In contrast, in the early phase of FBLD, libraries with a few thousand compounds with molecular weights of around 200 Da may be screened, and millimolar affinities can be considered useful.

Library Design

In analogy to the rule of five, it has been proposed that ideal fragments should follow the "rule of three" (molecular weight < 300, ClogP < 3, the number of hydrogen bond donors and acceptors each should be < 3 and the number of rotatable bonds should be < 3). Since the fragments have relatively low affinity for their targets, they must have high water solubility so that they can be screened at higher concentrations.

Library Screening and Quantification

In fragment-based drug discovery, the low binding affinities of the fragments pose significant challenges for screening. Many biophysical techniques have been applied to address this issue. In particular, ligand-observe nuclear magnetic resonance (NMR) methods such as water-ligand observed via gradient spectroscopy (waterLOGSY), saturation transfer difference spectroscopy (STD-NMR), ^{19}F NMR spectroscopy and inter-ligand Overhauser effect (ILOE) spectroscopy,protein-observe NMR methods such as ^{1}H-^{15}N heteronuclear single quantum coherence (HSQC) that utilises isotopically-labelled proteins, surface plasmon resonance (SPR) and isothermal titration calorimetry (ITC) are routinely-used for ligand screening and for the quantification of fragment binding affinity to the target protein.

Once a fragment (or a combination of fragments) have been identified, protein X-ray crystallography are used to obtain structural models of the protein-fragment(s) complexes. Such information can then be used to guide organic synthesis for high-affinity protein ligands and enzyme inhibitors.

Advantages over Traditional Libraries

Advantages of screening low molecular weight fragment based libraries over traditional higher molecular weight chemical libraries are several. These include:

- More hydrophilic hits in which hydrogen bonding is more likely to contribute to affinity (enthalpically driven binding). It is generally much easier to increase affinity by adding hydrophobic groups (entropically driven binding), starting with a hydrophilic ligand increases the chances that the final optimized ligand will not be too hydrophobic (log P < 5).
- Higher ligand efficiency so that the final optimized ligand will more likely be relatively low in molecular weight (MW < 500).
- Since two to three fragments in theory can be combined to form an optimized ligand, screening a fragment library of N compounds is equivalent to screening N^2- N^3 compounds in a traditional library.

- Fragments are less likely to contain sterically blocking groups that interfere with an otherwise favorable ligand-protein interaction, increasing the combinatorial advantage of a fragment library even further.

Hit to Lead

Hit to lead (H2L) also known as lead generation is a stage in early drug discovery where small molecule hits from a high throughput screen (HTS) are evaluated and undergo limited optimization to identify promising lead compounds. These lead compounds undergo more extensive optimization in a subsequent step of drug discovery called lead optimization (LO). The drug discovery process generally follows the following path that includes a hit to lead stage:

- target validation (TV) → assay development → high-throughput screening → hit to lead (H2L) → lead optimization (LO) → preclinical drug development → clinical drug development

The hit to lead stage starts with confirmation and evaluation of the initial screening hits and is followed by synthesis of analogs (hit expansion). Typically the initial screening hits display binding affinities for their biological target in the micromolar (10^{-6} molar concentration) range. Through limited H2L optimization, the affinities of the hits are often improved by several orders of magnitude to the nanomolar (10^{-9} M) range. The hits also undergo limited optimization to improve metabolic half life so that the compounds can be tested in animal models of disease and also to improve selectivity against other biological targets binding that may result in undesirable side effects.

On average, only one in every 5,000 compounds that enters drug discovery to the stage of pre-clinical development becomes an approved drug.

Hit Confirmation

After hits are identified from a high throughput screen, the hits are confirmed and evaluated using the following methods:

- Confirmatory testing: compounds that were found active against the selected target are re-tested using the same assay conditions used during the HTS to make sure that the activity is reproducible.
- Dose response curve: the compound is tested over a range of concentrations to determine the concentration that results in half maximal binding or activity (IC_{50}or EC_{50} value respectively).
- Orthogonal testing: confirmed hits are assayed using a different assay which is usually closer to the target physiological condition or using a different technology.
- Secondary screening: confirmed hits are tested in a functional cellular assay to determine efficacy.
- Synthetic tractability: medicinal chemists evaluate compounds according to their synthesis feasibility and other parameters such as up-scaling or cost of goods.

- Biophysical testing: nuclear magnetic resonance (NMR), isothermal titration calorimetry (ITC), dynamic light scattering (DLS), surface plasmon resonance (SPR), dual polarisation interferometry (DPI), microscale thermophoresis (MST) are commonly used to assess whether the compound binds effectively to the target, the kinetics, thermodynamics, and stoichiometry of binding, any associated conformational change and to rule out promiscuous binding.
- Hit ranking and clustering: Confirmed hit compounds are then ranked according to the various hit confirmation experiments.
- Freedom to operate evaluation: hit structures are checked in specialized databases to determine if they are patentable.

Hit Expansion

Following hit confirmation, several compound clusters will be chosen according to their characteristics in the previously defined tests. An Ideal compound cluster will contain members that possess:

- high affinity towards the target (less than 1 μM);
- selectivity versus other targets;
- significant efficacy in a cellular assay;
- druglikeness (moderate molecular weight and lipophilicity usually estimated as ClogP). Affinity, molecular weight and lipophilicity can be linked in single parameter such as ligand efficiency and lipophilic efficiency;
- low to moderate binding to human serum albumin;
- low interference with P450 enzymes and P-glycoproteins;
- low cytotoxicity;
- metabolic stability;
- high cell membrane permeability;
- high water solubility (above 10 μM);
- chemical stability;
- synthetic tractability and
- patentability.

The project team will usually select between three and six compound series to be further explored. The next step will allow the testing of analogous compounds to determine a quantitative structure-activity relationship (QSAR). Analogs can be quickly selected from an internal library or purchased from commercially available sources ("SAR by catalog"). Medicinal chemists will also start synthesizing related compounds using different methods such as combinatorial chemistry, high-throughput chemistry, or more classical organic chemistry synthesis.

Lead Optimization Phase

The objective of this drug discovery phase is to synthesize lead compounds, new analogs with improved potency, reduced off-target activities, and physiochemical/metabolic properties suggestive of reasonable *in vivo* pharmacokinetics. This optimization is accomplished through chemical modification of the hit structure, with modifications chosen by employing knowledge of the structure-activity relationship (SAR) as well as structure-based design if structural information about the target is available.

Lead optimization is concerned with experimental testing and confirmation of the compound based on animal efficacy models and ADMET (*in vitro* and *in situ*) tools.

Application of ADME-Tox tools has increased the success rate of drug development as well as helped in reducing the cost and time factors. The use of *in silico* and *in vitro* ADME-Tox has found universal acceptance. *In silico* tools provide a much higher throughput, but they suffer from adequate predictability, which limits their use. However, the reliance on *in silico* models is due to their ability to predict which compounds should be synthesized based on confirmed hits and structural modifications since it helps in selecting a drug-like compound. The best way to implement the ADME-Tox property prediction is the integration of both *in silico* and *in vitro* approaches to supplement each other for the production of candidate drugs.

REFERENCES

1. Anson D, Ma J, He JQ (1 May 2009). "Identifying Cardiotoxic Compounds". Genetic Engineering & Biotechnology News. TechNote. 29 (9). Mary Ann Liebert. pp. 34–35. ISSN 1935-472X. OCLC 77706455. Archived from the original on 25 July 2009. Retrieved 25 July 2009.
2. Paul SM, Mytelka DS, Dunwiddie CT, Persinger CC, Munos BH, Lindborg SR, Schacht AL (March 2010). "How to improve R&D productivity: the pharmaceutical industry's grand challenge". Nature Reviews. Drug Discovery. 9 (3): 203–14. doi:10.1038/nrd3078. PMID 20168317.
3. Warren J (April 2011). "Drug discovery: lessons from evolution". British Journal of Clinical Pharmacology. 71 (4): 497–503. doi:10.1111/j.1365-2125.2010.03854.x. PMC 3080636Freely accessible. PMID 21395642.
4. Takenaka T (September 2001). "Classical vs reverse pharmacology in drug discovery". BJU International. 88 Suppl 2: 7–10; discussion 49–50. doi:10.1111/j.1464-410X.2001.00112.x. PMID 11589663.
5. Lee JA, Uhlik MT, Moxham CM, Tomandl D, Sall DJ (May 2012). "Modern phenotypic drug discovery is a viable, neoclassic pharma strategy". Journal of Medicinal Chemistry. 55 (10): 4527–38. doi:10.1021/jm201649s. PMID 22409666.
6. Elion GB (1993). "The quest for a cure". Annual Review of Pharmacology and Toxicology. 33: 1–23. doi:10.1146/annurev.pa.33.040193.000245. PMID 8494337.
7. Elion GB. "The purine path to chemotherapy. Nobel Lecture 1988.".
8. Black J. "Drugs from emasculated hormones: the principles of synoptic antagonism.

Nobel Lecture 1988.". Retrieved 28 February 2014.

9. Endo A. "The discovery of the statins and their development.". Retrieved 28 February 2014.
10. Watts G (2012). "Obituary: Sir David Jack" (PDF). The Lancet. 379 (9811): 116. doi:10.1016/S0140-6736(12)60053-1.
11. Swinney DC, Anthony J (July 2011). "How were new medicines discovered?". Nature Reviews. Drug Discovery. 10 (7): 507–19. doi:10.1038/nrd3480. PMID 21701501.
12. Rask-Andersen M, Almén MS, Schiöth HB (August 2011). "Trends in the exploitation of novel drug targets". Nature Reviews. Drug Discovery. 10 (8): 579–90. doi:10.1038/nrd3478. PMID 21804595.
13. Hopkins AL, Groom CR, Alex A (May 2004). "Ligand efficiency: a useful metric for lead selection". Drug Discovery Today. 9 (10): 430–1. doi:10.1016/S1359-6446(04)03069-7. PMID 15109945.
14. Ryckmans T, Edwards MP, Horne VA, Correia AM, Owen DR, Thompson LR, Tran I, Tutt MF, Young T (August 2009). "Rapid assessment of a novel series of selective CB(2) agonists using parallel synthesis protocols: A Lipophilic Efficiency (LipE) analysis". Bioorganic & Medicinal Chemistry Letters. 19 (15): 4406–9. doi:10.1016/j.bmcl.2009.05.062. PMID 19500981.
15. Leeson PD, Springthorpe B (November 2007). "The influence of drug-like concepts on decision-making in medicinal chemistry". Nature Reviews. Drug Discovery. 6 (11): 881–90. doi:10.1038/nrd2445. PMID 17971784.
16. Rester U (July 2008). "From virtuality to reality - Virtual screening in lead discovery and lead optimization: a medicinal chemistry perspective". Current Opinion in Drug Discovery & Development. 11 (4): 559–68. PMID 18600572.
17. Rollinger JM, Stuppner H, Langer T (2008). "Virtual screening for the discovery of bioactive natural products". Progress in Drug Research. Progress in Drug Research. 65 (211): 211, 213–49. doi:10.1007/978-3-7643-8117-2_6. ISBN 978-3-7643-8098-4. PMID 18084917.
18. Barcellos GB, Pauli I, Caceres RA, Timmers LF, Dias R, de Azevedo WF (December 2008). "Molecular modeling as a tool for drug discovery". Current Drug Targets. 9 (12): 1084–91. doi:10.2174/138945008786949388. PMID 19128219.
19. Durrant JD, McCammon JA (Oct 2011). "Molecular dynamics simulations and drug discovery". BMC Biology. 9: 71. doi:10.1186/1741-7007-9-71. PMC 3203851Freely accessible. PMID 22035460.
20. Borhani DW, Shaw DE (January 2012). "The future of molecular dynamics simulations in drug discovery". Journal of Computer-Aided Molecular Design. 26 (1): 15–26. doi:10.1007/s10822-011-9517-y. PMC 3268975Freely accessible. PMID 22183577.
21. Erlanson DA, McDowell RS, O'Brien T (July 2004). "Fragment-based drug discovery". Journal of Medicinal Chemistry. 47 (14): 3463–82. doi:10.1021/

jm040031v. PMID 15214773.

22. Folkers G, Jahnke W, Erlanson DA, Mannhold R, Kubinyi H (2006). Fragment-based Approaches in Drug Discovery (Methods and Principles in Medicinal Chemistry). Weinheim: Wiley-VCH. ISBN 3-527-31291-9.
23. Erlanson DA (June 2011). "Introduction to fragment-based drug discovery". Topics in Current Chemistry. 317: 1–32. doi:10.1007/128_2011_180. PMID 21695633.
24. Zartler E, Shapiro M (2008). Fragment-based drug discovery a practical approach. Wiley.
25. Greaney MF, Bhat VT (2010). "Chapter 2: Protein-directed dynamic combinatorial chemistry". In Miller BL. Dynamic combinatorial chemistry: in drug discovery, bioinorganic chemistry, and materials sciences. New Jersey: John Wiley & Sons. pp. 43–82.
26. Huang R, Leung IK (Jul 2016). "Protein-directed dynamic combinatorial chemistry: a guide to protein ligand and inhibitor discovery". Molecules. 21 (7): 910. doi:10.3390/molecules21070910. PMID 27438816.
27. Mondal M, Hirsch AK (April 2015). "Dynamic combinatorial chemistry: a tool to facilitate the identification of inhibitors for protein targets". Chemical Society Reviews. 44 (8): 2455–88. doi:10.1039/c4cs00493k. PMID 25706945.
28. Herrmann A (March 2014). "Dynamic combinatorial/covalent chemistry: a tool to read, generate and modulate the bioactivity of compounds and compound mixtures". Chemical Society Reviews. 43 (6): 1899–933. doi:10.1039/c3cs60336a. PMID 24296754.
29. Hochgürtel M, Lehn JM (2006). "Chapter 16: Dynamic combinatorial diversity in drug discovery". In Jahnke W, Erlanson DA. Fragment-based approaches in drug discovery. Weinheim: Wiley-VCH. pp. 341–364.
30. Caliandro R, Belviso DB, Aresta BM, de Candia M, Altomare CD (June 2013). "Protein crystallography and fragment-based drug design". Future Medicinal Chemistry. 5 (10): 1121–40. doi:10.4155/fmc.13.84. PMID 23795969.
31. Chilingaryan Z, Yin Z, Oakley AJ (Oct 2012). "Fragment-based screening by protein crystallography: successes and pitfalls". International Journal of Molecular Sciences. 13 (10): 12857–79. doi:10.3390/ijms131012857. PMC 3497300Freely accessible. PMID 23202926.
32. Valade A, Urban D, Beau JM (Jan–Feb 2007). "Two galactosyltransferases' selection of different binders from the same uridine-based dynamic combinatorial library". Journal of Combinatorial Chemistry. 9 (1): 1–4. doi:10.1021/cc060033w. PMID 17206823.
33. Roger MJ, Reigosa MJ, Pedrol N, González L (2006), Allelopathy: a physiological process with ecological implications, Springer, p. 1, ISBN 1-4020-4279-5
34. Feher M, Schmidt JM (2003). "Property distributions: differences between drugs, natural products, and molecules from combinatorial chemistry". Journal of Chemical Information and Computer Sciences. 43 (1): 218–27. doi:10.1021/ci0200467. PMID 12546556.

35. Newman DJ, Cragg GM (March 2007). "Natural products as sources of new drugs over the last 25 years". Journal of Natural Products. 70 (3): 461–77. doi:10.1021/np068054v. PMID 17309302.

36. von Nussbaum F, Brands M, Hinzen B, Weigand S, Häbich D (August 2006). "Antibacterial natural products in medicinal chemistry--exodus or revival?". Angewandte Chemie. 45 (31): 5072–129. doi:10.1002/anie.200600350. PMID 16881035. The handling of natural products is cumbersome, requiring nonstandardized workflows and extended timelines. Revisiting natural products with modern chemistry and target-finding tools from biology (reversed genomics) is one option for their revival.

37. John Faulkner D, Newman DJ, Cragg GM (February 2004). "Investigations of the marine flora and fauna of the Islands of Palau". Natural Product Reports. 21 (1): 50–76. doi:10.1039/b300664f. PMID 15039835.

38. Jakoby WB, Ziegler DM (December 1990). "The enzymes of detoxication". J. Biol. Chem. 265 (34): 20715–8. PMID 2249981.

39. Mizuno N, Niwa T, Yotsumoto Y, Sugiyama Y (September 2003). "Impact of drug transporter studies on drug discovery and development". Pharmacol. Rev. 55 (3): 425–61. doi:10.1124/pr.55.3.1. PMID 12869659.

40. Thornalley PJ (July 1990). "The glyoxalase system: new developments towards functional characterization of a metabolic pathway fundamental to biological life". Biochem. J. 269 (1): 1–11. PMC 1131522Freely accessible. PMID 2198020.

41. Sies H (March 1997). "Oxidative stress: oxidants and antioxidants" (PDF). Exp. Physiol. 82 (2): 291–5. doi:10.1113/expphysiol.1997.sp004024. PMID 9129943.

42. Guengerich FP (June 2001). "Common and uncommon cytochrome P450 reactions related to metabolism and chemical toxicity". Chem. Res. Toxicol. 14 (6): 611–50. doi:10.1021/tx0002583. PMID 11409933.

43. Schlichting I, Berendzen J, Chu K, Stock AM, Maves SA, Benson DE, Sweet RM, Ringe D, Petsko GA, Sligar SG (March 2000). "The catalytic pathway of cytochrome p450cam at atomic resolution". Science. 287 (5458): 1615–22. doi:10.1126/science.287.5458.1615. PMID 10698731.

44. Akagah B, Lormier AT, Fournet A, Figadère B (December 2008). "Oxidation of antiparasitic 2-substituted quinolines using metalloporphyrin catalysts: scale-up of a biomimetic reaction for metabolite production of drug candidates". Org. Biomol. Chem. 6 (24): 4494–7. doi:10.1039/b815963g. PMID 19039354.

45. Liston HL, Markowitz JS, DeVane CL (October 2001). "Drug glucuronidation in clinical psychopharmacology". J Clin Psychopharmacol. 21 (5): 500–15. doi:10.1097/00004714-200110000-00008. PMID 11593076.

46. Boyland E, Chasseaud LF (1969). "The role of glutathione and glutathione S-transferases in mercapturic acid biosynthesis". Adv. Enzymol. Relat. Areas Mol. Biol. Advances in Enzymology – and Related Areas of Molecular Biology. 32: 173–219. doi:10.1002/9780470122778.ch5. ISBN 9780470122778. PMID 4892500.

47. Homolya L, Váradi A, Sarkadi B (2003). "Multidrug resistance-associated proteins: Export pumps for conjugates with glutathione, glucuronate or sulfate". BioFactors. 17 (1–4): 103–14. doi:10.1002/biof.5520170111. PMID 12897433.

48. König J, Nies AT, Cui Y, Leier I, Keppler D (December 1999). "Conjugate export pumps of the multidrug resistance protein (MRP) family: localization, substrate specificity, and MRP2-mediated drug resistance". Biochim. Biophys. Acta. 1461 (2): 377–94. doi:10.1016/S0005-2736(99)00169-8. PMID 10581368.

49. Commandeur JN, Stijntjes GJ, Vermeulen NP (June 1995). "Enzymes and transport systems involved in the formation and disposition of glutathione S-conjugates. Role in bioactivation and detoxication mechanisms of xenobiotics". Pharmacol. Rev. 47 (2): 271–330. PMID 7568330.

50. Rostami-Hodjegan A, Tucker GT (February 2007). "Simulation and prediction of in vivo drug metabolism in human populations from in vitro data". Nat Rev Drug Discov. 6 (2): 140–8. doi:10.1038/nrd2173. PMID 17268485.

51. Murphy PJ (June 2001). "Xenobiotic metabolism: a look from the past to the future". Drug Metab. Dispos. 29 (6): 779–80. PMID 11353742.

52. Neuberger A, Smith RL (1983). "Richard Tecwyn Williams: the man, his work, his impact". Drug Metab. Rev. 14 (3): 559–607. doi:10.3109/03602538308991399. PMID 6347595.

53. Booth J, Boyland E, Sims P (June 1961). "An enzyme from rat liver catalysing conjugations with glutathione". Biochem. J. 79 (3): 516–24. PMC 1205680Freely accessible. PMID 16748905.

54. Omura T, Sato R (April 1962). "A new cytochrome in liver microsomes". J. Biol. Chem. 237: 1375–6. PMID 14482007.

55. Estabrook RW (December 2003). "A passion for P450s (remembrances of the early history of research on cytochrome P450)". Drug Metab. Dispos. 31 (12): 1461–73. doi:10.1124/dmd.31.12.1461. PMID 14625342.

56. Estabrook RW, Cooper DY, Rosenthal O (1963). "The light reversible carbon monoxide inhibition of steroid C-21 hydroxylase system in adrenal cortex". Biochem Z. 338: 741–55. PMID 14087340.

CHAPTER 4

Personalized Medicine

Chapter Contents

Personalized medicine is a form of medicine that uses information about a person's genes, proteins, and environment to prevent, diagnose, and treat disease. In cancer, personalized medicine uses specific information about a person's tumor to help diagnose, plan treatment, find out how well treatment is working, or make a prognosis. Examples of personalized medicine include using targeted therapies to treat specific types of cancer cells, such as HER2-positive breast cancer cells, or using tumor marker testing to help diagnose cancer. Also called precision medicine.

INTRODUCTION

Personalized medicine is a medical procedure that separates patients into different groups—with medical decisions, practices, interventions and/or products being tailored to the individual patient based on their predicted response or risk of disease. The terms personalized medicine, precision medicine, *stratified medicine* and P4 medicine are used interchangeably to describe this concept though some authors and organizations use these expressions separately to indicate particular nuances.

While the tailoring of treatment to patients dates back at least to the time of Hippocrates, the term has risen in usage in recent years given the growth of new diagnostic and informatics approaches that provide understanding of the molecular basis of disease, particularly genomics. This provides a clear evidence base on which to stratify (group) related patients.

DEVELOPMENT OF CONCEPT

In personalized medicine, diagnostic testing is often employed for selecting appropriate and optimal therapies based on the context of a patient's genetic content or other molecular or cellular analysis. The use of genetic information has played a major role in certain aspects of personalized medicine (e.g. pharmacogenomics), and the term was first coined in the context of genetics, though it has since broadened to encompass all sorts of personalization measures.

Background

Basics

Every person has a unique variation of the human genome. Although most of the variation between individuals has no effect on health, an individual's health stems from genetic variation with behaviors and influences from the environment.

One way that biological variation manifests itself is responsiveness to drugs for example, ADHD medicine works only for one of ten preschoolers, cancer drugs are effective for 25% of patients, and depression drugs work with 6 of 10 patients.

Modern advances in personalized medicine rely on technology that confirms a patient's fundamental biology, DNA, RNA, or protein, which ultimately leads to confirming disease. For example, personalized techniques such as genome sequencing can reveal mutations in DNA that influence diseases ranging from cystic fibrosis to cancer. Another method, called RNA-seq, can show which RNA molecules are involved with specific diseases. Unlike DNA, levels of RNA can change in response to the environment. Therefore, sequencing RNA can provide a broader understanding of a person's state of health. Recent studies have linked genetic differences between individuals to RNA expression, translation, and protein levels.

The concepts of personalized medicine can be applied to new and transformative approaches to health care. Personalized health care is based on the dynamics of systems biology and uses predictive tools to evaluate health risks and to design personalized health plans to help patients mitigate risks, prevent disease and to treat it with precision when it occurs. The concepts of personalized health care are receiving increasing acceptance with the Veterans Administration committing to personalized, proactive patient driven care for all veterans.

METHOD

In order for physicians to know if a mutation is connected to a certain disease, researchers often do a study called a "genome-wide association study" (GWAS). A GWAS study will look at one disease, and then sequence the genome of many patients with that particular disease to look for shared mutations in the genome. Mutations that are determined to be related to a disease by a GWAS study can then be used to diagnose that disease in future patients, by looking at their genome sequence to find that same mutation. The first GWAS, conducted in 2005, studied patients with age-related macular degeneration (ARMD). It found two different mutations, each containing only a variation in only one nucleotide (called single nucleotide polymorphisms, or SNPs), which were associated with ARMD. GWAS studies like this have been very successful in identifying common genetic variations associated with diseases. As of early 2014, over 1,300 GWAS studies have been completed.

Disease Risk Assessment

Multiple genes collectively influence the likelihood of developing many common and complex diseases. Personalized medicine can also be used to predict a person's risk for a particular disease, based on one or even several genes. This approach uses the same sequencing technology to focus on the evaluation of disease risk, allowing the physician to initiate preventative treatment before the disease presents itself in their patient. For example, if it is found that a DNA mutation increases a person's risk of developing Type 2 Diabetes, this individual can begin lifestyle changes that will lessen their chances of developing Type 2 Diabetes later in life.

APPLICATIONS

Advances in personalized medicine will create a more unified treatment approach specific to the individual and their genome. Personalized medicine may provide better diagnoses with earlier intervention, and more efficient drug development and therapies.

Diagnosis and Intervention

Having the ability to look at a patient on an individual basis will allow for a more accurate diagnosis and specific treatment plan. Genotyping is the process of obtaining an individual's DNA sequence by using biological assays. By having a detailed account of an individual's DNA sequence, their genome can then be compared to a reference genome, like that of the Human Genome Project, to assess the existing genetic variations that can account for possible diseases. A number of private companies, such as 23 and ME, Navigenics, and Illumina, have created Direct-to-Consumer genome sequencing accessible to the public. Having this information from individuals can then be applied to effectively treat them. An individual's genetic make-up also plays a large role in how well they respond to a certain treatment, and therefore, knowing their genetic content can change the type of treatment they receive.

An aspect of this is pharmacogenomics, which uses an individual's genome to provide a more informed and tailored drug prescription. Often, drugs are prescribed with the idea that it will work relatively the same for everyone, but in the application of drugs, there are a number of factors that must be considered. The detailed account of genetic information from the individual will help prevent adverse events, allow for appropriate dosages, and create maximum efficacy with drug prescriptions. The pharmacogenomic process for discovery of genetic variants that predict adverse events to a specific drug has been termed toxgnostics.

In addition to specific treatment, personalized medicine can greatly aid the advancements of preventive care. For instance, many women are already being genotyped for certain mutations in the BRCA1 and BRCA2 gene if they are predisposed because of a family history of breast cancer or ovarian cancer. As more causes of diseases are mapped out according to mutations that exist within a genome, the easier they can be identified in an individual. Measures can then be taken to prevent a disease from developing. Even if mutations were found within a genome, having the details of their DNA can reduce the impact or delay the onset of certain diseases. Having the genetic content of an individual will allow better guided decisions in determining the source of the disease and thus treating it or preventing its progression. This will be extremely useful for diseases like Alzheimer's or cancers that are thought to be linked to certain mutations in our DNA.

A tool that is being used now to test efficacy and safety of a drug specific to a targeted patient group/sub-group is companion diagnostics. This technology is an assay that is developed during or after a drug is made available on the market and is helpful in enhancing the therapeutic treatment available based on the individual. These companion diagnostics have incorporated the pharmacogenomic information related to the drug into their prescription label in an effort to assist in making the most optimal treatment decision possible for the patient.

Drug Development and Usage

Having an individual's genomic information can be significant in the process of developing drugs as they await approval from the FDA for public use. Having a detailed account of an individual's genetic make-up can be a major asset in deciding if a patient can be chosen for inclusion or exclusion in the final stages of a clinical trial. Being able to identify patients who will benefit most from a clinical trial will increase the safety of patients from adverse outcomes caused by the product in testing, and will allow smaller and faster trials that lead to lower overall costs. In addition, drugs that are deemed ineffective for the larger population can gain approval by the FDA by using personal genomes to qualify the effectiveness and need for that specific drug or therapy even though it may only be needed by a small percentage of the population.,

Today in medicine, it is common that physicians often use a trial and error strategy until they find the treatment therapy that is most effective for their patient. With personalized medicine, these treatments can be more specifically tailored to an individual and give insight into how their body will respond to the drug and if that drug will work based on their genome. The personal genotype can allow physicians to have more detailed information that will guide them in their decision in treatment prescriptions, which will be more cost-effective and accurate. As quoted from the article *Pharmacogenomics: The Promise of Personalized Medicine*, "therapy with the right drug at the right dose in the right patient" is a description of how personalized medicine will affect the future of treatment. For instance, Tamoxifen used to be a drug commonly prescribed to women with ER+ breast cancer, but 65% of women initially taking it developed resistance. After some research by people such as David Flockhart, it was discovered that women with certain mutation in their CYP2D6 gene, a gene that encodes the metabolizing enzyme, were not able to efficiently break down Tamoxifen, making it an ineffective treatment for their cancer. Since then, women are now genotyped for those specific mutations, so that immediately these women can have the most effective treatment therapy.

Screening for these mutations is carried out via high-throughput screening or phenotypic screening. Several drug discovery and pharmaceutical companies are currently utilizing these technologies to not only advance the study of personalized medicine, but also to amplify genetic research and these companies included are: Alacris Theranostics, Persomics, Flatiron Health, Novartis, OncoDNA and Foundation Medicine, among others. Alternative multi-target approaches to the traditional approach of "forward" transfection library screening can entail reverse transfection or chemogenomics.

Pharmacy compounding is yet another application of personalized medicine. Though not necessarily utilizing genetic information, the customized production of a drug whose various properties (e.g. dose level, ingredient selection, route of administration, etc.) are selected and crafted for an individual patient is accepted as an area of personalized medicine (in contrast to mass-produced unit doses or fixed-dose combinations).

Cancer Genomics

Over recent decades cancer research has discovered a great deal about the genetic variety of types of cancer that appear the same in traditional pathology. There has also been increasing awareness of tumour heterogeneity, or genetic diversity within a single tumour. Among other prospects, these discoveries raise the possibility of finding that drugs that have not given good results applied to a general population of cases may yet be successful for a proportion of cases with particular genetic profiles.

Cancer Genomics, or "Oncogenomics," is the application of genomics and personalized medicine to cancer research and treatment. High-throughput sequencing methods are used to characterize genes associated with cancer to better understand disease pathology and improve drug development. Oncogenomics is one of the most promising branches of genomics, particularly because of its implications in drug therapy. Examples of this include:

- Trastuzumab (trade names Herclon, Herceptin) is a monoclonal antibody drug that interferes with the HER2/neu receptor. Its main use is to treat certain breast cancers. This drug is only used if a patient's cancer is tested for over-expression of the HER2/neu receptor. Two tissue-typing tests are used to screen patients for possible benefit from Herceptin treatment. The tissue tests are immunohistochemistry(IHC) and Fluorescence In Situ Hybridization(FISH) Only Her2+ patients will be treated with Herceptin therapy (trastuzumab)

- Tyrosine kinase inhibitors such as imatinib (marketed as Gleevec) have been developed to treat chronic myeloid leukemia (CML), in which the BCR-ABL fusion gene (the product of a reciprocal translocation between chromosome 9 and chromosome 22) is present in >95% of cases and produces hyperactivated abl-driven protein signaling. These medications specifically inhibit the Ableson tyrosine kinase (ABL) protein and are thus a prime example of "*rational drug design*" based on knowledge of disease pathophysiology.

Challenges

As personalized medicine is practiced more widely, a number of challenges arise. The current approaches to intellectual property rights, reimbursement policies, patient privacy and confidentiality as well as regulatory oversight will have to be redefined and restructured to accommodate the changes personalized medicine will bring to healthcare. Furthermore, the analysis of acquired diagnostic data is a recent challenge of personalized medicine and its adoption. For example, genetic data obtained from next-generation sequencing requires computer-intensive data processing prior to its analysis. In the future, adequate tools will be required to accelerate the adoption of personalized medicine to further fields of medicine, which requires the interdisciplinary cooperation of experts from specific fields of research, such as medicine, clinical oncology, biology, and software engineering.

Regulatory Oversight

The FDA has already started to take initiatives to integrate personalized medicine into their regulatory policies. They developed a report in October 2013 entitled, "*Paving the Way for Personalized Medicine: FDA's role in a New Era of Medical Product Development*," in which they outlined steps they would have to take to integrate genetic and biomarker information for clinical use and drug development. They determined that they would have to develop specific regulatory science standards, research methods, reference material and other tools in order to incorporate personalized medicine into their current regulatory practices. For example, they are working on a "genomic reference library" for regulatory agencies to compare and test the validity of different sequencing platforms in an effort to uphold reliability.

Intellectual Property Rights

As with any innovation in medicine, investment and interest in personalized medicine is influenced by intellectual property rights. There has been a lot of controversy regarding patent protection for diagnostic tools, genes, and biomarkers. In June 2013, the U.S Supreme Court ruled that natural occurring genes cannot be patented, while "synthetic DNA" that is edited or artificially- created can still be patented. The Patent Office is currently reviewing a number of issues related to patent laws for personalized medicine, such as whether "confirmatory" secondary genetic tests post initial diagnosis, can have full immunity from patent laws. Those who oppose patents argue that patents on DNA sequences are an impediment to ongoing research while proponents point to research exemption and stress that patents are necessary to entice and protect the financial investments required for commercial research and the development and advancement of services offered.

Reimbursement Policies

Reimbursement policies will have to be redefined to fit the changes that personalized medicine will bring to the healthcare system. Some of the factors that should be considered are the level of efficacy of various genetic tests in the general population, cost-effectiveness relative to benefits, how to deal with payment systems for extremely rare conditions, and how to redefine the insurance concept of "shared risk" to incorporate the effect of the newer concept of "individual risk factors".

Patient Privacy and Confidentiality

Perhaps the most critical issue with the commercialization of personalized medicine is the protection of patients. One of the largest issues is the fear and potential consequences for patients who are predisposed after genetic testing or found to be non-responsive towards certain treatments. This includes the psychological effects on patients due to genetic testing results. The right of family members who do not directly consent is another issue, considering that genetic predispositions and risks are inheritable. The implications for certain ethnic groups and presence of a common allele would also have to be considered. In 2008, the Genetic Information Nondiscrimination Act (GINA) was passed in an effort to minimize the fear of patients participating in genetic research by ensuring that their genetic information will not be misused by employers or insurers. On February 19, 2015 FDA issued a press release titled: "FDA permits marketing of first direct-to-consumer genetic carrier test for Bloom syndrome.

REFERENCES

1. Stratified, personalised or P4 medicine: a new direction for placing the patient at the centre of healthcare and health education (Technical report). Academy of Medical Sciences. May 2015. Retrieved 6 Jan 2016.
2. "Many names for one concept or many concepts in one name?". PHG Foundation. Retrieved 6 Jan 2015.
3. Egnew, Thomas (1 Mar 2009). "Suffering, Meaning, and Healing: Challenges of Contemporary Medicine". Annals of Family Medicine. 7 (2): 170–175. doi:10.1370/afm.943. Retrieved 6 January 2016.
4. "The Case for Personalized Medicine" (PDF). Personalized Medicine Coalition. 2014. Retrieved 6 Jan 2016.
5. Smith, Richard (15 Oct 2012). "Stratified, personalised, or precision medicine". British Medical Journal. Retrieved 6 January 2016.
6. "Personalized Medicine 101". Personalized Medicine Coalition. Retrieved 26 April 2014.

7. Dudley, J; Karczewski, K. (2014). Exploring Personal Genomics. Oxford: Oxford University Press.
8. "Personalized Medicine 101: The Science". Personalized Medicine Coalition. Retrieved 26 April 2014.
9. Lu, YF; Goldstein, DB; Angrist, M; Cavalleri, G (24 July 2014). "Personalized medicine and human genetic diversity". Cold Spring Harbor perspectives in medicine. 4 (9): a008581. doi:10.1101/cshperspect.a008581. PMID 25059740.
10. Alexis Battle, Sara Mostafavi, Xiaowei Zhu, James B. Potash, Myrna M. Weissman, Courtney McCormick, Christian D. Haudenschild, Kenneth B. Beckman, Jianxin Shi, Rui Mei, Alexander E. Urban, Stephen B. Montgomery, Douglas F. Levinson & Daphne Koller (2014). "Characterizing the genetic basis of transcriptome diversity through RNA-sequencing of 922 individuals". Genome research. 24 (1): 14–24. doi:10.1101/gr.155192.113. PMID 24092820.
11. Cenik, Can; Cenik, Elif Sarinay; Byeon, Gun W; Candille, Sophie P.; Spacek, Damek; Araya, Carlos L; Tang, Hua; Ricci, Emiliano; Snyder, Michael P. (Nov 2015). "Integrative analysis of RNA, translation, and protein levels reveals distinct regulatory variation across humans.". Genome Research. 25: 1610–21. doi:10.1101/gr.193342.115. PMID 26297486.
12. Linfeng Wu; Sophie I. Candille; Yoonha Choi; Dan Xie; Lihua Jiang; Jennifer Li-Pook-Than; Hua Tang; Michael Snyder (2013). "Variation and genetic control of protein abundance in humans". Nature. 499 (7456): 79–82. doi:10.1038/nature12223. PMC 3789121Freely accessible. PMID 23676674.
13. Snyderman, R. Personalized Health Care from Theory to Practice, Biotechnology J. 2012, 7
14. Haines, J.L. (Apr 15, 2005). "Complement Factor H Variant Increases the Risk of Age-Related Macular Degeneration". Science. 308 (5720): 419–21. doi:10.1126/science.1110359. PMID 15761120.
15. "A Catalog of Published Genome-Wide Association Studies". Retrieved 28 June 2015.
16. "Personalized Medicine 101: The Promise". Personalized Medicine Coalition. Retrieved April 26, 2014.
17. "Research Portfolio Online Reporting Tools: Human Genome Project". National Institutes of Health (NIH). Retrieved April 28, 2014.
18. "Genetics Home Reference: What is pharmacogenomics?". National Institutes of Health (NIH). Retrieved April 28, 2014.
19. Church D, Kerr R, Domingo E, Rosmarin D, Palles C, Maskell K, Tomlinson I, Kerr D (2014). "'Toxgnostics': an unmet need in cancer medicine". Nat Rev Cancer (6):440-5
20. "Fact Sheet: BRCA1 and BRCA2: Cancer and Genetic Testing". National Cancer Institute (NCI). Retrieved April 28, 2014.
21. "BIOMARKER TOOLKIT: Companion Diagnostics" (PDF). Amgen. Archived from the original (PDF) on August 1, 2014. Retrieved May 2, 2014.

22. "Paving the Way for Personalized Medicine: FDA's Role in a New Era of Medical Product Development" (PDF). Federal Drug Administration (FDA). Retrieved April 28, 2014.
23. "The Path to Personalized Medicine". New England Journal of Medicine (NEJM). 363: 301–304. July 22, 2010. doi:10.1056/nejmp1006304. Retrieved April 28, 2014.
24. Mancinelli L, Cronin M, Sadée W (2000). "Pharmacogenomics. The Promise of Personalized Medicine". AAPS PharmSci. 2 (1): E4. PMC 2750999Freely accessible. PMID 11741220.
25. "Breast Cancer in the Personal Genomics Era". Current Genomics: Bentham Science. Retrieved April 28, 2014.
26. Carney, Walter (2006). "HER2/neu Status is an Important Biomarker in Guiding Personalized HER2/neu Therapy" (PDF). Connection. 9: 25–27.
27. Telli, M. L.; Hunt, S. A.; Carlson, R. W.; Guardino, A. E. (2007). "Trastuzumab-Related Cardiotoxicity: Calling Into Question the Concept of Reversibility". Journal of Clinical Oncology. 25 (23): 3525–3533. doi:10.1200/JCO.2007.11.0106. ISSN 0732-183X. PMID 17687157.
28. Saglio G; Morotti A; Mattioli G; et al. (December 2004). "Rational approaches to the design of therapeutics targeting molecular markers: the case of chronic myelogenous leukemia". Ann. N. Y. Acad. Sci. 1028 (1): 423–31. Bibcode:2004NYASA1028..423S. doi:10.1196/annals.1322.050. PMID 15650267.
29. "Personalized Medicine 101: The Challenges". Personalized Medicine Coalition. Retrieved April 26, 2014.
30. Huser, V; Sincan, M; Cimino, J. J. (2014). "Developing genomic knowledge bases and databases to support clinical management: Current perspectives". Pharmacogenomics and Personalized Medicine. 7: 275–83. doi:10.2147/PGPM.S49904. PMC 4175027Freely accessible. PMID 25276091.
31. "Analyze Genomes: Motivation". Schapranow, Matthieu-P. Retrieved July 20, 2014.
32. "Paving the Way for Personalized Medicine: FDA's Role in a New Era of Medical Product Development" (PDF). U.S Food and Drug Administration. Retrieved April 26, 2014.
33. "Intellectual Property Issues Impacting the Future of Personalized Medicine". American Intellectual Property Law Association. Retrieved April 26, 2014

CHAPTER 5

Drug Design

Chapter Contents

- **Introduction**
- **Drug Targets**
- **Retrometabolic Drug Design**
- **Drug Development**
- **Drug Repositioning**
- **Generic Drug**

The vast majority of drugs are small molecules designed to bind, interact, and modulate the activity of specific biological receptors. Receptors are proteins that bind and interact with other molecules to perform the numerous functions required for the maintenance of life. They include an immense array of cell-surface receptors (hormone receptors, cell-signaling receptors, neurotransmitter receptors, etc.), enzymes, and other functional proteins. Due to genetic abnormalities, physiologic stressors, or some combination thereof, the function of specific receptors and enzymes may become altered to the point that our well-being is diminished. These alterations may manifest as minor physical symptoms, as in the case of a runny nose due to allergies, or as life threatening and debilitating events, such as sepsis or depression. The role of drugs is to correct the functioning of these receptors to remedy the resulting medical condition.

INTRODUCTION

Drug design, often referred to as rational drug design or simply rational design, is the inventive process of finding new medications based on the knowledge of a biological target. The drug is most commonly an organic small molecule that activates or inhibits the function of a biomolecule such as a protein, which in turn results in a therapeutic benefit to the patient. In the most basic sense, drug design involves the design of molecules that are complementary in shape and charge to the biomolecular target with which they interact and therefore will bind to it. Drug design frequently but not necessarily relies on computer modeling techniques. This type of modeling is sometimes referred to as computer-aided drug design. Finally, drug design that relies on the knowledge of the three-dimensional structure of the biomolecular target is known as structure-based drug design. In addition to small molecules, biopharmaceuticals and especially therapeutic antibodies are an increasingly important class of drugs and computational methods for improving the affinity, selectivity, and stability of these protein-based therapeutics have also been developed.

The phrase "drug design" is to some extent a misnomer. A more accurate term is ligand design (i.e., design of a molecule that will bind tightly to its target). Although design techniques for prediction of binding affinity are reasonably successful, there are many other properties, such as bioavailability, metabolic half-life, side effects, etc., that first must be optimized before a ligand can become a safe and efficacious drug. These other characteristics are often difficult to predict with rational design techniques. Nevertheless, due to high attrition rates, especially during clinical phases of drug development, more attention is being focused early in the drug design process on selecting candidate drugs whose physicochemical properties are predicted to result in fewer complications during development and hence more likely to lead to an approved, marketed drug. Furthermore, in vitro experiments complemented with computation methods are increasingly used in early drug discovery to select compounds with more favorable ADME (absorption, distribution, metabolism, and excretion) and toxicological profiles.

DRUG TARGETS

A biomolecular target (most commonly a protein or nucleic acid) is a key molecule involved in a particular metabolic or signaling pathway that is associated with a specific disease condition or pathology or to the infectivity or survival of a microbial pathogen. Potential drug targets are not necessarily disease causing but must by definition be disease modifying. In some cases, small molecules will be designed to enhance or inhibit the target function in the specific disease modifying pathway. Small molecules (for example receptor agonists, antagonists, inverse agonists, or modulators; enzyme activators or inhibitors; or ion channel openers or blockers) will be designed that are complementary to the binding site of target. Small molecules (drugs) can be designed so as not to affect any other important "off-target" molecules (often referred to as antitargets) since drug interactions with off-target molecules may lead to undesirable side effects. Due to similarities in binding sites, closely related targets identified through sequence homology have the highest chance of cross reactivity and hence highest side effect potential.

Most commonly, drugs are organic small molecules produced through chemical synthesis, but biopolymer-based drugs (also known as biopharmaceuticals) produced through biological processes are becoming increasingly more common. In addition, mRNA-based gene silencing technologies may have therapeutic applications.

Rational Drug Discovery

In contrast to traditional methods of drug discovery (known as forward pharmacology), which rely on trial-and-error testing of chemical substances on cultured cells or animals, and matching the apparent effects to treatments, rational drug design (also called reverse pharmacology) begins with a hypothesis that modulation of a specific biological target may have therapeutic value. In order for a biomolecule to be selected as a drug target, two essential pieces of information are required. The first is evidence that modulation of the target will be disease modifying. This knowledge may come from, for example, disease linkage studies that show an association between mutations in the biological target and certain disease states. The second is that the target is "druggable". This means that it is capable of binding to a small molecule and that its activity can be modulated by the small molecule.

Once a suitable target has been identified, the target is normally cloned and produced and purified. The purified protein is then used to establish a screening assay. In addition, the three-dimensional structure of the target may be determined.

The search for small molecules that bind to the target is begun by screening libraries of potential drug compounds. This may be done by using the screening assay (a "wet screen"). In addition, if the structure of the target is available, a virtual screen may be performed of candidate drugs. Ideally the candidate drug compounds should be "drug-like", that is they should possess properties that are predicted to lead to oral bioavailability, adequate chemical and metabolic stability, and minimal toxic effects. Several methods are available to estimate druglikeness such as Lipinski's Rule of Five and a range of scoring methods such as lipophilic efficiency. Several methods for predicting drug metabolism have also been proposed in the scientific literature.

Due to the large number of drug properties that must be simultaneously optimized during the design process, multi-objective optimization techniques are sometimes employed. Finally because of the limitations in the current methods for prediction of activity, drug design is still very much reliant on serendipity and bounded rationality.

Computer-Aided Drug Design

The most fundamental goal in drug design is to predict whether a given molecule will bind to a target and if so how strongly. Molecular mechanics or molecular dynamics is most often used to estimate the strength of the intermolecular interaction between the small molecule and its biological target. These methods are also used to predict the conformation of the small molecule and to model conformational changes in the target that may occur when the small molecule binds to it. Semi-empirical, ab initio quantum chemistry methods, or density functional theory are often used to provide optimized parameters for the molecular mechanics calculations and also provide an estimate of the electronic properties (electrostatic potential, polarizability, etc.) of the drug candidate that will influence binding affinity.

Molecular mechanics methods may also be used to provide semi-quantitative prediction of the binding affinity. Also, knowledge-based scoring function may be used to provide binding affinity estimates. These methods use linear regression, machine learning, neural nets or other statistical techniques to derive predictive binding affinity equations by fitting experimental affinities to computationally derived interaction energies between the small molecule and the target.

Ideally, the computational method will be able to predict affinity before a compound is synthesized and hence in theory only one compound needs to be synthesized, saving enormous time and cost. The reality is that present computational methods are imperfect and provide, at best, only qualitatively accurate estimates of affinity. In practice it still takes several iterations of design, synthesis, and testing before an optimal drug is discovered. Computational methods have accelerated discovery by reducing the number of iterations required and have often provided novel structures.

Drug design with the help of computers may be used at any of the following stages of drug discovery:

- hit identification using virtual screening (structure- or ligand-based design);
- hit-to-lead optimization of affinity and selectivity (structure-based design, QSAR, etc.) and
- lead optimization of other pharmaceutical properties while maintaining affinity.

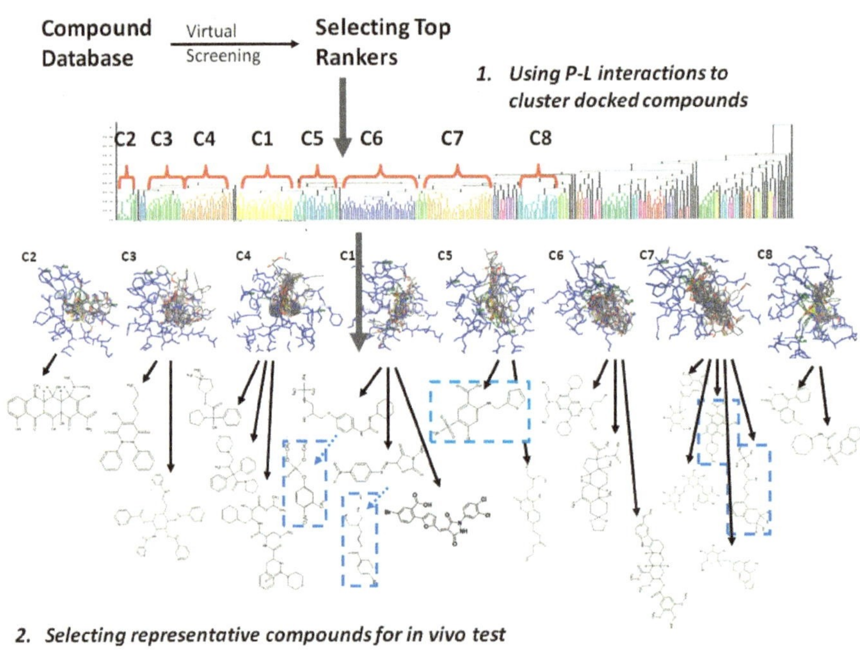

Flowchart of a Usual Clustering Analysis for Structure-Based Drug Design

In order to overcome the insufficient prediction of binding affinity calculated by recent scoring functions, the protein-ligand interaction and compound 3D structure information are used for analysis. For structure-based drug design, several post-screening analyses focusing on protein-ligand interaction have been developed for improving enrichment and effectively mining potential candidates:

- Consensus scoring
  - Selecting candidates by voting of multiple scoring functions and
  - May lose the relationship between protein-ligand structural information and scoring criterion.
- Cluster analysis
  - Represent and cluster candidates according to protein-ligand 3D information and
  - Needs meaningful representation of protein-ligand interactions.

Types

Drug discovery cycle highlighting both ligand-based (indirect) and structure-based (direct) drug design strategies.

There are two major types of drug design. The first is referred to as ligand-based drug design and the second, structure-based drug design.

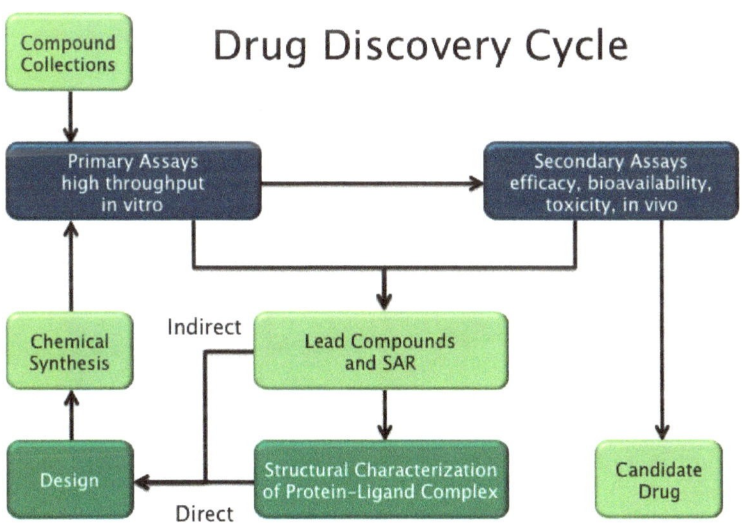

Ligand-based

Ligand-based drug design (or indirect drug design) relies on knowledge of other molecules that bind to the biological target of interest. These other molecules may be used to derive a pharmacophore model that defines the minimum necessary structural characteristics a molecule must possess in order to bind to the target. In other words, a model of the biological target may be built based on the knowledge of what binds to it, and this model in turn may be used to design new molecular entities that interact with the target. Alternatively, a quantitative structure-activity relationship (QSAR), in which a correlation between calculated properties of molecules and their experimentally determined biological activity, may be derived. These QSAR relationships in turn may be used to predict the activity of new analogs.

Structure-based

Structure-based drug design (or direct drug design) relies on knowledge of the three dimensional structure of the biological target obtained through methods such as x-ray crystallography or NMR spectroscopy. If an experimental structure of a target is not available, it may be possible to create a homology model of the target based on the experimental structure of a related protein. Using the structure of the biological target, candidate drugs that are predicted to bind with high affinity and selectivity to the target may be designed using interactive graphics and the intuition of a medicinal chemist. Alternatively various automated computational procedures may be used to suggest new drug candidates.

Current methods for structure-based drug design can be divided roughly into three main categories. The first method is identification of new ligands for a given receptor by searching large databases of 3D structures of small molecules to find those fitting the binding pocket of the receptor using fast approximate docking programs. This method is known as virtual screening. A second category is de novo design of new ligands. In this method, ligand molecules are built up within the constraints of the binding pocket by assembling small pieces in a stepwise manner. These pieces can be either individual atoms or molecular fragments. The key advantage of such a method is that novel structures, not contained in any database, can be suggested. A third method is the optimization of known ligands by evaluating proposed analogs within the binding cavity.

Binding Site Identification

Binding site identification is the first step in structure based design. If the structure of the target or a sufficiently similar homolog is determined in the presence of a bound ligand, then the ligand should be observable in the structure in which case location of the binding site is trivial. However, there may be unoccupied allosteric binding sites that may be of interest. Furthermore, it may be that only apoprotein (protein without ligand) structures are available and the reliable identification of unoccupied sites that have the potential to bind ligands with high affinity is non-trivial. In brief, binding site identification usually relies on identification of concave surfaces on the protein that can accommodate drug sized molecules that also possess appropriate "hot spots" (hydrophobic surfaces, hydrogen bonding sites, etc.) that drive ligand binding.

Scoring Functions

Structure-based drug design attempts to use the structure of proteins as a basis for designing new ligands by applying the principles of molecular recognition. Selective high affinity binding to the target is generally desirable since it leads to more efficacious drugs with fewer side effects. Thus, one of the most important principles for designing or obtaining potential new ligands is to predict the binding affinity of a certain ligand to its target (and known antitargets) and use the predicted affinity as a criterion for selection.

One early general-purposed empirical scoring function to describe the binding energy of ligands to receptors was developed by Böhm. This empirical scoring function took the form:

$$\Delta G_{\text{bind}} = \Delta G_0 + \Delta G_{\text{hb}} \Sigma_{h-bonds} + \Delta G_{\text{ionic}} \Sigma_{ionic-int} + \Delta G_{\text{lipophilic}} |A| + \Delta G_{\text{rot}} NROT$$

where:

- ΔG_0 – empirically derived offset that in part corresponds to the overall loss of translational and rotational entropy of the ligand upon binding.
- ΔG_{hb} – contribution from hydrogen bonding
- ΔG_{ionic} – contribution from ionic interactions
- ΔG_{lip} – contribution from lipophilic interactions where $|A_{lipo}|$ is surface area of lipophilic contact between the ligand and receptor
- ΔG_{rot} – entropy penalty due to freezing a rotatable in the ligand bond upon binding

A more general thermodynamic "master" equation is as follows:

$$\Delta G_{\text{bind}} = -RT \ln K_{\text{d}}$$

$$K_{\text{d}} = \frac{[\text{Ligand}][\text{Receptor}]}{[\text{Complex}]}$$

$$\Delta G_{\text{bind}} = \Delta G_{\text{desolvation}} + \Delta G_{\text{motion}} + \Delta G_{\text{configuration}} + \Delta G_{\text{interaction}}$$

where:

- desolvation – enthalpic penalty for removing the ligand from solvent
- motion – entropic penalty for reducing the degrees of freedom when a ligand binds to its receptor
- configuration – conformational strain energy required to put the ligand in its "active" conformation
- interaction – enthalpic gain for "resolvating" the ligand with its receptor

The basic idea is that the overall binding free energy can be decomposed into independent components that are known to be important for the binding process. Each component reflects a certain kind of free energy alteration during the binding process between a ligand and its target receptor. The Master Equation is the linear combination of these components. According to Gibbs free energy equation, the relation between dissociation equilibrium constant, K_d, and the components of free energy was built.

Various computational methods are used to estimate each of the components of the master equation. For example, the change in polar surface area upon ligand binding can be used to estimate the desolvation energy. The number of rotatable bonds frozen upon ligand binding is proportional to the motion term. The configurational or strain energy can be estimated using molecular mechanics calculations. Finally the interaction energy can be estimated using methods such as the change in non polar surface, statistically derived potentials of mean force, the number of hydrogen bonds formed, etc. In practice, the components of the master equation are fit to experimental data using multiple linear regression. This can be done with a diverse training set including many types of ligands and receptors to produce a less accurate but more general "global" model or a more restricted set of ligands and receptors to produce a more accurate but less general "local" model.

Examples

A particular example of rational drug design involves the use of three-dimensional information about biomolecules obtained from such techniques as X-ray crystallography and NMR spectroscopy. Computer-aided drug design in particular becomes much more tractable when there is a high-resolution structure of a target protein bound to a potent ligand. This approach to drug discovery is sometimes referred to as structure-based drug design. The first unequivocal example of the application of structure-based drug design leading to an approved drug is the carbonic anhydrase inhibitor dorzolamide, which was approved in 1995.

Another important case study in rational drug design is imatinib, a tyrosine kinase inhibitor designed specifically for the *bcr-abl* fusion protein that is characteristic for Philadelphia chromosome-positive leukemias (chronic myelogenous leukemia and occasionally acute lymphocytic leukemia). Imatinib is substantially different from previous drugs for cancer, as most agents of chemotherapy simply target rapidly dividing cells, not differentiating between cancer cells and other tissues.

Additional examples include:

- Many of the atypical antipsychotics;
- Cimetidine, the prototypical H_2-receptor antagonist from which the later members of the class were developed;
- Selective COX-2 inhibitor NSAIDs;
- Enfuvirtide, a peptide HIV entry inhibitor;
- Nonbenzodiazepines like zolpidem and zopiclone;
- Raltegravir, an HIV integrase inhibitor;
- SSRIs (selective serotonin reuptake inhibitors), a class of antidepressants and
- Zanamivir, an antiviral drug.

Criticism

It has been argued that the highly rigid and focused nature of rational drug design suppresses serendipity in drug discovery. Because many of the most significant medical discoveries have been inadvertent, the recent focus on rational drug design may limit the progress of drug discovery. Furthermore, the rational design of a drug may be limited by a crude or incomplete understanding of the underlying molecular processes of the disease it is intended to treat.

RETROMETABOLIC DRUG DESIGN

In the field of drug discovery, retrometabolic drug design is a strategy for the design of safer drugs using either a soft drug or targeted drug delivery approaches. The phrase retrometabolic drug design was coined by Nicholas Bodor (2007). The method is analogous to retrosynthetic analysis where the synthesis of a target molecule is planned backwards. In retrometabolic drug design, metabolic reaction information of drugs is used to design parent drugs whose metabolism and distribution can be controlled to target and eliminate the drug to increase efficacy and minimize undesirable side effects. The new drugs designed had achieved a selective organ and/or therapeutic site drug targeting and produce safe therapeutic agents and safe environmental chemicals. These approaches represent systematic methodologies that thoroughly integrate structure-activity (SAR) and structure-metabolism (SMR) relationships and are aimed at designing safe, locally active compounds with improved therapeutic index (ratio of benefit vs. side effect).

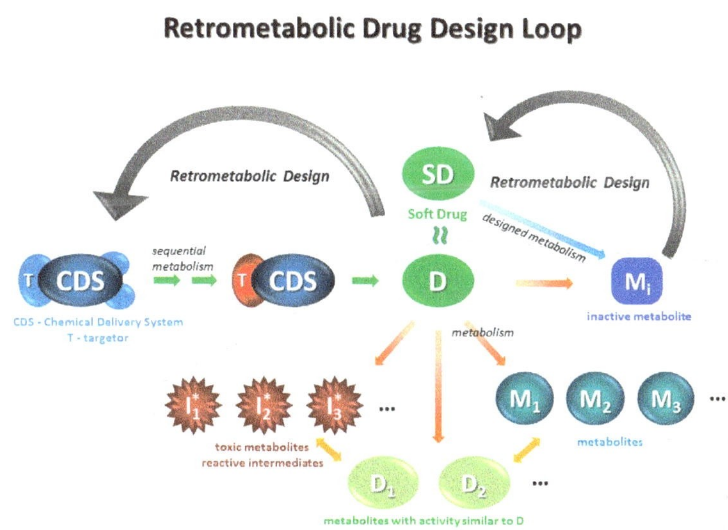

Retrometabolic drug design loop that includes chemical delivery systems (CDS) design and soft drug (SD) design. Possible metabolic pathways for drugs (D) in general are indicated within the dashed box.

Classification

The concept of retrometabolic drug design encompasses two distinct approaches. One approach is the design of soft drugs (SDs), new, active therapeutic agents, often isosteric or isolelectronic analogs of a lead compound, with a chemical structure specifically designed to allow predictable metabolism into inactive metabolites after exerting their desired therapeutic effect(s). The other approach is the design of chemical delivery systems (CDSs). CDSs are biologically inert molecules intended to enhance drug delivery to a particular organ or site and requiring several conversion steps before releasing the active drug.

Although both retrometabolic design approaches involve chemical modifications of the molecular structure and both require enzymatic reactions to fulfill drug targeting, the principles of SD and CDS design are distinctly different. While CDSs are inactive as administered and sequential enzymatic reactions provide the differential distribution and ultimately release the active drug, SDs are active as administered and are designed to be easily metabolized into inactive species. Assuming an ideal situation, with a CDS the drug is present at the site and nowhere else in the body because enzymatic processes destroy the drug at those sites. Whereas, CDSs are designed to achieve drug targeting at a selected organ or site, SDs are designed to afford a differential distribution that can be regarded as reverse targeting.

Soft Drugs

Since its introduction by Nicholas Bodor in the late 1970s, the soft drug concept generated considerable research both in academic and in industrial settings and there are several rationally designed soft drugs that have either already reached the market such as:

- esmolol (Breviblock);
- landiolol (Onoact);
- remifentanil (Ultiva);
- loteprednol etabonate (Lotemax, Alrex, Zylet) and
- clevidipine (Cleviprex)or are in late-stage development (remimazolam, budiodarone, celivarone, AZD3043, tecafarin). There are also compounds that can be considered as soft chemicals (e.g., malathion) or soft drugs (e.g., articaine, methylphenidate)even though they were not developed as such.

Chemical Delivery Systems

Since their introduction in the early 1980's, CDSs have also generated considerable research work, especially for brain and eye targeting of various therapeutic agents, including those that cannot cross the blood-brain barrier or the blood-retinal barrier on their own. Within this approach, three major general CDS classes have been identified:

- *Enzymatic physicochemical-based (e.g., brain-targeting) CDSs:* exploit site-specific traffic properties by sequential metabolic conversions that result in considerably altered properties;
- *Site-specific enzyme-activated (e.g., eye-targeting) CDSs:* exploit specific enzymes found primarily, exclusively, or at higher activity at the site of action;

- *Receptor-based transient anchor-type (e.g., lung-targeting) CDSs:* provide enhanced selectivity and activity through transient, reversible binding at the receptor.

This concept has been extended to many drugs and peptides, its importance illustrated by the fact that its first applications and uses were published in *Science* in 1975, 1981 and 1983. Its extension to the targeted brain-delivery of neuropeptides was included by the *Harvard Health Letter* as one of the top 10 medical advances of 1992. Several compounds have reached advanced clinical development phase, such as

- E_2-CDS (Estredox) for the brain-targeted delivery of estradiol and
- betaxoxime for the eye-targeted delivery of betaxolol.

In the first example above, brain-targeted CDSs employ a sequential metabolic conversion of a redox-based targetor moiety, which is closely related to the ubiquitous NAD(P)H $\rightleftharpoons$ NAD(P)$^+$ coenzyme system, to exploit the unique properties of the blood-brain barrier (BBB). After enzymatic oxidation of the NADH type drug conjugate to its corresponding NAD$^+$- drug, the still inactive precursor, "locks-in" behind the BBB to provide targeted and sustained CNS-delivery of the compound of interest.

The second example involves eye-specific delivery of betaxoxime, the oxime derivative of betaxolol. The administered, inactive β-amino-ketoxime is converted to the corresponding ketone via oxime hydrolase, an enzyme recently identified with preferential activity in the eye, and then stereospecifically reduced to its alcohol form. IOP-lowering activity is demonstrated without producing the active β-blockers systemically, making them void of any cardiovascular activity, a major drawback of classical antiglaucoma agents. Because of the advantages provided by this unique eye-targeting profile, oxime-based eye-targeting CDSs could replace the β-blockers currently used for ophthalmic applications.

History and Significance

These retrometabolic design strategies were introduced by Nicholas Bodor, one of the first and most prominent advocates for the early integration of metabolism, pharmacokinetic and general physicochemical considerations in the drug design process. These drug design concepts recognize the importance of design-controlled metabolism and directly focus not on the increase of activity alone but on the increase of the activity/toxicity ratio (therapeutic index) in order to deliver the maximum benefit while also reducing or eliminating unwanted side effects. The importance of this field is reviewed in a book dedicated to the subject (Bodor, N.; Buchwald, P.; *Retrometabolic Drug Design and Targeting*, 1st ed., Wiley & Sons, 2012), as well as by a full chapter of *Burger's Medicinal Chemistry and Drug Design*, 7th ed. (2010) with close to 150 chemical structures and more than 450 references. At the time of its introduction, the idea of designed-in metabolism represented a significant novelty and was against mainstream thinking then in place that instead focused on minimizing or entirely eliminating drug metabolism. Bodor's work on these design concepts developed during the late 1970's and early 1980's and came to prominence during the mid-1990's. Loteprednol etabonate, a soft corticosteroid designed and patented by Bodor received final Food and Drug Administration (FDA) approval in 1998 as the active ingredient of two ophthalmic preparations (Lotemax and Alrex), currently the only corticosteroid approved by the FDA for use in all inflammatory and allergy-related ophthalmic disorders. Its safety for long-term use further supports the soft drug concept, and in 2004, loteprednol etabonate was also approved as part of a combination product (Zylet). A second generation of soft corticosteroids such as etiprednol dicloacetate is in development for a full spectrum of other possible applications such as nasal spray for rhinitis or inhalation products for asthma.

The soft drug concept ignited research work in both academic (e.g., Aston University, Göteborg University, Okayama University, Uppsala University, University of Iceland, University of Florida, Université Louis Pasteur, Yale University) and industrial (e.g., AstraZeneca, DuPont, GlaxoSmithKline, IVAX, Janssen Pharmaceutica, Nippon Organon, Novartis, ONO Pharmaceutical, Schering AG) settings. Besides corticosteroids, various other therapeutic areas have been pursued such as soft beta-blockers, soft opioid analgetics, soft estrogens, soft beta-agonists, soft anticholinergics, soft antimicrobials, soft antiarrhythmic agents, soft angiotensin converting enzyme (ACE) inhibitors, soft dihydrofolate reductase (DHFR) inhibitors, soft cancineurin inhibitors (soft immunosuppressants), soft matrix metalloproteinase (MMP) inhibitors, soft cytokine inhibitors, soft cannabinoids, soft Ca^{2+} channel blockers.

Following the introduction of the CDS concepts, work along those lines started in numerous pharmaceutical centers around the world, and brain-targeting CDSs were explored for many therapeutic agents such as steroids (testosterone, progestins, estradiol, dexamethasone), anti-infective agents (penicillins, sulfonamides), antivirals (acyclovir, trifluorothymidine, ribavirin), antiretrovirals (AZT, ganciclovir), anticancer agents (Lomustine, chlorambucil), neurotransmitters (dopamine, GABA), nerve growth factor (NGF) inducers, anticonvulsants (Phenytoin, valproate, stiripentol), Ca^{2+} antagonists (felodipine), MAO inhibitors, NSAIDs and neuropeptides (tryptophan, Leu-enkephalin analogs, TRH analogs, kyotorphin analogs). A number of new chemical entities (NCE) were developed based on these principles, such as E_2-CDS (Estredox or betaxoxime are in advanced clinical development phases.

DRUG DEVELOPMENT

Drug development is the process of bringing a new pharmaceutical drug to the market once a lead compound has been identified through the process of drug discovery. It includes pre-clinical research on microorganisms and animals, filing for regulatory status, such as via the United States Food and Drug Administration for an investigational new drug to initiate clinical trials on humans, and may include the step of obtaining regulatory approval with a new drug application to market the drug.

New Chemical Entity Development

Broadly, the process of drug development can be divided into pre-clinical and clinical work.

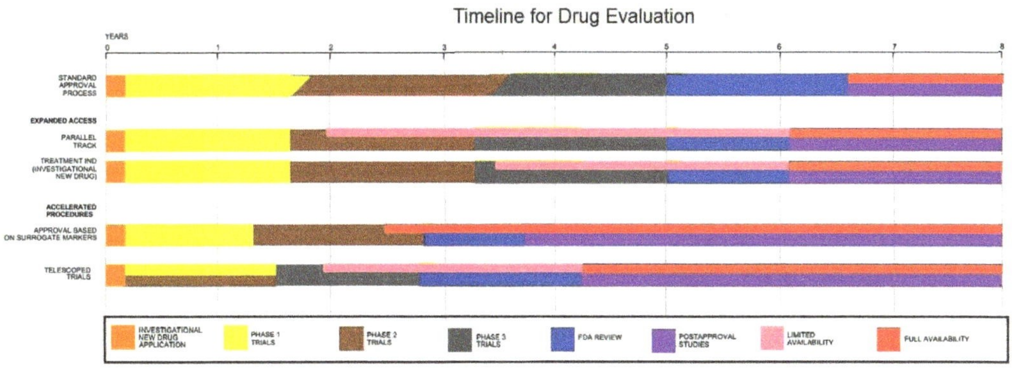

Timeline showing the various drug approval tracks and research phases

Pre-Clinical

New chemical entities (NCEs, also known as new molecular entities or NMEs) are compounds that emerge from the process of drug discovery. These have promising activity against a particular biological target that is important in disease. However, little is known about the safety, toxicity, pharmacokinetics, and metabolism of this NCE in humans. It is the function of drug development to assess all of these parameters prior to human clinical trials. A further major objective of drug development is to recommend the dose and schedule for the first use in a human clinical trial ("first-in-man" [FIM] or First Human Dose [FHD]).

In addition, drug development must establish the physicochemical properties of the NCE: its chemical makeup, stability, and solubility. Manufacturers must optimize the process they use to make the chemical so they can scale up from a medicinal chemist producing milligrams, to manufacturing on the kilogram and ton scale. They further examine the product for suitability to package as capsules, tablets, aerosol, intramuscular injectable, subcutaneous injectable, or intravenousformulations. Together, these processes are known in preclinical development as *chemistry, manufacturing, and control* (CMC).

Many aspects of drug development focus on satisfying the regulatory requirements of drug licensing authorities. These generally constitute a number of tests designed to determine the major toxicities of a novel compound prior to first use in humans. It is a legal requirement that an assessment of major organ toxicity be performed (effects on the heart and lungs, brain, kidney, liver and digestive system), as well as effects on other parts of the body that might be affected by the drug (e.g., the skin if the new drug is to be delivered through the skin). Increasingly, these tests are made using *in vitro* methods (e.g., with isolated cells), but many tests can only be made by using experimental animals to demonstrate the complex interplay of metabolism and drug exposure on toxicity.

The information is gathered from this pre-clinical testing, as well as information on CMC, and submitted to regulatory authorities (in the US, to the FDA), as an Investigational New Drug application or IND. If the IND is approved, development moves to the clinical phase.

Clinical Phase

Clinical trials involve three or four steps:

- Phase I trials, usually in healthy volunteers, determine safety and dosing.
- Phase II trials are used to get an initial reading of efficacy and further explore safety in small numbers of patients having the disease targeted by the NCE.
- Phase III trials are large, pivotal trials to determine safety and efficacy in sufficiently large numbers of patients with the targeted disease. If safety and efficacy are adequately proved, clinical testing may stop at this step and the NCE advances to the new drug application (NDA) stage.
- Phase IV trials are post-approval trials that are sometimes a condition attached by the FDA, also called post-market surveillance studies.

The process of defining characteristics of the drug does not stop once an NCE begins human clinical trials. In addition to the tests required to move a novel drug into the clinic for the first time, manufacturers must ensure that any long-term or chronic toxicities are well-defined, including effects on systems not previously monitored (fertility, reproduction, immune system, among others). They must also test the compound for its potential to cause cancer (carcinogenicity testing).

If a compound emerges from these tests with an acceptable toxicity and safety profile, and the company can further show it has the desired effect in clinical trials, then the NCE portfolio of evidence can be submitted for marketing approval in the various countries where the manufacturer plans to sell it. In the United States, this process is called a "new drug application" or NDA.

Most NCEs fail during drug development, either because they have unacceptable toxicity or because they simply do not have the intended effect on the targeted disease as shown in clinical trials.

Cost

The full cost of bringing a new drug (i.e., new chemical entity) to market – from discovery through clinical trials to approval – is complex and controversial. Typically, companies spend tens to hundreds of millions of U.S. dollars. One element of the complexity is that the much-publicized final numbers often not only include the out-of-pocket expenses for conducting a series of Phase I-III clinical trials, but also the *capital costs* of the long period (10 or more years) during which the company must cover out-of-pocket costs for preclinical drug discovery. Additionally, companies often do not report whether a given figure includes the capitalized cost or comprises only out-of-pocket expenses, or both.

Another element of complexity is that all estimates are based on confidential information controlled by drug companies, released by them voluntarily, leading to inability to verify costs. The numbers are controversial, as drug companies use them to justify the prices of their drugs and various advocates for lower drug prices have challenged them. The controversy is not only between "high" and "low", but also the high numbers may vary considerably for the manifold factors in drug development.

One study assessed both capitalized and out-of-pocket costs as about US$1.8 billion and $870 million, respectively.

In an analysis of the drug development costs for 98 companies over a decade, the average cost per drug developed and approved by a single-drug company was $350 million. But for companies that approved between eight and 13 drugs over 10 years, the cost per drug went as high as $5.5 billion, due mainly to geographic expansion for marketing and ongoing costs for Phase IV trials and continuous monitoring for safety.

Alternatives to conventional drug development have the objective for universities, governments and pharmaceutical industry to collaborate and optimize resources.

Valuation

The nature of a drug development project is characterized by high attrition rates, large capital expenditures, and long timelines. This makes the valuation of such projects and companies a challenging task. Not all valuation methods can cope with these particularities. The most commonly used valuation methods are risk-adjusted net present value (rNPV), decision trees, real options, or comparables.

The most important value drivers are the cost of capital or discount rate that is used, phase attributes such as duration, success rates, and costs, and the forecasted sales, including cost of goods and marketing and sales expenses. Less objective aspects like quality of the management or novelty of the technology should be reflected in the cash flows estimation.

Success Rate

Candidates for a new drug to treat a disease might, theoretically, include from 5,000 to 10,000 chemical compounds. On average about 250 of these show sufficient promise for further evaluation using laboratory tests, mice and other test animals. Typically, about ten of these qualify for tests on humans. A study conducted by the Tufts Center for the Study of Drug Development covering the 1980's and 1990's found that only 21.5 percent of drugs that started Phase I trials were eventually approved for marketing. In the time period of 2006 to 2015, the success rate was 9.6%. The high failure rates associated with pharmaceutical development are referred to as the "attrition rate" problem. Careful decision making during drug development is essential to avoid costly failures. In many cases, intelligent programme and clinical trial design can prevent false negative results. Well-designed, dose-finding studies and comparisons against both a placebo and a gold-standard treatment arm play a major role in achieving reliable data.

Novel initiatives to boost development

Novel initiatives include partnering between governmental organizations and industry. The world's largest such initiative is the Innovative Medicines Initiative (IMI), and examples of major national initiatives are Top Institute Pharma in the Netherlands and Biopeople in Denmark. In 2004, the FDA created the "Critical Path Initiative" to guide the new drug development process.

Pre-Clinical Development

In drug development, preclinical development, also named preclinical studies and nonclinical studies, is a stage of research that begins before clinical trials (testing in humans) can begin, and during which important feasibility, iterative testing and drug safety data are collected.

The main goals of pre-clinical studies are to determine the safe dose for first-in-man study and assess a product's safety profile. Products may include new medical devices, drugs, gene therapy solutions and diagnostic tools.

On average, only one in every 5,000 compounds that enters drug discovery to the stage of preclinical development becomes an approved drug.

Types of Preclinical Research

Each class of product may undergo different types of preclinical research. For instance, drugs may undergo pharmacodynamics (what the drug does to the body)(PD), pharmacokinetics (what the body does to the drug) (PK), ADME, and toxicology testing. This data allows researchers to allometrically estimate a safe starting dose of the drug for clinical trials in humans. Medical devices that do not have drug attached will not undergo these additional tests and may go directly to good laboratory practices (GLP) testing for safety of the device and its components. Some medical devices will also undergo biocompatibility testing which helps to show whether a component of the device or all components are sustainable in a living model. Most preclinical studies must adhere to GLPs in ICH Guidelines to be acceptable for submission to regulatory agencies such as the Food & Drug Administration in the United States.

Typically, both *in vitro* and *in vivo* tests will be performed. Studies of a drug's toxicity include which organs are targeted by that drug, as well as if there are any long-term carcinogenic effects or toxic effects on mammalian reproduction.

Animal Testing

The information collected from these studies is vital so that safe human testing can begin. Typically, in drug development studies animal testing involves two species. The most commonly used models are murine and canine, although primate and porcine are also used.

Choice of Species

The choice of species is based on which will give the best correlation to human trials. Differences in the gut, enzyme activity, circulatory system, or other considerations make certain models more appropriate based on the dosage form, site of activity, or noxious metabolites. For example, canines may not be good models for solid oral dosage forms because the characteristic carnivore intestine is underdeveloped compared to the omnivore's, and gastric emptying rates are increased. Also, rodents can not act as models for antibiotic drugs because the resulting alteration to their intestinal flora causes significant adverse effects. Depending on a drug's functional groups, it may be metabolized in similar or different ways between species, which will affect both efficacy and toxicology.

Medical device studies also use this basic premise. Most studies are performed in larger species such as dogs, pigs and sheep which allow for testing in a similar sized model as that of a human. In addition, some species are used for similarity in specific organs or organ system physiology (swine for dermatological and coronary stent studies; goats for mammary implant studies; dogs for gastric and cancer studies; etc.).

Importantly, the regulatory guidelines of FDA, EMA, and other similar international and regional authorities usually require safety testing in at least two mammalian species, including one non-rodent species, prior to human trials authorization.

Ethical Issues

Animal testing in the research-based pharmaceutical industry has been reduced in recent years both for ethical and cost reasons. However, most research will still involve animal based testing for the need of similarity in anatomy and physiology that is required for diverse product development.

No observable effect levels

Based on preclinical trials, No Observable Adverse Effect Levels (NOAEL) on drugs are established, which are used to determine initial phase 1 clinical trial dosage levels on a mass API per mass patient basis. Generally a 1/100 uncertainty factor or "safety margin" is included to account for interspecies (1/10) and inter-individual (1/10) differences.

DRUG REPOSITIONING

Drug repositioning (also known as drug repurposing, re-profiling, re-tasking or therapeutic switching) is the application of known drugs and compounds to treat new indications (i.e., new diseases).

A significant advantage of drug repositioning over traditional drug development is that since the repositioned drug has already passed a significant number of toxicity and other tests, its safety is known and the risk of failure for reasons of adverse toxicology are reduced. More than 90% of drugs fail during development, and this is the most significant reason for the high costs of pharmaceutical R&D. In addition, repurposed drugs can bypass much of the early cost and time needed to bring a drug to market. It significantly reduces the transition of bench research work to treatment at bedside. On the other hand, drug repositioning faces some challenges itself since the intellectual property issues surrounding the original drug may be complex and from a commercial point of view it may not always make sense to take such a drug to market.

Drug repositioning has been growing in importance in the last few years as an increasing number of drug development and pharmaceutical companies see their drug pipelines drying up and realize that many previously promising technologies have failed to deliver 'as advertised'. Computational approaches based on virtual screening of comprehensive libraries of approved and other human use compounds against large numbers of protein targets simultaneously have been developed to enhance the efficiency and success rates of drug repositioning, particularly in terms of high-throughput shotgun repurposing.

Commercialization

Smaller companies, including Ore Pharmaceuticals, Biovista, GVK BIO (GVK (conglomerate)), Numedicus, Melior Discovery and SOM Biotech are also performing drug repositioning on a systematic basis. These companies use a combination of approaches including in silico biology and *in vivo/in vitro* experimentation to assess a compound and develop and confirm hypotheses concerning its usage for new indications.

Examples

Using drug repositioning, pharmaceutical companies have achieved a number successes, for example Pfizer's Viagra in erectile dysfunction and Celgene's thalidomide in severe erythema nodosum leprosum.

One notable example of drug repurposing is taking the partial mu-opioid receptor agonist buprenorphine - which has been prescribed for control of moderate pain for decades in low dosages in the form of Temgesic 200mcg sublingual tablets, Buprenex 300mcg/mL ampoules - and marketing a high-dosage formulation (Subutex 2 mg and 8 mg) for the interruption and maintenance of heroin and other opioid addictions, which it has proven very beneficial for, with over 200,000 people in the United States alone on buprenorphine maintenance. Some of the reasons for this are that the drug has a ceiling effect - higher doses do not cause further activation of opioid receptors - and a very long half-life in >2 mg dosages. It also has an extremely high binding affinity for opioid receptors, which keeps the drug from being displaced by opioids like Dilaudid, heroin, morphine, and oxycodone, with the result that a user maintained on it can not get high no matter what dosage taken of most opioids. The only opioids that may be able to break through the buprenorphine blockade (which are required in an acute care setting if a buprenorphine patient requires pain relief, as no standard opioids are strong enough) - drugs with similar or higher binding affinities to buprenorphine itself - are the fentanil-class opioids, and the Bentley-series opioids (cf. etorphine, dihydroetorphine), which are rarely primary drugs of abuse and not often found on the streets. Buprenorphine itself is a modified Bentley-series opioid.

Requip is another notable example of drug repurposing. Originally developed as an anti-Parkinsonian agent, it has found application in the treatment of both Restless Legs Syndrome and SSRI-induced sexual dysfunction.

Colesevelam is another example of drug repurposing. Originally developed as an adjunct to diet and exercise to reduce elevated low-density lipoprotein cholesterol (LDL-C) in patients with primary hyperlipidemia as monotherapy, it has also gained approval to improve glycemic control in adults with type 2 diabetes mellitus.

Another example of drug repurposing is that of gabapentin, and its chemical cousin pregabalin. Originally developed as anti-epileptics, they have found more use treating anxiety disorders and neuropathic pain than as seizure medications.

Plerixafor, initially developed as an HIV drug to block viral entry in the cell via the chemokine co-receptor CXCR4, failed in its initial medical indication. Nevertheless, it was noticed that the drug induced peripheral blood leukocytosis within which peripheral blood CD34 hematopoietic stem cells were found. On basis of this observation, the drug has been re-purposed as a stem cell mobilizing drug.

GENERIC DRUG

A generic drug is a pharmaceutical drug that is equivalent to a brand-name product in dosage, strength, route of administration, quality, performance, and intended use. The term may also refer to any drug marketed under its chemical name without advertising, or to the chemical makeup of a drug rather than the brand name under which the drug is sold.

Although they may not be associated with a particular company, generic drugs are usually subject to government regulations in the countries where they are dispensed. They are labeled with the name of the manufacturer and a generic nonproprietary name such as the United States Adopted Name or international nonproprietary name of the drug. A generic drug must contain the same active ingredients as the original brand-name formulation. The U.S. Food and Drug Administration (FDA) requires that generics be identical to, or within an acceptable bioequivalent range of, their brand-name counterparts with respect to pharmacokinetic and pharmacodynamic properties. (The FDA's use of the word "identical" is a legal interpretation, not literal.)

Biopharmaceuticals such as monoclonal antibodies differ biologically from small molecule drugs. Generic versions of these drugs, known as biosimilars, are typically regulated under an extended set of rules. In most cases, generic products become available after the patent protections afforded to a drug's original developer expire. Once generic drugs enter the market, competition often leads to substantially lower prices for both the original brand-name product and its generic equivalents. In most countries, patents give 20 years of protection. However, many countries and regions, such as the European Union and the United States, may grant up to five years of additional protection ("patent term restoration") if manufacturers meet specific goals, such as conducting clinical trials for pediatric patients. Manufacturers, wholesalers, insurers, and drugstores can each increase prices at various stages of production and distribution.

In 2014, according to an analysis by the Generic Pharmaceutical Association, generic drugs accounted for 88% of the 4.3 billion prescriptions filled in the United States.

Nomenclature

Generic drug names are constructed using standardized affixes that distinguish drugs between and within classes and suggest their action.

Economics

When a pharmaceutical company first markets a drug, it is usually under a patent that, until it expires, the company can use to exclude competitors by suing them for patent infringement. Pharmaceutical companies that develop new drugs generally only invest in drug candidates with strong patent protection as a strategy to recoup their costs to develop the drug (include the costs of the drug candidates that fail) and to make a profit. The average cost to a brand-name company of discovering, testing, and obtaining regulatory approval for a new drug, with a new chemical entity, was estimated to be as much as $800 million in 2003 and $2.6 billion in 2014. Drug companies that bring new products have several product line extension strategies they use to extend their exclusivity, some of which are seen as gaming the system and referred to by critics as "evergreening", but at some point there is no patent protection available. For as long as a drug patent lasts, a brand-name company enjoys a period of market exclusivity, or monopoly, in which the company is able to set the price of the drug at a level that maximizes profit. This profit often greatly exceeds the development and production costs of the drug, allowing the company to offset the cost of research and development of other drugs that are not profitable or do not pass clinical trials.

Large pharmaceutical companies often spend millions of dollars protecting their patents from generic competition. Apart from litigation, they may reformulate a drug or license a subsidiary (or another company) to sell generics under the original patent. Generics sold under license from the patent holder are known as authorized generics.

Generic drugs are usually sold for significantly lower prices than their branded equivalents and at lower profit margins. One reason for this is that competition increases among producers when a drug is no longer protected by patents. Generic companies incur fewer costs in creating generic drugs—only the cost of manufacturing, without the costs of drug discovery and drug development—and are therefore able to maintain profitability at a lower price. The prices are often low enough for users in less-prosperous countries to afford them. For example, Thailand has imported millions of doses of a generic version of the blood-thinning drug Plavix (used to help prevent heart attacks) from India, the leading manufacturer of generic drugs, at a cost of 3 US cents per dose.

Generic drug companies may also receive the benefit of the previous marketing efforts of the brand-name company, including advertising, presentations by drug representatives, and distribution of free samples. Many drugs introduced by generic manufacturers have already been on the market for a decade or more and may already be well known to patients and providers, although often under their branded name.

In the United Kingdom, generic drug pricing is controlled by the government's reimbursement rate. The price paid by pharmacists and doctors is determined mainly by the number of license holders, the sales value of the original brand, and the ease of manufacture. A typical price decay graph will show a "scalloped" curve, which usually starts at the brand-name price on the day of generic launch and then falls as competition intensifies. After some years, the graph typically flattens out at approximately 20% of the original brand price. In about 20% of cases, the price "bounces": Some license holders withdraw from the market when the selling price dips below their cost of goods, and the price then rises for a while until the license holders re-enter the market with new stock.

In 2012, 84% of prescriptions in the US were filled with generic drugs, and in 2014, the use of generic drugs in the United States led to $254 billion in health care savings

Regulation

Most nations require generic drug manufacturers to prove that their formulations are bioequivalent to their brand name counterparts.

Bioequivalence does not mean generic drugs must be exactly the same as the brand name product ("pharmaceutical equivalent"). Chemical differences may exist; a different salt or ester may be used, for instance. However, the therapeutic effect of the drug must be the same ("pharmaceutical alternative"). Most small molecule drugs are accepted as bioequivalent if their pharmacokinetic parameters of AUC (area under concentration) and Cmax (maximum concentration) are within a 90% confidence interval of 80–125%; most approved generics are well within this limit. For more complex products—such as inhalers, patch delivery systems, liposomal preparations, or biosimilar drugs—demonstrating pharmacodynamic or clinical equivalence is more challenging.

United States

Enacted in 1984, the Drug Price Competition and Patent Term Restoration Act, informally known as the Hatch-Waxman Act, standardized procedures for recognition of generic drugs. In 2007, the FDA launched the Generic Initiative for Value and Efficiency (GIVE): an effort to modernize and streamline the generic drug approval process, and to increase the number and variety of generic products available.

Before a company can market a generic drug, it needs to file an Abbreviated New Drug Application (ANDA) with the Food and Drug Administration, seeking to demonstrate therapeutic equivalence to a previously approved "reference-listed drug" and proving that it can manufacture the drug safely and consistently. For an ANDA to be approved, the FDA requires the bioequivalence of a generic drug to be between 80% and 125% of the innovator product. (This range is part of a statistical calculation, and does not mean that generic drugs are allowed to differ from their brand-name counterparts by up to 25 percent.) The FDA evaluated 2,070 studies conducted between 1996 and 2007 that compared the absorption of brand-name and generic drugs into a person's body. The average difference in absorption between the generic and the brand-name drug was 3.5 percent, comparable to the difference between two batches of a brand-name drug. Generic versions of biologic drugs, or biosimilars, require clinical trials for immunogenicity in addition to tests establishing bioequivalency. These products cannot be entirely identical because of batch-to-batch variability and their biological nature, and they are subject to extra rules.

When an application is approved, the FDA adds the generic drug to its Approved Drug Products with Therapeutic Equivalence Evaluations list and annotates the list to show equivalence between the reference-listed drug and the generic. The FDA also recognizes drugs that use the same ingredients with different bioavailability, and divides them into therapeutic equivalence groups. For example, as of 2006, diltiazem hydrochloride had four equivalence groups, all using the same active ingredient, but considered equivalent only within each group.

In order to start selling a drug promptly after the patent on innovator drug expires, a generic company has to file its ANDA well before the patent expires. This puts the generic company at risk of being sued for patent infringement, since the act of filing the ANDA is considered "constructive infringement" of the patent. In order to incentivize generic companies to take that risk the Hatch-Waxman act granted a 180-day administrative exclusivity period to generic drug manufacturers who are the first to file an ANDA.

When faced with patent litigation from the drug innovator, generic companies will often counter-sue, challenging the validity of the patent. Like any litigation between private parties, the innovator and generic companies may choose to settle the litigation. Some of these settlement agreements have been stuck down by courts when they took the form of reverse payment patent settlement agreements, in which the generic company basically accepts a payment to drop the litigation, delaying the introduction of the generic product and frustrating the purpose of the Hatch-Waxman Act.

Innovator companies sometimes try to maintain some of the revenue from their drug after patents expire by allowing another company to sell an authorized generic; a 2011 FTC report found that consumers benefitted from lower costs when an authorized generic was introduced during the 180 exclusivity period, as it created competition.

Innovator companies may also present arguments to the FDA that the ANDA should not be accepted by filing a "citizen petition" with the FDA. Citizen petitions are part of the basic law governing everything the FDA does - at any time, any "interested person" can request that the FDA "issue, amend, or revoke a regulation or order," or "take or refrain from taking any other form of administrative action." Originally there was no deadline by which the FDA had to respond to citizen petitions filed to protest ANDAs, leading to significant delays in approving generics. In 2007 the law was amended to include a new section, Section 505(q), in the part of the federal code created by the Hatch-Waxman Act; this section said that the FDA could not delay approving an ANDA due to concerns raised in a citizen petition unless the delay was "necessary to protect public health"; it also mandated that the FDA needed to respond to a petition within 180 days - this was shorted to 150 days in a 2011 amendment. In 2014 the FDA issued guidance to industry about submitting citizen petitions and how it would consider them.

Acceptance

A series of scandals around the approval of generic drugs in the late 1980's shook public confidence in generic drugs and there were several instances in which companies obtained bioequivalence data fraudulently, by using the branded drug in their tests instead of their own product, and a congressional investigation found corruption at the FDA, where employees were accepting bribes to approve some generic companies' applications and delaying or denying others.

Some generic drugs are viewed with suspicion by doctors. For example, warfarin (Coumadin) has a narrow therapeutic window and requires frequent blood tests to make sure patients do not have a subtherapeutic or a toxic level. A study performed in Ontario showed that replacing Coumadin with generic warfarin was safe,but many physicians are not comfortable with their patients taking branded generic equivalents. In some countries (for example, Australia) where a drug is prescribed under more than one brand name, doctors may choose not to allow pharmacists to substitute a brand different from the one prescribed unless the consumer requests it.

Recalls

In 2007, North Carolina Public Radio's *The People's Pharmacy* began reporting on consumer's complaints that generic versions of bupropion (Wellbutrin) were yielding unexpected effects. Subsequently, Impax Laboratories's 300 mg extended-release tablets, marketed by Teva Pharmaceutical Industries, were withdrawn from the US market after the FDA determined in 2012 that they were not bioequivalent.

Litigation

Two women, each claiming to have suffered severe medical complications from a generic version of metoclopramide, lost their Supreme Court appeal on June 23, 2011. In a 5-4 ruling in PLIVA, Inc. v. Mensing, in which the court held that generic companies cannot be held liable for information, or the lack of information, on the originator's label.

India

The Indian government began encouraging more drug manufacturing by Indian companies in the early 1960's and with the Patents Act in 1970. The Patents Act removed composition patents for foods and drugs, and though it kept process patents, these were shortened to a period of five to seven years. The resulting lack of patent protection created a niche in both the Indian and global markets that Indian companies filled by reverse-engineering new processes for manufacturing low-cost drugs. Mumbai, India headquartered Sun Pharmaceutical's consolidated revenues for the 12 months ending March 2015 are US$4.5 billion.

China

Generic drug production is a large part of the pharmaceutical industry in China. Western observers have said that China lacks administrative protection for patents. However, entry to the World Trade Organization has brought a stronger patent system.

REFERENCES

1. Madsen U, Krogsgaard-Larsen P, Liljefors T (2002). Textbook of Drug Design and Discovery. Washington, DC: Taylor & Francis. ISBN 0-415-28288-8.
2. Reynolds CH, Merz KM, Ringe D, eds. (2010). Drug Design: Structure- and Ligand-Based Approaches (1 ed.). Cambridge, UK: Cambridge University Press. ISBN 978-0521887236.
3. Shirai H, Prades C, Vita R, Marcatili P, Popovic B, Xu J, Overington JP, Hirayama K, Soga S, Tsunoyama K, Clark D, Lefranc MP, Ikeda K (Nov 2014). "Antibody informatics for drug discovery". Biochimica et Biophysica Acta. 1844 (11): 2002–2015. doi:10.1016/j.bbapap.2014.07.006. PMID 25110827.
4. Tollenaere JP (Apr 1996). "The role of structure-based ligand design and molecular modelling in drug discovery". Pharmacy World & Science. 18 (2):

56–62. doi:10.1007/BF00579706. PMID 8739258.

5. Waring MJ, Arrowsmith J, Leach AR, Leeson PD, Mandrell S, Owen RM, Pairaudeau G, Pennie WD, Pickett SD, Wang J, Wallace O, Weir A (2015). "An analysis of the attrition of drug candidates from four major pharmaceutical companies". Nature Reviews Drug Discovery. 14: 475–86. doi:10.1038/nrd4609. PMID 26091267.
6. Yu H, Adedoyin A (Sep 2003). "ADME-Tox in drug discovery: integration of experimental and computational technologies". Drug Discovery Today. 8 (18): 852–61. doi:10.1016/S1359-6446(03)02828-9. PMID 12963322.
7. Dixon SJ, Stockwell BR (Dec 2009). "Identifying druggable disease-modifying gene products". Current Opinion in Chemical Biology. 13 (5-6): 549–55. doi:10.1016/j.cbpa.2009.08.003. PMC 2787993Freely accessible. PMID 19740696.
8. Imming P, Sinning C, Meyer A (Oct 2006). "Drugs, their targets and the nature and number of drug targets". Nature Reviews. Drug Discovery. 5 (10): 821–34. doi:10.1038/nrd2132. PMID 17016423.
9. Anderson AC (Sep 2003). "The process of structure-based drug design". Chemistry & Biology. 10 (9): 787–97. doi:10.1016/j.chembiol.2003.09.002. PMID 14522049.
10. Recanatini M, Bottegoni G, Cavalli A (Dec 2004). "In silico antitarget screening". Drug Discovery Today. Technologies. 1 (3): 209–15. doi:10.1016/j.ddtec.2004.10.004. PMID 24981487.
11. Wu-Pong S, Rojanasakul Y (2008). Biopharmaceutical drug design and development (2nd ed.). Totowa, NJ Humana Press: Humana Press. ISBN 978-1-59745-532-9.
12. Scomparin A, Polyak D, Krivitsky A, Satchi-Fainaro R (Apr 2015). "Achieving successful delivery of oligonucleotides - From physico-chemical characterization to in vivo evaluation". Biotechnology Advances. 33: 1294–309. doi:10.1016/j.biotechadv.2015.04.008. PMID 25916823.
13. Ganellin CR, Jefferis R, Roberts SM (2013). "The small molecule drug discovery process — from target selection to candidate selection". Introduction to Biological and Small Molecule Drug Research and Development: theory and case studies. Elsevier. ISBN 9780123971760.
14. Yuan Y, Pei J, Lai L (Dec 2013). "Binding site detection and druggability prediction of protein targets for structure-based drug design". Current Pharmaceutical Design. 19 (12): 2326–33. doi:10.2174/1381612811319120019. PMID 23082974.
15. Rishton GM (Jan 2003). "Nonleadlikeness and leadlikeness in biochemical screening". Drug Discovery Today. 8 (2): 86–96. doi:10.1016/s1359644602025722. PMID 12565011.
16. Hopkins AL (2011). "Chapter 25: Pharmacological space". In Wermuth CG. The Practice of Medicinal Chemistry (3 ed.). Academic Press. pp. 521–527. ISBN 978-0-12-374194-3.
17. Kirchmair J (2014). Drug Metabolism Prediction. Wiley's Methods and Principles in Medicinal Chemistry. 63. Wiley-VCH. ISBN 978-3-527-67301-8.

18. Nicolaou CA, Brown N (Sep 2013). "Multi-objective optimization methods in drug design". Drug Discovery Today. Technologies. 10 (3): 427–35. doi:10.1016/j.ddtec.2013.02.001. PMID 24050140.
19. Ban TA (2006). "The role of serendipity in drug discovery". Dialogues in Clinical Neuroscience. 8 (3): 335–44. PMC 3181823Freely accessible. PMID 17117615.
20. Ethiraj SK, Levinthal D (Sep 2004). "Bounded Rationality and the Search for Organizational Architecture: An Evolutionary Perspective on the Design of Organizations and Their Evolvability". Administrative Science Quarterly. Sage Publications, Inc. on behalf of the Johnson Graduate School of Management, Cornell University. 49 (3): 404–437. JSTOR 4131441.
21. Lewis RA (2011). "Chapter 4: The Development of Molecular Modelling Programs: The Use and Limitations of Physical Models". In Gramatica P, Livingstone DJ, Davis AM. Drug Design Strategies: Quantitative Approaches. Royal Society of Chemistry. pp. 88–107. doi:10.1039/9781849733410-00088. ISBN 978-1849731669.
22. Rajamani R, Good AC (May 2007). "Ranking poses in structure-based lead discovery and optimization: current trends in scoring function development". Current Opinion in Drug Discovery & Development. 10 (3): 308–15. PMID 17554857.
23. de Azevedo WF, Dias R (Dec 2008). "Computational methods for calculation of ligand-binding affinity". Current Drug Targets. 9 (12): 1031–9. doi:10.2174/138945008786949405. PMID 19128212.
24. Singh J, Chuaqui CE, Boriack-Sjodin PA, Lee WC, Pontz T, Corbley MJ, Cheung HK, Arduini RM, Mead JN, Newman MN, Papadatos JL, Bowes S, Josiah S, Ling LE (Dec 2003). "Successful shape-based virtual screening: the discovery of a potent inhibitor of the type I TGFbeta receptor kinase (TbetaRI)". Bioorganic & Medicinal Chemistry Letters. 13 (24): 4355–9. doi:10.1016/j.bmcl.2003.09.028. PMID 14643325.
25. Becker OM, Dhanoa DS, Marantz Y, Chen D, Shacham S, Cheruku S, Heifetz A, Mohanty P, Fichman M, Sharadendu A, Nudelman R, Kauffman M, Noiman S (Jun 2006). "An integrated in silico 3D model-driven discovery of a novel, potent, and selective amidosulfonamide 5-HT1A agonist (PRX-00023) for the treatment of anxiety and depression". Journal of Medicinal Chemistry. 49 (11): 3116–35. doi:10.1021/jm0508641. PMID 16722631.
26. Liang S, Meroueh SO, Wang G, Qiu C, Zhou Y (May 2009). "Consensus scoring for enriching near-native structures from protein-protein docking decoys". Proteins. 75 (2): 397–403. doi:10.1002/prot.22252. PMC 2656599Freely accessible. PMID 18831053.
27. Oda A, Tsuchida K, Takakura T, Yamaotsu N, Hirono S (2006). "Comparison of consensus scoring strategies for evaluating computational models of protein-ligand complexes". Journal of Chemical Information and Modeling. 46 (1): 380–91. doi:10.1021/ci050283k. PMID 16426072.
28. Deng Z, Chuaqui C, Singh J (Jan 2004). "Structural interaction fingerprint

(SIFt): a novel method for analyzing three-dimensional protein-ligand binding interactions". Journal of Medicinal Chemistry. 47 (2): 337–44. doi:10.1021/jm030331x. PMID 14711306.

29. Amari S, Aizawa M, Zhang J, Fukuzawa K, Mochizuki Y, Iwasawa Y, Nakata K, Chuman H, Nakano T (2006). "VISCANA: visualized cluster analysis of protein-ligand interaction based on the ab initio fragment molecular orbital method for virtual ligand screening". Journal of Chemical Information and Modeling. 46 (1): 221–30. doi:10.1021/ci050262q. PMID 16426058.
30. Guner OF (2000). Pharmacophore Perception, Development, and use in Drug Design. La Jolla, Calif: International University Line. ISBN 0-9636817-6-1.
31. Tropsha A (2010). "QSAR in Drug Discovery". In Reynolds CH, Merz KM, Ringe D. Drug Design: Structure- and Ligand-Based Approaches (1 ed.). Cambridge, UK: Cambridge University Press. pp. 151–164. ISBN 978-0521887236.
32. Leach, Andrew R.; Harren, Jhoti (2007). Structure-based Drug Discovery. Berlin: Springer. ISBN 1-4020-4406-2.
33. Mauser H, Guba W (May 2008). "Recent developments in de novo design and scaffold hopping". Current Opinion in Drug Discovery & Development. 11 (3): 365–74. PMID 18428090.
34. Klebe G (2000). "Recent developments in structure-based drug design". Journal of Molecular Medicine. 78 (5): 269–81. doi:10.1007/s001090000084. PMID 10954199.
35. Wang R, Gao Y, Lai L (2000). "LigBuilder: A Multi-Purpose Program for Structure-Based Drug Design". Journal of Molecular Modeling. 6 (7–8): 498–516. doi:10.1007/s0089400060498.
36. Schneider G, Fechner U (Aug 2005). "Computer-based de novo design of drug-like molecules". Nature Reviews. Drug Discovery. 4 (8): 649–63. doi:10.1038/nrd1799. PMID 16056391.
37. Jorgensen WL (Mar 2004). "The many roles of computation in drug discovery". Science. 303 (5665): 1813–8. Bibcode:2004Sci...303.1813J. doi:10.1126/science.1096361. PMID 15031495.
38. Leis S, Schneider S, Zacharias M (2010). "In silico prediction of binding sites on proteins". Current Medicinal Chemistry. 17 (15): 1550–62. doi:10.2174/092986710790979944. PMID 20166931.
39. Warren GL, Warren SD (2011). "Chapter 16: Scoring Drug-Receptor Interactions". In Gramatica P, Livingstone DJ, Davis AM. Drug Design Strategies: Quantitative Approaches. Royal Society of Chemistry. pp. 440–457. doi:10.1039/9781849733410-00440. ISBN 978-1849731669.
40. Böhm HJ (Jun 1994). "The development of a simple empirical scoring function to estimate the binding constant for a protein-ligand complex of known three-dimensional structure". Journal of Computer-Aided Molecular Design. 8 (3): 243–56. Bibcode:1994JCAMD...8..243B. doi:10.1007/BF00126743. PMID 7964925.

41. Liu J, Wang R (23 March 2015). "Classification of Current Scoring Functions". Journal of Chemical Information and Modeling. 55 (3): 475–482. doi:10.1021/ci500731a.

42. Ajay, Murcko MA (1995). "Computational methods to predict binding free energy in ligand-receptor complexes". J. Med. Chem. 38 (26): 4953–67. doi:10.1021/jm00026a001. PMID 8544170.

43. Gramatica P (2011). "Chapter 17: Modeling Chemicals in the Environment". In Gramatica P, Livingstone DJ, Davis AM. Drug Design Strategies: Quantitative Approaches. Royal Society of Chemistry. p. 466. doi:10.1039/9781849733410-00458. ISBN 978-1849731669.

44. Greer J, Erickson JW, Baldwin JJ, Varney MD (Apr 1994). "Application of the three-dimensional structures of protein target molecules in structure-based drug design". Journal of Medicinal Chemistry. 37 (8): 1035–54. doi:10.1021/jm00034a001. PMID 8164249.

45. Timmerman H, Gubernator K, Böhm H, Mannhold R, Kubinyi H (1998). Structure-based Ligand Design (Methods and Principles in Medicinal Chemistry). Weinheim: Wiley-VCH. ISBN 3-527-29343-4.

46. Capdeville R, Buchdunger E, Zimmermann J, Matter A (Jul 2002). "Glivec (STI571, imatinib), a rationally developed, targeted anticancer drug". Nature Reviews. Drug Discovery. 1 (7): 493–502. doi:10.1038/nrd839. PMID 12120256.

47. "AutoDock's role in Developing the First Clinically-Approved HIV Integrase Inhibitor". Press Release. The Scripps Research Institute. 2007-12-17.

48. Klein DF (Mar 2008). "The loss of serendipity in psychopharmacology". JAMA. 299 (9): 1063–5. doi:10.1001/jama.299.9.1063. PMID 18319418.

CHAPTER 6

Targeted Drug Delivery: Methods and Applications

Chapter Contents

- **Introduction**
- **Drug Targets**
- **Retrometabolic Drug Design**
- **Drug Development**
- **Drug Repositioning**
- **Generic Drug**

Targeted drug delivery is a kind of smart drug delivery system which is miraculous in delivering the drug to a patient. This conventional drug delivery system is done by the absorption of the drug across a biological membrane, whereas the targeted release system is that drug is released in a dosage form.

Targeted drug delivery system is based on a method that delivers a certain amount of a therapeutic agent for a prolonged period of time to a targeted diseased area within the body. This helps maintain the required plasma and tissue drug levels in the body; therefore avoiding any damage to the healthy tissue via the drug. The drug delivery system is highly integrated and requires various disciplines, such as chemists, biologist and engineers, to join forces to optimize this system. When implementing a targeted release system, the following design criteria for the system need to take into account: the drug properties, side effects of the drugs, the route taken for the delivery of the drug, the targeted site, and the disease.

INTRODUCTION

Targeted drug delivery, sometimes called smart drug delivery, is a method of delivering medication to a patient in a manner that increases the concentration of the medication in some parts of the body relative to others. This means of delivery is largely founded on nanomedicine, which plans to employ nanoparticle-mediated drug delivery in order to combat the downfalls of conventional drug delivery. These nanoparticles would be loaded with drugs and targeted to specific parts of the body where there is solely diseased tissue, thereby avoiding interaction with healthy tissue. The goal of a targeted drug delivery system is to prolong, localize, target and have a protected drug interaction with the diseased tissue. The conventional drug delivery system is the absorption of the drug across a biological membrane, whereas the *targeted release system* releases the drug in a dosage form. The advantages to the targeted release system is the reduction in the frequency of the dosages taken by the patient, having a more uniform effect of the drug, reduction of drug side-effects, and reduced fluctuation in circulating drug levels. The disadvantage of the system is high cost, which makes productivity more difficult and the reduced ability to adjust the dosages.

Targeted drug delivery systems have been developed to optimize regenerative techniques. The system is based on a method that delivers a certain amount of a therapeutic agent for a prolonged period of time to a targeted diseased area within the body. This helps maintain the required plasma and tissue drug levels in the body, thereby preventing any damage to the healthy tissue via the drug. The drug delivery system is highly integrated and requires various disciplines, such as chemists, biologists, and engineers, to join forces to optimize this system.

BACKGROUND

In traditional drug delivery systems such as oral ingestion or intravascular injection, the medication is distributed throughout the body through the systemic blood circulation. For most therapeutic agents, only a small portion of the medication reaches the organ to be affected, such as in chemotherapy where roughly 99% of the drugs administered do not reach the tumor site. Targeted drug delivery seeks to concentrate the medication in the tissues of interest while reducing the relative concentration of the medication in the remaining tissues. For example, by avoiding the host's defense mechanisms and inhibiting non-specific distribution in the liver and spleen, a system can reach the intended site of action in higher concentrations. Targeted delivery is believed to improve efficacy while reducing side-effects.

When implementing a targeted release system, the following design criteria for the system must be taken into account: the drug properties, side effects of the drugs, the route taken for the delivery of the drug, the targeted site, and the disease.

Increasing developments to novel treatments requires a controlled microenvironment that is accomplished only through the implementation of therapeutic agents whose side-effects can be avoided with targeted drug delivery. Advances in the field of targeted drug delivery to cardiac tissue will be an integral component to regenerate cardiac tissue.

There are two kinds of targeted drug delivery: active targeted drug delivery, such as some antibody medications, and passive targeted drug delivery, such as the enhanced permeability and retention effect (EPR-effect).

TARGETING METHODS

This ability for nanoparticles to concentrate in areas of solely diseased tissue is accomplished through either one or both means of targeting: passive or active.

Passive Targeting

In passive targeting, the drug's success is directly related to circulation time. This is achieved by cloaking the nanoparticle with some sort of coating. Several substances can achieve this, with one of them being polyethylene glycol (PEG). By adding PEG to the surface of the nanoparticle, it is rendered hydrophilic, thus allowing water molecules to bind to the oxygen molecules on PEG via hydrogen bonding. The result of this bond is a film of hydration around the nanoparticle which makes the substance antiphagocytic. The particles obtain this property due to the hydrophobic interactions that are natural to the reticuloendothelial system (RES), thus the drug-loaded nanoparticle is able to stay in circulation for a longer period of time. To work in conjunction with this mechanism of passive targeting, nanoparticles that are between 10 and 100 nanometers in size have been found to circulate systemically for longer periods of time.

Active Targeting

Active targeting of drug-loaded nanoparticles enhances the effects of passive targeting to make the nanoparticle more specific to a target site. There are several ways that active targeting can be accomplished. One way to actively target solely diseased tissue in the body is to know the nature of a receptor on the cell for which the drug will be targeted to. Researchers can then utilize cell-specific ligands that will allow for the nanoparticle to bind specifically to the cell that has the complimentary receptor. This form of active targeting was found to be successful when utilizing transferrin as the cell-specific ligand. The transferrin was conjugated to the nanoparticle to target tumor cells that possess transferrin-receptor mediated endocytosis mechanisms on their membrane. This means of targeting was found to increase uptake, as opposed to non-conjugated nanoparticles.

Active targeting can also be achieved by utilizing magnetoliposomes, which usually serves as a contrast agent in magnetic resonance imaging. Thus, by grafting these liposomes with a desired drug to deliver to a region of the body, magnetic positioning could aid with this process.

Furthermore, a nanoparticle could possess the capability to be activated by a trigger that is specific to the target site, such as utilizing materials that are pH responsive. Most of the body has a consistent, neutral pH. However, some areas of the body are naturally more acidic than others, and, thus, nanoparticles can take advantage of this ability by releasing the drug when it encounters a specific pH. Another specific triggering mechanism is based on the redox potential. One of the side effects of tumors is hypoxia, which alters the redox potential in the vicinity of the tumor. By modifying the redox potential that triggers the payload release the vesicles can by selective to different types of tumors.

By utilizing both passive and active targeting, a drug-loaded nanoparticle has a heightened advantage over a conventional drug. It is able to circulate throughout the body for an extended period of time until it is successfully attracted to its target through the use of cell-specific ligands, magnetic positioning, or pH responsive materials. Because of these advantages, side effects from conventional drugs will be largely reduced as a result of the drug-loaded nanoparticles affecting only diseased tissue. However, an emerging field known as nanotoxicology has concerns that the nanoparticles themselves could pose a threat to both the environment and human health with side effects of their own. Active targeting can be also be achieved through peptide based drug targeting system.

DELIVERY VEHICLES

There are different types of drug delivery vehicles, such as polymeric micelles, liposomes, lipoprotein-based drug carriers, nano-particle drug carriers, dendrimers, etc. An ideal drug delivery vehicle must be non-toxic, biocompatible, non-immunogenic, biodegradable, and must avoid recognition by the host's defense mechanisms

Liposomes

Liposomes are composite structures made of phospholipids and may contain small amounts of other molecules. Though liposomes can vary in size from low micrometer range to tens of micrometers, unilamellar liposomes, as pictured here, are typically in the lower size range, with various targeting ligands attached to their surface, allowing for their surface-attachment and accumulation in pathological areas for treatment of disease.

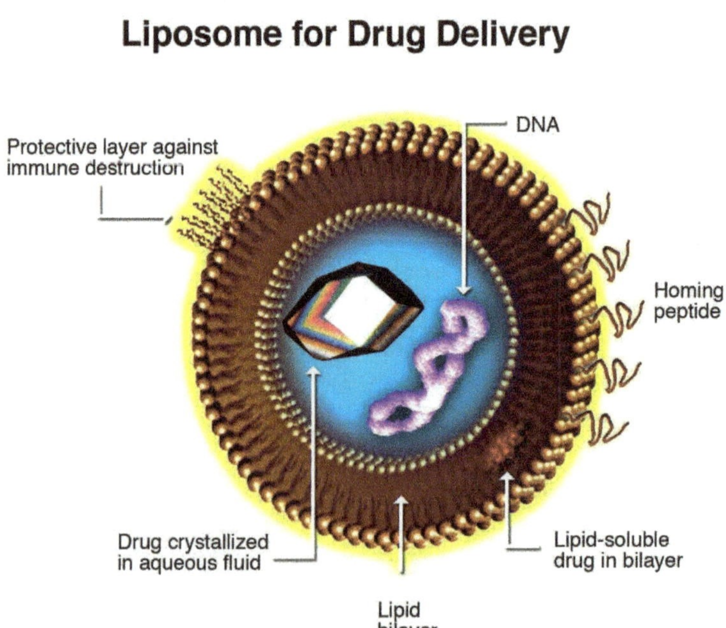

The most common vehicle currently used for targeted drug delivery is the liposome. Liposomes are non-toxic, non-hemolytic, and non-immunogenic even upon repeated injections; they are biocompatible and biodegradable and can be designed to avoid clearance

mechanisms (reticuloendothelial system (RES), renal clearance, chemical or enzymatic inactivation, etc.) Lipid-based, ligand-coated nanocarriers can store their payload in the hydrophobic shell or the hydrophilic interior depending on the nature of the drug/contrast agent being carried.

The only problem to using liposomes *in vivo* is their immediate uptake and clearance by the RES system and their relatively low stability in vitro. To combat this, polyethylene glycol (PEG) can be added to the surface of the liposomes. Increasing the mole percent of PEG on the surface of the liposomes by 4-10% significantly increased circulation time *in vivo* from 200 to 1000 minutes.

PEGylation of the liposomal nanocarrier elongates the half-life of the construct while maintaining the passive targeting mechanism that is commonly conferred to lipid-based nanocarriers. When used as a delivery system, the ability to induce instability in the construct is commonly exploited allowing the selective release of the encapsulated therapeutic agent in close proximity to the target tissue/cell *in vivo*. This nanocarrier system is commonly used in anti-cancer treatments as the acidity of the tumour mass caused by an over-reliance on glycolysis triggers drug release.

Micelles and Dendrimers

Another type of drug delivery vehicle used is polymeric micelles. They are prepared from certain amphiphilic co-polymers consisting of both hydrophilic and hydrophobic monomer units. They can be used to carry drugs that have poor solubility. This method offers little in the terms of size control or function malleability. Techniques that utilize reactive polymers along with a hydrophobic additive to produce a larger micelle that create a range of sizes have been developed.

Dendrimers are also polymer-based delivery vehicles. They have a core that branches out in regular intervals to form a small, spherical, and very dense nanocarrier.

Biodegradable Particles

Biodegradable particles have the ability to target diseased tissue as well as deliver their payload as a controlled-release therapy. Biodegradable particles bearing ligands to P-selectin, endothelial selectin (E-selectin) and ICAM-1 have been found to adhere to inflamed endothelium. Therefore, the use of biodegradable particles can also be used for cardiac tissue.

Artificial DNA Nanostructures

The success of DNA nanotechnology in constructing artificially designed nanostructures out of nucleic acids such as DNA, combined with the demonstration of systems for DNA computing, has led to speculation that artificial nucleic acid nanodevices can be used to target drug delivery based upon directly sensing its environment. These methods make use of DNA solely as a structural material and a chemical, and do not make use of its biological role as the carrier of genetic information. Nucleic acid logic circuits that could potentially be used as the core of a system that releases a drug only in response to a stimulus such as a specific mRNA have been demonstrated. In addition, a DNA "box" with a controllable lid has been synthesized using the DNA origami method. This structure could encapsulate a drug in its closed state, and open to release it only in response to a desired stimulus.

Applications

Targeted drug delivery can be used to treat many diseases, such as the cardiovascular diseases and diabetes. However, the most important application of targeted drug delivery is to treat cancerous tumors. In doing so, the passive method of targeting tumors takes advantage of the enhanced permeability and retention (EPR) effect. This is a situation specific to tumors that results from rapidly forming blood vessels and poor lymphatic drainage. When the blood vessels form so rapidly, large fenestrae result that are 100 to 600 nanometers in size, which allows enhanced nanoparticle entry. Further, the poor lymphatic drainage means that the large influx of nanoparticles are rarely leaving, thus, the tumor retains more nanoparticles for successful treatment to take place.

The American Heart Association rates cardiovascular disease as the number one cause of death in the United States. Each year 1.5 million myocardial infarctions (MI), also known as heart attacks, occur in the United States, with 500,000 leading to deaths. The costs related to heart attacks exceed $60 billion per year. Therefore, there is a need to come up with an optimum recovery system. The key to solving this problem lies in the effective use of pharmaceutical drugs that can be targeted directly to the diseased tissue. This technique can help develop many more regenerative techniques to cure various diseases. The development of a number of regenerative strategies in recent years for *curing* heart disease represents a paradigm shift away from conventional approaches that aim to *manage* heart disease.

Stem cell therapy can be used to help regenerate myocardium tissue and return the contractile function of the heart by creating/supporting a microenvironment before the MI. Developments in targeted drug delivery to tumors have provided the groundwork for the burgeoning field of targeted drug delivery to cardiac tissue. Recent developments have shown that there are different endothelial surfaces in tumors, which has led to the concept of endothelial cell adhesion molecule-mediated targeted drug delivery to tumors.

Liposomes can be used as drug delivery for the treatment of tuberculosis. The traditional treatment for TB is skin to chemotherapy which is not overly effective, which may be due to the failure of chemotherapy to make a high enough concentration at the infection site. The liposome delivery system allows for better microphage penetration and better builds a concentration at the infection site. The delivery of the drugs works intravenously and by inhalation. Oral intake is not advised because the liposomes break down in the Gastrointestinal System.

3D printing is also used by doctors to investigate how to target cancerous tumors in a more efficient way. By printing a plastic 3D shape of the tumor and filling it with the drugs used in the treatment the flow of the liquid can be observed allowing the modification of the doses and targeting location of the drugs.

TARGETED THERAPY

Targeted therapy or molecularly targeted therapy is one of the major modalities of medical treatment (pharmacotherapy) for cancer, others being hormonal therapy and cytotoxic chemotherapy. As a form of molecular medicine, targeted therapy blocks the growth of cancer cells by interfering with specific targeted molecules needed for carcinogenesis and tumor growth, rather than by simply interfering with all rapidly dividing cells (e.g. with traditional chemotherapy). Because most agents for targeted therapy are biopharmaceuticals, the term *biologic therapy* is sometimes synonymous with *targeted therapy* when used in the context of cancer therapy (and thus distinguished from chemotherapy, that is, cytotoxic therapy). However, the modalities can be combined; antibody-drug conjugates combine biologic and cytotoxic mechanisms into one targeted therapy.

Another form of targeted therapy involves use of nanoengineered enzymes to bind to a tumor cell such that the body's natural cell degradation process can digest the cell, effectively eliminating it from the body. The basic biological mechanism behind such research techniques are under investigation in a limited form with drugs derived from medicinal cannabis (drug) today in the United States. One example includes reduction and elimination of brain tumors with intake of small amounts of oil derived from engineered strains of medicinal cannabis.

Targeted cancer therapies are expected to be more effective than older forms of treatments and less harmful to normal cells. Many targeted therapies are examples of immunotherapy (using immune mechanisms for therapeutic goals) developed by the field of cancer immunology. Thus, as immunomodulators, they are one type of biological response modifiers.

The most successful targeted therapies are chemical entities that target or preferentially target a protein or enzyme that carries a mutation or other genetic alteration that is specific to cancer cells and not found in normal host tissue. One of the most successful molecular targeted therapeutic is Gleevec, which is a kinase inhibitor with exceptional affinity for the oncofusion protein BCR-Abl which is a strong driver of tumorigenesis in Chronic Myelogenous Leukemia. Although employed in other indications, Gleevec is most effective targeting BCR-Abl. Other examples of molecular targeted therapeutics targeting mutated oncogenes, include PLX27892 which targets mutant B-raf in melanoma.

There are targeted therapies for colorectal cancer, head and neck cancer, breast cancer, multiple myeloma, lymphoma, prostate cancer, melanoma and other cancers.

The definitive experiments that showed that targeted therapy would reverse the malignant phenotype of tumor cells involved treating Her2/neu transformed cells with monoclonal antibodies in vitro and in vivo by Mark Greene's laboratory and reported from 1985.

Some have challenged the use of the term, stating that drugs usually associated with the term are insufficiently selective. The phrase occasionally appears in scare quotes: "targeted therapy". Targeted therapies may also be described as "chemotherapy" or "non-cytotoxic chemotherapy", as "chemotherapy" strictly means only "treatment by chemicals". But in typical medical and general usage "chemotherapy" is now mostly used specifically for "traditional" cytotoxic chemotherapy.

Types

The main categories of targeted therapy are currently *small molecules* and *monoclonal antibodies.*

Small Molecules

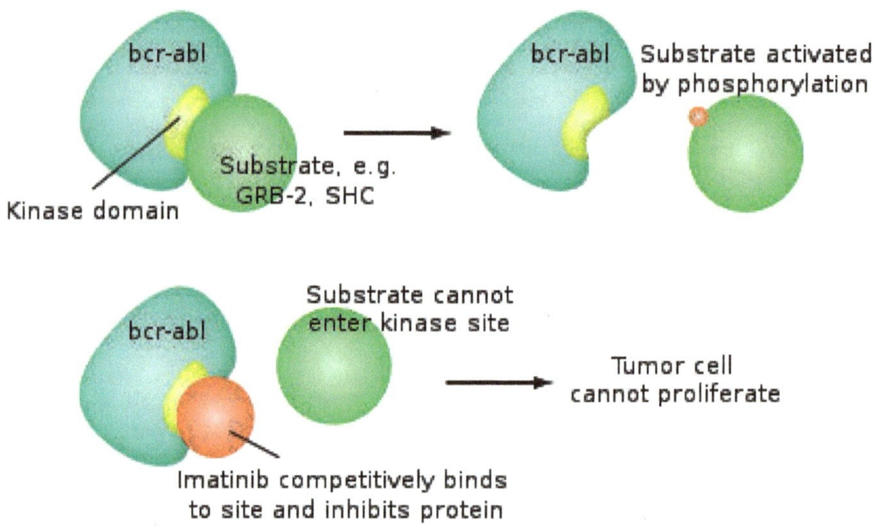

Mechanism of imatinib

Many are tyrosine-kinase inhibitors.

- Imatinib mesylate (Gleevec, also known as STI–571) is approved for chronic myelogenous leukemia, gastrointestinal stromal tumor and some other types of cancer. Early clinical trials indicate that imatinib may be effective in treatment of dermatofibrosarcoma protuberans.
- Gefitinib (Iressa, also known as ZD1839), targets the epidermal growth factor receptor (EGFR) tyrosine kinase and is approved in the U.S. for non small cell lung cancer.
- Erlotinib (marketed as Tarceva). Erlotinib inhibits epidermal growth factor receptor, and works through a similar mechanism as gefitinib. Erlotinib has been shown to increase survival in metastatic non small cell lung cancer when used as second line therapy. Because of this finding, erlotinib has replaced gefitinib in this setting.
- Sorafenib (Nexavar)
- Sunitinib (Sutent)
- Dasatinib (Sprycel)

- Lapatinib (Tykerb)
- Nilotinib (Tasigna)
- Bortezomib (Velcade) is an apoptosis-inducing proteasome inhibitor drug that causes cancer cells to undergo cell death by interfering with proteins. It is approved in the U.S. to treat multiple myeloma that has not responded to other treatments.
- The selective estrogen receptor modulator tamoxifen has been described as the foundation of targeted therapy.
- Janus kinase inhibitors, e.g. FDA approved tofacitinib
- ALK inhibitors, e.g. crizotinib
- Bcl-2 inhibitors (e.g. obatoclax in clinical trials, navitoclax, and gossypol.
- PARP inhibitors (e.g. Iniparib, Olaparib in clinical trials)
- PI3K inhibitors (e.g. perifosine in a phase III trial)
- Apatinib is a selective VEGF Receptor 2 inhibitor which has shown encouraging anti-tumor activity in a broad range of malignancies in clinical trials. Apatinib is currently in clinical development for metastatic gastric carcinoma, metastatic breast cancer and advanced hepatocellular carcinoma.
- AN-152, (AEZS-108) doxorubicin linked to [D-Lys(6)]- LHRH, Phase II results for ovarian cancer.
- Braf inhibitors (vemurafenib, dabrafenib, LGX818) used to treat metastatic melanoma that harbors BRAF V600E mutation
- MEK inhibitors (trametinib, MEK162) are used in experiments, often in combination with BRAF inhibitors to treat melanoma
- CDK inhibitors, e.g. PD-0332991, LEE011 in clinical trials
- Hsp90 inhibitors, some in clinical trials
- salinomycin has demonstrated potency in killing cancer stem cells in both laboratory-created and naturally occurring breast tumors in mice.

Small Molecule Drug Conjugates

- Vintafolide is a small molecule drug conjugate consisting of a small molecule targeting the folate receptor. It is currently in clinical trials for platinum-resistant ovarian cancer (PROCEED trial) and a Phase 2b study(TARGET trial) in non-small-cell lung carcinoma (NSCLC).

Serine/Threonine Kinase Inhibitors (Small Molecules)

- Temsirolimus (Torisel)
- Everolimus (Afinitor)
- Vemurafenib (Zelboraf)

- Trametinib (Mekinist)
- Dabrafenib (Tafinlar)

Monoclonal Antibodies

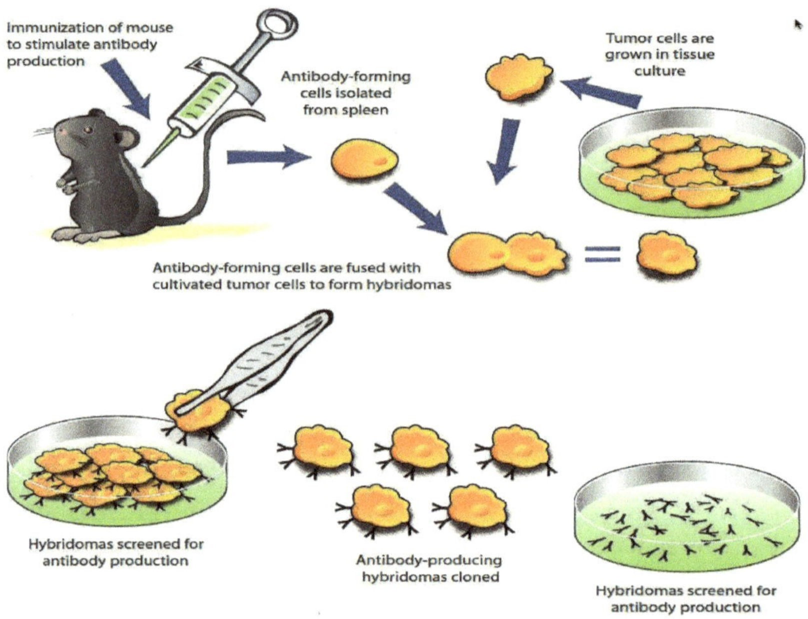

Monoclonal Antibody

Several are in development and a few have been licensed by the FDA and the European Commission. Examples of licensed monoclonal antibodies include:

- Rituximab targets CD20 found on B cells. It is used in non Hodgkin lymphoma;
- Trastuzumab targets the Her2/neu (also known as ErbB2) receptor expressed in some types of breast cancer;
- Alemtuzumab;
- Cetuximab target the epidermal growth factor receptor (EGFR). It is approved for use in the treatment of metastatic colorectal cancer, and squamous cell carcinoma of the head and neck;
- Panitumumab also targets the EGFR. It is approved for the use in the treatment of metastatic colorectal cancer;
- Bevacizumab targets circulating VEGF ligand. It is approved for use in the treatment of colon cancer, breast cancer, non-small cell lung cancer, and is investigational in the treatment of sarcoma. Its use for the treatment of brain tumors has been recommended;
- Ipilimumab (Yervoy) and

Many antibody-drug conjugates (ADCs) are being developed.

Progress and Future

In the U.S., the National Cancer Institute's *Molecular Targets Development Program* (MTDP) aims to identify and evaluate molecular targets that may be candidates for drug development.

NANOMEDICINE

Nanomedicine is the medical application of nanotechnology. Nanomedicine ranges from the medical applications of nanomaterials and biological devices, to nanoelectronic biosensors, and even possible future applications of molecular nanotechnology such as biological machines. Current problems for nanomedicine involve understanding the issues related to toxicity and environmental impact of nanoscale materials (materials whose structure is on the scale of nanometers, i.e. billionths of a meter).

Functionalities can be added to nanomaterials by interfacing them with biological molecules or structures. The size of nanomaterials is similar to that of most biological molecules and structures; therefore, nanomaterials can be useful for both in vivo and in vitro biomedical research and applications. Thus far, the integration of nanomaterials with biology has led to the development of diagnostic devices, contrast agents, analytical tools, physical therapy applications, and drug delivery vehicles.

Nanomedicine seeks to deliver a valuable set of research tools and clinically useful devices in the near future. The National Nanotechnology Initiative expects new commercial applications in the pharmaceutical industry that may include advanced drug delivery systems, new therapies, and in vivo imaging. Nanomedicine research is receiving funding from the US National Institutes of Health, including the funding in 2005 of a five-year plan to set up four nanomedicine centers.

Nanomedicine sales reached $16 billion in 2015, with a minimum of $3.8 billion in nanotechnology R&D being invested every year. Global funding for emerging nanotechnology increased by 45% per year in recent years, with product sales exceeding $1 trillion in 2013. As the nanomedicine industry continues to grow, it is expected to have a significant impact on the economy.

Drug Delivery

Nanotechnology has provided the possibility of delivering drugs to specific cells using nanoparticles.

The overall drug consumption and side-effects may be lowered significantly by depositing the active agent in the morbid region only and in no higher dose than needed. Targeted drug delivery is intended to reduce the side effects of drugs with concomitant decreases in consumption and treatment expenses. Drug delivery focuses on maximizing bioavailability both at specific places in the body and over a period of time. This can potentially be achieved by molecular targeting by nanoengineered devices. More than

$65 billion are wasted each year due to poor bioavailability. A benefit of using nanoscale for medical technologies is that smaller devices are less invasive and can possibly be implanted inside the body, plus biochemical reaction times are much shorter. These devices are faster and more sensitive than typical drug delivery. The efficacy of drug delivery through nanomedicine is largely based upon: a) efficient encapsulation of the drugs, b) successful delivery of drug to the targeted region of the body, and c) successful release of the drug.

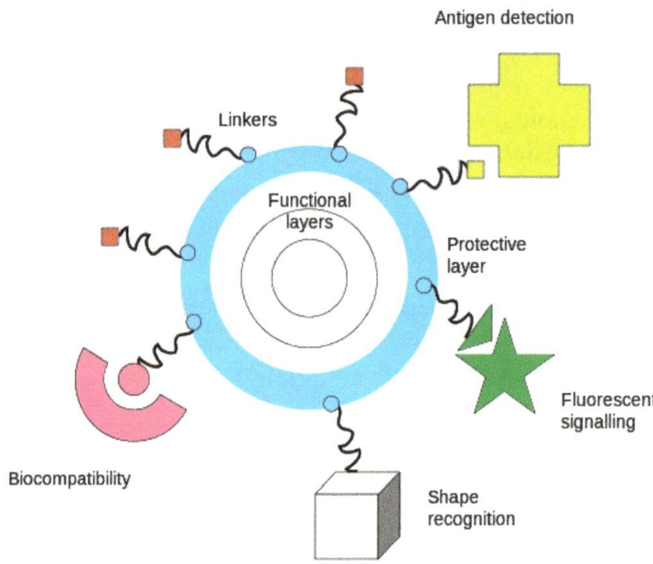

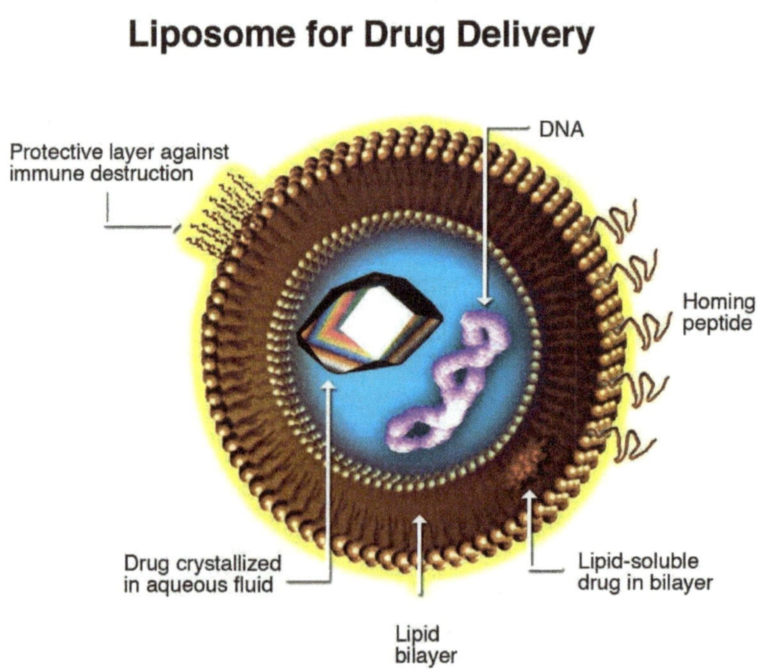

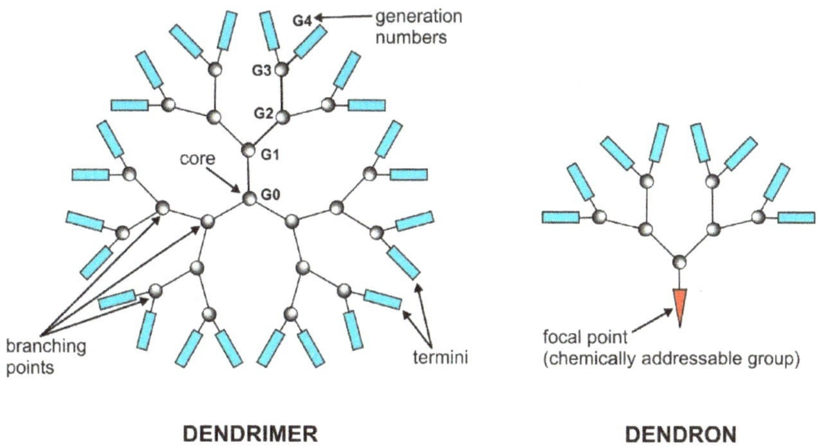

Nanoparticles *(top)*, liposomes*(middle)*, and dendrimers *(bottom)*are some nanomaterials being investigated for use in nanomedicine.

Drug delivery systems, lipid- or polymer-based nanoparticles, can be designed to improve the pharmacokinetics and biodistribution of the drug. However, the pharmacokinetics and pharmacodynamics of nanomedicine is highly variable among different patients. When designed to avoid the body's defence mechanisms, nanoparticles have beneficial properties that can be used to improve drug delivery. Complex drug delivery mechanisms are being developed, including the ability to get drugs through cell membranes and into cell cytoplasm. Triggered response is one way for drug molecules to be used more efficiently. Drugs are placed in the body and only activate on encountering a particular signal. For example, a drug with poor solubility will be replaced by a drug delivery system where both hydrophilic and hydrophobic environments exist, improving the solubility. Drug delivery systems may also be able to prevent tissue damage through regulated drug release; reduce drug clearance rates; or lower the volume of distribution and reduce the effect on non-target tissue. However, the biodistribution of these nanoparticles is still imperfect due to the complex host's reactions to nano- and microsized materials and the difficulty in targeting specific organs in the body. Nevertheless, a lot of work is still ongoing to optimize and better understand the potential and limitations of nanoparticulate systems. While advancement of research proves that targeting and distribution can be augmented by nanoparticles, the dangers of nanotoxicity become an important next step in further understanding of their medical uses.

Nanoparticles can be used in combination therapy for decreasing antibiotic resistance or for their antimicrobial properties. Nanoparticles might also used to circumvent multidrug resistance (MDR) mechanisms.

Types of Systems Used

Two forms of nanomedicine that have already been tested in mice and are awaiting human trials that will be using gold nanoshells to help diagnose and treat cancer, and using liposomes as vaccine adjuvants and as vehicles for drug transport. Similarly, drug detoxification is also another application for nanomedicine which has shown promising results in rats. Advances in Lipid nanotechnology was also instrumental in engineering medical nanodevices and novel drug delivery systems as well as in developing sensing applications. Another example can be found in dendrimers and nanoporous materials. Another example is to use block co-polymers, which form micelles for drug encapsulation.

Polymeric nano-particles are a competing technology to lipidic (based mainly on Phospholipids) nano-particles. There is an additional risk of toxicity associated with polymers not widely studied or understood. The major advantages of polymers is stability, lower cost and predictable characterisation. However, in the patient's body this very stability (slow degradation) is a negative factor. Phospholipids on the other hand are membrane lipids (already present in the body and surrounding each cell), have a GRAS (Generally Recognised As Safe) status from FDA and are derived from natural sources without any complex chemistry involved. They are not metabolised but rather absorbed by the body and the degradation products are themselves nutrients (fats or micronutrients).

Protein and peptides exert multiple biological actions in the human body and they have been identified as showing great promise for treatment of various diseases and disorders. These macromolecules are called biopharmaceuticals. Targeted and/or controlled delivery of these biopharmaceuticals using nanomaterials like nanoparticles and Dendrimers is an emerging field called nanobiopharmaceutics, and these products are called nanobiopharmaceuticals.

Another highly efficient system for microRNA delivery for example are nanoparticles formed by the self-assembly of two different microRNAs deregulated in cancer.

Another vision is based on small electromechanical systems; nanoelectromechanical systems are being investigated for the active release of drugs. Some potentially important applications include cancer treatment with iron nanoparticles or gold shells.Nanotechnology is also opening up new opportunities in implantable delivery systems, which are often preferable to the use of injectable drugs, because the latter frequently display first-order kinetics (the blood concentration goes up rapidly, but drops exponentially over time). This rapid rise may cause difficulties with toxicity, and drug efficacy can diminish as the drug concentration falls below the targeted range.

Applications

Some nanotechnology-based drugs that are commercially available or in human clinical trials include:

- Abraxane, approved by the U.S. Food and Drug Administration (FDA) to treat breast cancer, non-small- cell lung cancer (NSCLC) and pancreatic cancer, is the nanoparticle albumin bound paclitaxel.
- Doxil was originally approved by the FDA for the use on HIV-related Kaposi's sarcoma. It is now being used to also treat ovarian cancer and multiple myeloma. The drug is encased in liposomes, which helps to extend the life of the drug that is being distributed. Liposomes are self-assembling, spherical, closed colloidal structures that are composed of lipid bilayers that surround an aqueous space. The liposomes also help to increase the functionality and it helps to decrease the damage that the drug does to the heart muscles specifically.

- Onivyde, liposome encapsulated irinotecan to treat metastatic pancreatic cancer, was approved by FDA in October 2015.
- C-dots (Cornell dots) are the smallest silica-based nanoparticles with the size <10 nm. The particles are infused with organic dye which will light up with fluorescence. Clinical trial is underway since 2011 to use the C-dots as diagnostic tool to assist surgeons to identify the location of tumor cells.
- An early phase clinical trial using the platform of 'Minicell' nanoparticle for drug delivery have been tested on patients with advanced and untreatable cancer. Built from the membranes of mutant bacteria, the minicells were loaded with paclitaxel and coated with cetuximab, antibodies that bind the epidermal growth factor receptor (EGFR) which is often overexpressed in a number of cancers, as a 'homing' device to the tumor cells. The tumor cells recognize the bacteria from which the minicells have been derived, regard it as invading microorganism and engulf it. Once inside, the payload of anti-cancer drug kills the tumor cells. Measured at 400 nanometers, the minicell is bigger than synthetic particles developed for drug delivery. The researchers indicated that this larger size gives the minicells a better profile in side-effects because the minicells will preferentially leak out of the porous blood vessels around the tumor cells and do not reach the liver, digestive system and skin. This Phase 1 clinical trial demonstrated that this treatment is well tolerated by the patients. As a platform technology, the minicell drug delivery system can be used to treat a number of different cancers with different anti-cancer drugs with the benefit of lower dose and less side-effects.
- In 2014, a Phase 3 clinical trial for treating inflammation and pain after cataract surgery, and a Phase 2 trial for treating dry eye disease were initiated using nanoparticle loteprednol etabonate. In 2015, the product, KPI-121 was found to produce statistically significant positive results for the post-surgery treatment.

Cancer

Existing and potential drug nanocarriers have been reviewed.

Nanoparticles have high surface area to volume ratio. This allows for many functional groups to be attached to a nanoparticle, which can seek out and bind to certain tumor cells. Additionally, the small size of nanoparticles (10 to 100 nanometers), allows them to preferentially accumulate at tumor sites (because tumors lack an effective lymphatic drainage system). Limitations to conventional cancer chemotherapy include drug resistance, lack of selectivity, and lack of solubility. Nanoparticles have the potential to overcome these problems.

In photodynamic therapy, a particle is placed within the body and is illuminated with light from the outside. The light gets absorbed by the particle and if the particle is metal, energy from the light will heat the particle and surrounding tissue. Light may also be used to produce high energy oxygen molecules which will chemically react with and destroy most organic molecules that are next to them (like tumors). This therapy is appealing for many reasons. It does not leave a "toxic trail" of reactive molecules throughout the body (chemotherapy) because it is directed where only the light is shined and the particles exist. Photodynamic therapy has potential for a noninvasive procedure for dealing with diseases, growth and tumors. Kanzius RF therapy is one example of such therapy (nanoparticle hyperthermia) . Also, gold nanoparticles have the potential to join numerous therapeutic functions into a single platform, by targeting specific tumor cells, tissues and organs.

Visualization

In vivo imaging is another area where tools and devices are being developed. Using nanoparticle contrast agents, images such as ultrasound and MRI have a favorable distribution and improved contrast. This might be accomplished by self assembled biocompatible nanodevices that will detect, evaluate, treat and report to the clinical doctor automatically.

The small size of nanoparticles endows them with properties that can be very useful in oncology, particularly in imaging. Quantum dots (nanoparticles with quantum confinement properties, such as size-tunable light emission), when used in conjunction with MRI (magnetic resonance imaging), can produce exceptional images of tumor sites. Nanoparticles of cadmium selenide (quantum dots) glow when exposed to ultraviolet light. When injected, they seep into cancer tumors. The surgeon can see the glowing tumor, and use it as a guide for more accurate tumor removal.These nanoparticles are much brighter than organic dyes and only need one light source for excitation. This means that the use of fluorescent quantum dots could produce a higher contrast image and at a lower cost than today's organic dyes used as contrast media. The downside, however, is that quantum dots are usually made of quite toxic elements.

Tracking movement can help determine how well drugs are being distributed or how substances are metabolized. It is difficult to track a small group of cells throughout the body, so scientists used to dye the cells. These dyes needed to be excited by light of a certain wavelength in order for them to light up. While different color dyes absorb different frequencies of light, there was a need for as many light sources as cells. A way around this problem is with luminescent tags. These tags are quantum dots attached to proteins that penetrate cell membranes. The dots can be random in size, can be made of bio-inert material, and they demonstrate the nanoscale property that color is size-dependent. As a result, sizes are selected so that the frequency of light used to make a group of quantum dots fluoresce is an even multiple of the frequency required to make another group incandesce. Then both groups can be lit with a single light source. They have also found a way to insert nanoparticles into the affected parts of the body so that those parts of the body will glow showing the tumor growth or shrinkage or also organ trouble.

Sensing

Nanotechnology-on-a-chip is one more dimension of lab-on-a-chip technology. Magnetic nanoparticles, bound to a suitable antibody, are used to label specific molecules, structures or microorganisms. Gold nanoparticles tagged with short segments of DNA can be used for detection of genetic sequence in a sample. Multicolor optical coding for biological assays has been achieved by embedding different-sized quantum dots into polymeric microbeads.

Nanopore technology for analysis of nucleic acids converts strings of nucleotides directly into electronic signatures.

Sensor test chips containing thousands of nanowires, able to detect proteins and other biomarkers left behind by cancer cells, could enable the detection and diagnosis of cancer in the early stages from a few drops of a patient's blood. Nanotechnology is helping to advance the use of arthroscopes, which are pencil-sized devices that are used in surgeries with lights and cameras so surgeons can do the surgeries with smaller incisions. The smaller the incisions the faster the healing time which is better for the patients. It is also helping to find a way to make an arthroscope smaller than a strand of hair.

Research on nanoelectronics-based cancer diagnostics could lead to tests that can be done in pharmacies. The results promise to be highly accurate and the product promises to be inexpensive. They could take a very small amount of blood and detect cancer anywhere in the body in about five minutes, with a sensitivity that is a thousand times better than in a conventional laboratory test. These devices that are built with nanowires to detect cancer proteins; each nanowire detector is primed to be sensitive to a different cancer marker. The biggest advantage of the nanowire detectors is that they could test for anywhere from ten to one hundred similar medical conditions without adding cost to the testing device. Nanotechnology has also helped to personalize oncology for the detection, diagnosis, and treatment of cancer. It is now able to be tailored to each individual's tumor for better performance. They have found ways that they will be able to target a specific part of the body that is being affected by cancer.

Blood Purification

Magnetic micro particles are proven research instruments for the separation of cells and proteins from complex media. The technology is available under the name Magnetic-activated cell sorting or Dynabeads among others. More recently it was shown in animal models that magnetic nanoparticles can be used for the removal of various noxious compounds including toxins, pathogens, and proteins from whole blood in an extracorporeal circuit similar to dialysis. In contrast to dialysis, which works on the principle of the size related diffusion of solutes and ultrafiltration of fluid across a semi-permeable membrane, the purification with nanoparticles allows specific targeting of substances. Additionally larger compounds which are commonly not dialyzable can be removed.

The purification process is based on functionalized iron oxide or carbon coated metal nanoparticles with ferromagnetic or superparamagnetic properties. Binding agents such as proteins, antibodies, antibiotics, or synthetic ligands are covalently linked to the particle surface. These binding agents are able to interact with target species forming an agglomerate. Applying an external magnetic field gradient allows exerting a force on the nanoparticles. Hence the particles can be separated from the bulk fluid, thereby cleaning it from the contaminants.

The small size (< 100 nm) and large surface area of functionalized nanomagnets leads to advantageous properties compared to hemoperfusion, which is a clinically used technique for the purification of blood and is based on surface adsorption. These advantages are high loading and accessibility of the binding agents, high selectivity towards the target compound, fast diffusion, small hydrodynamic resistance, and low dosage.

This approach offers new therapeutic possibilities for the treatment of systemic infections such as sepsis by directly removing the pathogen. It can also be used to selectively remove cytokines or endotoxins or for the dialysis of compounds which are not accessible by traditional dialysis methods. However the technology is still in a preclinical phase and first clinical trials are not expected before 2017.

Tissue Engineering

Nanotechnology may be used as part of tissue engineering to help reproduce or repair or reshape damaged tissue using suitable nanomaterial-based scaffolds and growth factors. Tissue engineering if successful may replace conventional treatments like organ transplants or artificial implants. Nanoparticles such as graphene, carbon nanotubes, molybdenum disulfide and tungsten disulfide are being used as reinforcing agents to fabricate mechanically strong biodegradable polymeric nanocomposites for bone tissue engineering applications. The addition of these nanoparticles in the polymer matrix at low concentrations (~0.2 weight %) leads to significant improvements in the compressive and flexural mechanical properties of polymeric nanocomposites. Potentially, these nanocomposites may be used as a novel, mechanically strong, light weight composite as bone implants.

For example, a flesh welder was demonstrated to fuse two pieces of chicken meat into a single piece using a suspension of gold-coated nanoshells activated by an infrared laser. This could be used to weld arteries during surgery. Another example is nanonephrology, the use of nanomedicine on the kidney.

Medical Devices

Neuro-electronic interfacing is a visionary goal dealing with the construction of nanodevices that will permit computers to be joined and linked to the nervous system. This idea requires the building of a molecular structure that will permit control and detection of nerve impulses by an external computer. A refuelable strategy implies energy is refilled continuously or periodically with external sonic, chemical, tethered, magnetic, or biological electrical sources, while a nonrefuelable strategy implies that all power is drawn from internal energy storage which would stop when all energy is drained. A nanoscale enzymatic biofuel cell for self-powered nanodevices have been developed that uses glucose from biofluids including human blood and watermelons. One limitation to this innovation is the fact that electrical interference or leakage or overheating from power consumption is possible. The wiring of the structure is extremely difficult because they must be positioned precisely in the nervous system. The structures that will provide the interface must also be compatible with the body's immune system.

Molecular nanotechnology is a speculative subfield of nanotechnology regarding the possibility of engineering molecular assemblers, machines which could re-order matter at a molecular or atomic scale. Nanomedicine would make use of these nanorobots, introduced into the body, to repair or detect damages and infections. Molecular nanotechnology is highly theoretical, seeking to anticipate what inventions nanotechnology might yield and to propose an agenda for future inquiry. The proposed elements of molecular nanotechnology, such as molecular assemblers and nanorobots are far beyond current capabilities. Future advances in nanomedicine could give rise to life extension through the repair of many processes thought to be responsible for aging. K. Eric Drexler, one of the founders of nanotechnology, postulated cell repair machines, including ones operating within cells and utilizing as yet hypothetical molecular machines, in his 1986 book Engines of Creation, with the first technical discussion of medical nanorobots by Robert Freitas appearing in 1999. Raymond Kurzweil, a futurist and transhumanist, stated in his book *"The Singularity is Near"* that he believes that advanced medical nanorobotics could completely remedy the effects of aging by 2030. According to Richard Feynman, it was his former graduate student and collaborator Albert Hibbs who originally suggested to him (circa 1959) the idea of a *medical* use for Feynman's theoretical micromachines. Hibbs suggested that certain repair machines might one day be reduced in size to the point that it would, in theory, be possible to (as Feynman put it) "swallow the doctor". The idea was incorporated into Feynman's 1959 essay *"There's Plenty of Room at the Bottom"*.

ANTIBODY-DRUG CONJUGATE

Antibody-drug conjugates or ADCs are an important class of highly potent biopharmaceutical drugs designed as a targeted therapy for the treatment of people with cancer. Unlike chemotherapy, ADCs are intended to target and kill only the cancer cells and spare healthy cells. ADCs are complex molecules composed of an antibody linked to a biologically active cytotoxic (anticancer) payload or drug. Antibody-drug conjugates are examples of bioconjugates and immunoconjugates.

By combining the unique targeting capabilities of monoclonal antibodies with the cancer-killing ability of cytotoxic drugs, antibody-drug conjugates allow sensitive discrimination between healthy and diseased tissue. This means that, in contrast to traditional chemotherapeutic agents, antibody-drug conjugates target and attack the cancer cell so that healthy cells are less severely affected.

Mechanism of Action

In developing antibody-drug conjugates, an anticancer drug (e.g. a cell toxin or cytotoxin) is coupled to an antibody that specifically targets a certain tumor marker (e.g. a protein that, ideally, is only to be found in or on tumor cells). Antibodies track these proteins down in the body and attach themselves to the surface of cancer cells. The biochemical reaction between the antibody and the target protein (antigen) triggers a signal in the tumor cell, which then absorbs or internalizes the antibody together with the cytotoxin. After the ADC is internalized, the cytotoxic drug is released and kills the cancer. Due to this targeting, ideally the drug has lower side effects and gives a wider therapeutic window than other chemotherapeutic agents. These advantages have led to ADC technologies being featured in many publications, notably the New York Times, as well as numerous scientific journals.

Marketed ADC Products

To date, only three ADCs have received market approval. However, after a request from the U.S. Food and Drug Administration (FDA), Pfizer/Wyeth, the developer and marketer of the first ADC to receive marketing approval in 2001 for the treatment of patients with acute myelogenous leukemia (Gemtuzumab ozogamicin, trade name: Mylotarg®), withdrew the drug from the market in June 2010. As a result, only two ADC are marketed (2013), including Brentuximab vedotin (trade name: Adcetris®, marketed by Seattle Genetics and Millennium/Takeda) and Trastuzumab emtansine (trade name: Kadcyla, marketed by Genentech and Roche).

Brentuximab vedotin was granted accelerated approval by the U.S. Food and Drug Administration (FDA) on August 19, 2011 for relapsed HL and relapsed sALCL and conditional Marketing authorization from the European Medicines Agency in October 2012 for relapsed or refractory HL and relapsed or refractory sALCL. Trastuzumab emtansine (ado-trastuzumab emtansine or T-DM1) was approved in February 2013 for the treatment of people with HER2-positive metastatic breast cancer (mBC) who have received prior treatment with trastuzumab (Herceptin®, Genentech and Roche) and a taxane chemotherapy.

Cleavable and Non-Cleavable Linkers

A stable link between the antibody and cytotoxic (anti-cancer) agent is a crucial aspect of an ADC. A highly stable ADC linker will ensure that less of the cytotoxic payload falls off in circulation, driving an improved safety profile, and will also ensure that more of the payload arrives at the cancer cell, driving enhanced efficacy. Linkers are based on chemical motifs including disulfides, hydrazones or peptides (cleavable), or thioethers (noncleavable) and control the distribution and delivery of the cytotoxic agent to the target cell. Cleavable and noncleavable types of linkers have been proven to be safe in preclinical and clinical trials. Brentuximab vedotin includes an enzyme-sensitive *cleavable linker* that delivers the potent and highly toxic antimicrotubule agent monomethyl auristatin E or MMAE, a synthetic antineoplastic agent, to human specific CD30-positive malignant cells. Because of its high toxicity MMAE, which inhibits cell division by blocking the polymerization of tubulin, cannot be used as a single-agent chemotherapeutic drug. However, the combination of MMAE linked to an anti-CD30 monoclonal antibody (cAC10, a cell membrane protein of the tumor necrosis factor or TNF receptor) proved to be stable in extracellular fluid, cleavable by cathepsin and safe for therapy. Trastuzumab emtansine, the other approved ADC, is a combination of the microtubule-formation inhibitor mertansine (DM-1), a derivative of the Maytansine, and antibody trastuzumab (Herceptin/ Genentech/ Roche) attached by a stable, *non-cleavable linker*.

The availability of better and more stable linkers has changed the function of the chemical bond. The type of linker, *cleavable* or *noncleavable*, lends specific properties to the cytotoxic (anti-cancer) drug. For example, a *non-cleavable* linker keeps the drug within the cell. As a result, the entire antibody, linker and cytotoxic (anti-cancer) agent enter the targeted cancer cell where the antibody is degraded to the level of an amino acid. The resulting complex – amino acid, linker and cytotoxic agent – now becomes the active drug. In contrast, *cleavable linkers* are catalyzed by enzymes in the cancer cell where it releases the cytotoxic agent. The difference is that the cytotoxic payload delivered via a cleavable linker can escape from the targeted cell and, in a process called "bystander killing", attack neighboring cancer cells.

Another type of cleavable linker, currently in development, adds an extra molecule between the cytotoxic drug and the cleavage site. This linker technology allows researchers to create ADCs with more flexibility without worrying about changing cleavage kinetics. Researchers are also developing a new method of peptide cleavage based on Edman degradation, a method of sequencing amino acids in a peptide. Future direction in the development of ADCs also include the development of site-specific conjugation (TDCs) to further improve stability and therapeutic index and α emitting immunoconjugates and antibody-conjugated nanoparticles.

Non-Natural Amino Acids

The first generation of ADCs use linking technologies that conjugate drugs non-selectively to cysteine or lysine residues in the antibody, resulting in a heterogeneous mixture of ADCs. This approach leads to suboptimal safety and efficacy properties and makes optimization of the biological, physical and pharmacological properties of an ADC challenging. The site-specific incorporation of unnatural amino acids into the antibody generates a site for controlled and stable attachment of the drug. This enables the production of homogeneous ADCs with the antibody precisely linked to the drug and controlled ratios of antibody to drug, allowing the selection of a best-in-class ADC. An Escherichia coli based open cell-free synthesis (OCFS), developed by Stanford Professor James R. Swartz, allows the synthesis of proteins containing site-specifically incorporated non-natural amino acids and has been optimized for predictable high-yield protein synthesis and folding at any scale with straightforward downstream purification processes. The absence of a cell wall allows the addition of non-natural factors to the open system in order to manipulate transcription, translation and folding to provide precise modulation of the protein expression process.

Other disease areas

The majority of the ADCs currently under development or in clinical trials are for oncological and hematological indications. This is primarily driven by the availability of monoclonal antibodies targeting various types of cancer. However, some drug developers are also looking to expanding the application of ADCs beyond oncology and hematology to other important disease areas.

REFERENCES

1. Muller, R; Keck, C (2004). "Challenges and solutions for the delivery of biotech drugs – a review of drug nanocrystal technology and lipid nanoparticles". Journal of Biotechnology. 113 (1–3): 151–170. doi:10.1016/j.jbiotec.2004.06.007. PMID 15380654.

2. Saltzman, W. Mark; Torchilin, Vladimir P. (2008). "Drug delivery systems". AccessScience. McGraw-Hill Companies.
3. Trafton, A. Tumors Targeted Using Tiny Gold Particles. MIT Tech Talk. 2009, 53, 4–4.
4. Bertrand N, Leroux JC.; Leroux (2011). "The journey of a drug carrier in the body: an anatomo-physiological perspective". Journal of Controlled Release. 161 (2): 152–63. doi:10.1016/j.jconrel.2011.09.098. PMID 22001607.
5. Scott, Robert C; Crabbe, Deborah; Krynska, Barbara; Ansari, Ramin; Kiani, Mohammad F (2008). "Aiming for the heart: targeted delivery of drugs to diseased cardiac tissue". Expert Opinion on Drug Delivery. 5 (4): 459–70. doi:10.1517/17425247.5.4.459. PMID 18426386.
6. Sagnella, S.; Drummond, C. Drug Delivery: A Nanomedicine Approach. Australian Biochemist. [Online] 2012, 43, 5–8, 20. The Australian Society for Biochemistry and Molecular Biology.
7. Vlerken, L. E. V.; Vyas, T. K.; Amiji, M. M. Poly(Ethylene Glycol)-Modified Nanocarriers for Tumor-Targeted and Intracellular Delivery. Pharm. Res. 2007, 24, 1405–1414.
8. Gullotti, E.; Yeo, Y. Extracellularly Activated Nanocarriers: A New Paradigm of Tumor Targeted Drug Delivery. Mol. Pharm., [Online] 2009, 6, 1041-1051. ACS Publications.
9. Galvin, P.; Thompson, D.; Ryan, K. B.; Mccarthy, A.; Moore, A. C.; Burke, C. S.; Dyson, M.; Maccraith, B. D.; Gun'Ko, Y. K.; Byrne, M. T.; Volkov, Y.; Keely, C.; Keehan, E.; Howe, M.; Duffy, C.; Macloughlin, R. Nanoparticle-Based Drug Delivery: Case Studies for Cancer and Cardiovascular Applications. Cell. Mol. Life Sci. [Online] 2011, 69, 389–404.
10. Noyhouzer, Tomer; L'Homme, Chloé; Beaulieu, Isabelle; Mazurkiewicz, Stephanie; Kuss, Sabine; Kraatz, Heinz-Bernhard; Canesi, Sylvain; Mauzeroll, Janine (2016-05-03). "Ferrocene-Modified Phospholipid: An Innovative Precursor for Redox-Triggered Drug Delivery Vesicles Selective to Cancer Cells". Langmuir. 32 (17): 4169–4178. doi:10.1021/acs.langmuir.6b00511. ISSN 0743-7463.
11. Mitra, A. K.; Kwatra, D.; Vadlapudi, A. D. Drug Delivery; Jones & Bartlett Learning: Burlington, Massachusetts, 2015.
12. Jong, W. H. D.; Borm, P. J. A. Drug Delivery and Nanoparticles: Applications and Hazards. Int. J. Nanomedicine. [Online] 2008, 3, 133–149. The National Center for Biotechnology Information.
13. He, X; Bonaparte, N; Kim, S; Acharya, B; Lee, JY; Chi, L; Lee, HJ; Paik, YK; Moon, PG; Baek, MC; Lee, EK; KIM, JH; KIM, IS; Lee, BH (2012). "Enhanced delivery of T cells to tumor after chemotherapy using membrane-anchored, apoptosis-targeted peptide". Journal of Controlled Release. 162 (6): 521–8. doi:10.1016/j.jconrel.2012.07.023. PMID 22824781.
14. Torchilin, VP "Multifunctional Nanocarriers." Adv Drug Deliv Rev 2006 Dec; 58 (14): 1532-55 doi: 10.1016/j.addr.2006.09.009

15. Cobleigh, M; Langmuir, VK; Sledge, GW; Miller, KD; Haney, L; Novotny, WF; Reimann, JD; Vassel, A (2003). "A phase I/II dose-escalation trial of bevacizumab in previously treated metastatic breast cancer". Seminars in Oncology. 30 (5 Suppl 16): 117–24. doi:10.1053/j.seminoncol.2003.08.013. PMID 14613032.
16. Seidman, A.; Hudis, C; Pierri, MK; Shak, S; Paton, V; Ashby, M; Murphy, M; Stewart, SJ; Keefe, D (2002). "Cardiac Dysfunction in the Trastuzumab Clinical Trials Experience". Journal of Clinical Oncology. 20 (5): 1215–21. doi:10.1200/JCO.20.5.1215. PMID 11870163.
17. Brufsky, Adam (2009). "Trastuzumab-Based Therapy for Patients With HER2-Positive Breast Cancer". American Journal of Clinical Oncology. 33 (2): 186–95. doi:10.1097/COC.0b013e318191bfb0. PMID 19675448.
18. Lee, Jinhyun Hannah; Yeo, Yoon (2015-03-24). "Controlled drug release from pharmaceutical nanocarriers". Chemical Engineering Science. Pharmaceutical Particles and Processing. 125: 75–84. doi:10.1016/j.ces.2014.08.046. PMC 4322773Freely accessible. PMID 25684779.
19. Cho, Kwangjae; Wang, Xu; Nie, Shuming; Chen, Zhuo Georgia; Shin, Dong M. (2008-03-01). "Therapeutic nanoparticles for drug delivery in cancer". Clinical Cancer Research. 14 (5): 1310–1316. doi:10.1158/1078-0432.CCR-07-1441. ISSN 1078-0432. PMID 18316549.
20. Macosko, Cristopher W. "Polymer Nanoparticles Improve Delivery of Compounds" University of Minnesota Office for Technology Commercialization."Nanodeliv ery".
21. Pili, R.; Rosenthal, M. A.; Mainwaring, P. N.; Van Hazel, G.; Srinivas, S.; Dreicer, R.; Goel, S.; Leach, J.; et al. (2010). "Phase II Study on the Addition of ASA404 (Vadimezan; 5,6-Dimethylxanthenone-4-Acetic Acid) to Docetaxel in CRMPC". Clinical Cancer Research. 16 (10): 2906–14. doi:10.1158/1078-0432.CCR-09-3026. PMID 20460477.
22. Homsi, J.; Simon, G. R.; Garrett, C. R.; Springett, G.; De Conti, R.; Chiappori, A. A.; Munster, P. N.; Burton, M. K.; et al. (2007). "Phase I Trial of Poly-L-Glutamate Camptothecin (CT-2106) Administered Weekly in Patients with Advanced Solid Malignancies". Clinical Cancer Research. 13 (19): 5855–61. doi:10.1158/1078-0432.CCR-06-2821. PMID 17908979.
23. Vogel, V. G.; Costantino, JP; Wickerham, DL; Cronin, WM; Cecchini, RS; Atkins, JN; Bevers, TB; Fehrenbacher, L; et al. (2006). "Effects of Tamoxifen vs Raloxifene on the Risk of Developing Invasive Breast Cancer and Other Disease Outcomes: The NSABP Study of Tamoxifen and Raloxifene (STAR) P-2 Trial". JAMA. 295 (23): 2727–41. doi:10.1001/jama.295.23.joc60074. PMID 16754727.
24. Kahan, M; Gil, B; Adar, R; Shapiro, E (2008). "Towards Molecular Computers that Operate in a Biological Environment". Physica D: Nonlinear Phenomena. 237 (9): 1165–1172. doi:10.1016/j.physd.2008.01.027.
25. Andersen, Ebbe S.; Dong, Mingdong; Nielsen, Morten M.; Jahn, Kasper; Subramani, Ramesh; Mamdouh, Wael; Golas, Monika M.; Sander, Bjoern; et al. (2009). "Self-assembly of a nanoscale DNA box with a controllable lid".

Nature. 459 (7243): 73–6. doi:10.1038/nature07971. PMID 19424153.

26. Medscape from WebMD [Internet]. New York: WebMD LLC; 1994-2015. Liposomes as Drug Delivery Systems for the Treatment of TB; 2011 [cited 2015 May 8] Available from: http://www.medscape.com/viewarticle/752329_3
27. Hirschler B. 2014. 3D Printing Points Way to Smarter Cancer Treatment. London: Reuters. Dec,1.
28. Nanomedicine, Volume I: Basic Capabilities, by Robert A. Freitas Jr. 1999, ISBN 1-57059-645-X
29. Wagner V; Dullaart A; Bock AK; Zweck A. (2006). "The emerging nanomedicine landscape". Nat. Biotechnol. 24 (10): 1211–1217. doi:10.1038/nbt1006-1211. PMID 17033654.
30. Freitas RA Jr. (2005). "What is Nanomedicine?" (PDF). Nanomedicine: Nanotechnology, Biology and Medicine. 1 (1): 2–9. doi:10.1016/j.nano.2004.11.003. PMID 17292052.
31. Nanotechnology in Medicine and the Biosciences, by Coombs RRH, Robinson DW. 1996, ISBN 2-88449-080-9
32. "Market report on emerging nanotechnology now available". Market Report. US National Science Foundation. 25 February 2014. Retrieved 7 June 2016.
33. LaVan DA; McGuire T; Langer R. (2003). "Small-scale systems for in vivo drug delivery". Nat. Biotechnol. 21 (10): 1184–1191. doi:10.1038/nbt876. PMID 14520404.
34. Cavalcanti A; Shirinzadeh B; Freitas RA Jr.; Hogg T. (2008). "Nanorobot architecture for medical target identification". Nanotechnology. 19 (1): 015103(15pp). Bibcode:2008Nanot..19a5103C. doi:10.1088/0957-4484/19/01/015103.
35. Boisseau, P.; Loubaton, B. (2011). "Nanomedicine, nanotechnology in medicine". Comptes Rendus Physique. 12 (7): 620–636. doi:10.1016/j.crhy.2011.06.001.
36. Rao, Shasha; Tan, Angel; Thomas, Nicky; Prestidge, Clive. "Perspective and potential of oral lipid-based delivery to optimize pharmacological therapies against cardiovascular diseases". Journal of Controlled Release. 193: 174–187. doi:10.1016/j.jconrel.2014.05.013.
37. University of Waterloo, Nanotechnology in Targeted Cancer Therapy, https://www.youtube.com/watch?v=RBjWwlnq3cA 15 January 2010
38. Allen TM; Cullis PR (2004). "Drug Delivery Systems: Entering the Mainstream". Science. 303 (5665): 1818–1822. Bibcode:2004Sci...303.1818A. doi:10.1126/science.1095833. PMID 15031496.
39. Walsh MD; Hanna SK; Sen J; Rawal S; Cabral CB; Yurkovetskiy AV; Fram RJ; Lowinger TB; et al. (2012). "Pharmacokinetics and antitumor efficacy of XMT-1001, a novel, polymeric topoisomerase I inhibitor, in mice bearing HT-29 human colon carcinoma xenografts". Clin. Cancer Res. 18 (9): 2591–602. doi:10.1158/1078-0432.CCR-11-1554. PMID 22392910.
40. Chu KS; Hasan W; Rawal S; Walsh MD; Enlow EM; Luft JC; Bridges AS; Kuijer JL; et al. (Jul 2013). "Plasma, tumor and tissue pharmacokinetics of

Docetaxel delivered via nanoparticles of different sizes and shapes in mice bearing SKOV-3 human ovarian carcinoma xenograft". Nanomedicine. 9 (5): 686–93. doi:10.1016/j.nano.2012.11.008. PMID 23219874.

41. Caron WP; Song G; Kumar P; Rawal S; Zamboni WC (2012). "Interpatient pharmacokinetic and pharmacodynamic variability of carrier-mediated anticancer agents". Clin. Pharmacol. Ther. 91 (5): 802–12. doi:10.1038/clpt.2012.12. PMID 22472987.

42. Bertrand N; Leroux JC (2011). "The journey of a drug carrier in the body: an anatomo-physiological perspective". Journal of Controlled Release. 161 (2): 152–63. doi:10.1016/j.jconrel.2011.09.098. PMID 22001607.

43. Nagy ZK, Zsombor K.; Balogh A; Vajna B; Farkas A; Patyi G; Kramarics A; Marosi G (2011). "Comparison of Electrospun and Extruded Soluplus-Based Solid Dosage Forms of Improved Dissolution". Journal of Pharmaceutical Sciences. 101 (1): n/a. doi:10.1002/jps.22731. PMID 21918982.

44. Minchin, Rod (2008). "Sizing up targets with nanoparticles". Nature Nanotechnology. 3 (1): 12–13. Bibcode:2008NatNa...3...12M. doi:10.1038/nnano.2007.433. PMID 18654442.

45. Banoee, M.; Seif, S.; Nazari, Z. E.; Jafari-Fesharaki, P.; Shahverdi, H. R.; Moballegh, A.; Moghaddam, K. M.; Shahverdi, A. R. (2010). "ZnO nanoparticles enhanced antibacterial activity of ciprofloxacin against Staphylococcus aureus and Escherichia coli". J Biomed Mater Res B Appl Biomater. 93 (2): 557–61. doi:10.1002/jbm.b.31615. PMID 20225250.

46. Seil JT; Webster TJ (2012). "Antimicrobial applications of nanotechnology: methods and literature". Int J Nanomedicine. 7: 2767–81. doi:10.2147/IJN.S24805. PMID 22745541.

47. Borzabadi-Farahani A; Borzabadi E; Lynch E. (2013). "Nanoparticles in orthodontics, a review of antimicrobial and anti-caries applications". Acta Odontol Scand. 72 (6): 413–417. doi:10.3109/00016357.2013.859728. PMID 24325608.

48. Conde, J.; de la Fuente, JM; Baptista, PV. "Nanomaterials for reversion of multidrug resistance in cancer: a new hope for an old idea?." Front. Pharmacol.2013. Vol 4 No 134.

49. Sanjeev Soni, Himanshu Tyagi, Robert A. Taylor, Amod Kumar, Role of optical coefficients and healthy tissue-sparing characteristics in gold nanorod-assisted thermal therapy, International Journal of Hyperthermia, 2013, Vol. 29, No. 1 , Pages 87-97

50. Nanospectra Biosciences, Inc. – Publications (http://www.nanospectra.com/clinicians/spublications.html)

51. Mozafari, M.R. (ed), (2006) Nanocarrier Technologies: Frontiers of Nanotherapy (Chapters 1 and 2) pages 10–11, 25–34

52. Bertrand N; Bouvet C; Moreau P & Leroux JC (2010). "Transmembrane pH-Gradient Liposomes To Treat Cardiovascular Drug Intoxication". ACS Nano. 4 (12): 7552–7558. doi:10.1021/nn101924a. PMID 21067150.

53. Mashaghi S.; Jadidi T.; Koenderink G.; Mashaghi A. (2013). "Lipid Nanotechnology". Int. J. Mol. Sci. 2013 (14): 4242–4282. doi:10.3390/ijms14024242. PMC 3588097Freely accessible. PMID 23429269.

54. Conde, J; Oliva, N; Atilano, M; Song, HS; Artzi, N (2015). "Self-assembled RNA-triple-helix hydrogel scaffold for microRNA modulation in the tumour microenvironment". Nat Mater. doi:10.1038/nmat4497.

55. FDA (October 2012). "Highlights of Prescribing Information, Abraxane for Injectable Suspension" (PDF).

56. "Paclitaxel (Abraxane)". U.S. Food and Drug Administration. 11 October 2012. Retrieved 10 December 2012.

57. FDA Press Announcements (6 September 2013). "FDA approves Abraxane for late-stage pancreatic cancer". FDA.

58. Martis, Elvis A.; Badve, Rewa R.; Degwekar, Mukta D. (January 2012). "Nanotechnology based devices and applications in medicine: An overview". Chronicles of Young Scientists. 3 (1): 68–73. doi:10.4103/2229-5186.94320.

59. News Release (22 October 2015). "FDA approves new treatment for advanced pancreatic cancer". FDA.

60. Gibney, Michael (18 April 2013). "Cornell nanosized 'dots' for diagnostics may now deliver drugs". fiercedrugdelivery.com. Retrieved 17 June 2013.

61. Elvidge, Suzanne (11 November 2012). "Bacterial 'minicells' deliver cancer drugs straight to the target". fiercedrugdelivery.com. Retrieved 10 December 2012.

62. "First trial in humans of 'minicells': a completely new way of delivering anti-cancer drugs". fiercedrugdelivery.com. 12 November 2012. Retrieved 10 December 2012.

63. Press Release (19 June 2014). "Kala Pharmaceuticals Initiates Phase3 Clinical Trial for Treatment of Post-Surgical Ocular Inflammation and Phase 2 Clinical Trial in Dry Eye Disease" (PDF). Kala Pharmaceuticals.

64. Press Release (1 April 2015). "Kala Pharmaceuticals Announces Positive Results from Phase 3 Trial of KPI-121 in Cataract Surgery" (PDF). Kala Pharmaceuticals.

65. Wang AZ, Langer R, Farokhzad OC (2012). "Nanoparticle delivery of cancer drugs". Annu. Rev. Med. 63: 185–98. doi:10.1146/annurev-med-040210-162544. PMID 21888516.

66. Pérez-Herrero E, Fernández-Medarde A (2015). "Advanced targeted therapies in cancer: Drug nanocarriers, the future of chemotherapy". Eur J Pharm Biopharm. 93: 52–79. doi:10.1016/j.ejpb.2015.03.018. PMID 25813885.

67. Nguyen-Ngoc T, Raymond E (2015). "Reinvention of chemotherapy: drug conjugates and nanoparticles". Curr Opin Oncol. 27: 232–42. doi:10.1097/CCO.0000000000000183. PMID 25783982.

68. Ghaz-Jahanian MA, Abbaspour-Aghdam F, Anarjan N, Berenjian A, Jafarizadeh-Malmiri H (2015). "Application of chitosan-based nanocarriers in tumor-targeted drug delivery". Mol. Biotechnol. 57 (3): 201–18. doi:10.1007/s12033-014-9816-3. PMID 25385004.

69. Nie, Shuming; Yun Xing; Gloria J. Kim & Jonathan W. Simmons (2007). "Nanotechnology Applications in Cancer". Annual Review of Biomedical Engineering. 9 (1): 257–88. doi:10.1146/annurev.bioeng.9.060906.152025. PMID 17439359.

70. Chidambaram, M.; Manavalan, R.; Kathiresan, K. (2011). "Nanotherapeutics to overcome conventional cancer chemotherapy limitations". Journal of pharmacy & pharmaceutical sciences : a publication of the Canadian Society for Pharmaceutical Sciences, Societe canadienne des sciences pharmaceutiques. 14 (1): 67–77. PMID 21501554.

71. Loo C; Lin A; Hirsch L; Lee MH; Barton J; Halas N; West J; Drezek R. (2004). "Nanoshell-enabled photonics-based imaging and therapy of cancer". Technol Cancer Res Treat. 3 (1): 33–40. doi:10.1177/153303460400300104. PMID 14750891.

72. Conde J, Tian F, Hernández Y, Bao C, Cui D, Janssen KP, Ibarra MR, Baptista PV, Stoeger T, de la Fuente JM. In vivo tumor targeting via nanoparticle-mediated therapeutic siRNA coupled to inflammatory response in lung cancer mouse models. Biomaterials. 2013;34(31):7744-53. doi:10.1016/j.biomaterials.2013.06.041

73. Yasitha L Hewakuruppu et al., Plasmonic " pump – probe " method to study semi-transparent nanofluids, Applied Optics, 52(24) 6041-6050.

74. Coffey, Rebecca (August 2010). "20 Things You Didn't Know About Nanotechnology". Discover. 31 (6): 96.

75. Zheng G; Patolsky F; Cui Y; Wang WU; Lieber CM (2005). "Multiplexed electrical detection of cancer markers with nanowire sensor arrays". Nat. Biotechnol. 23 (10): 1294–1301. doi:10.1038/nbt1138. PMID 16170313.

76. Hall, J. Storrs (2005). Nanofuture : what's next for nanotechnology. Amherst, NY: Prometheus Books. ISBN 978-1591022879.

77. "Drug Store Cancer Tests". Technology Review. 2005-10-31. Retrieved 2009-10-08.

78. Keller, John (2013). "Nanotechnology has also helped to personalize oncology for the detection, diagnosis, and treatment of cancer. It is now able to be tailored to each individual's tumor for better performance". Military & Aerospace Electronics. 23 (6): 27.

79. Herrmann, I. K. et al. Nanomagnet-based removal of lead and digoxin from living rats. Nanoscale 5, 8718–8723 (2013).

80. Kang J. H.; et al. (2014). "An extracorporeal blood-cleansing device for sepsis therapy". Nat. Med. 20: 1211–1216. doi:10.1038/nm.3640.

81. Berry C. C.; Curtis A. S. G. (2003). "Functionalisation of magnetic nanoparticles for applications in biomedicine". J. Phys. Appl. Phys. 36: R198. doi:10.1088/0022-3727/36/13/203.

82. Herrmann I. K.; et al. (2013). "Endotoxin Removal by Magnetic Separation-Based Blood Purification". Adv. Healthcare Mater. 2: 829–835. doi:10.1002/adhm.201200358.

83. Lee J.-J.; et al. (2014). "Synthetic Ligand-Coated Magnetic Nanoparticles for Microfluidic Bacterial Separation from Blood". Nano Lett. 14: 1–5. doi:10.1021/nl3047305.

84. Schumacher C. M.; et al. (2013). "Quantitative Recovery of Magnetic Nanoparticles from Flowing Blood: Trace Analysis and the Role of Magnetization". Adv. Funct. Mater. 23: 4888–4896. doi:10.1002/adfm.201300696.

85. Yung C. W.; Fiering J.; Mueller A. J.; Ingber D. E. (2009). "Micromagnetic–microfluidic blood cleansing device". Lab. Chip. 9: 1171–7. doi:10.1039/b816986a. PMID 19370233.

86. Herrmann, I. K., Grass, R. N. & Stark, W. J. High-strength metal nanomagnets for diagnostics and medicine: carbon shells allow long-term stability and reliable linker chemistry. Nanomed. 4, 787–798 (2009).

87. Stacy Shepherd,"Harvard Engineers Invented an Artificial Spleen to Treat Sepsis", Boston Magazine. Retrieved on 20 April 2015.

88. Lalwani Gaurav; Henslee Allan M.; Farshid Behzad; Lin Liangjun; Kasper F. Kurtis, Yi-; Qin Xian; Mikos Antonios G.; Sitharaman Balaji; et al. (2013). "Two-dimensional nanostructure-reinforced biodegradable polymeric nanocomposites for bone tissue engineering". Biomacromolecules. 14 (3): 900–909. doi:10.1021/bm301995s. PMC 3601907Freely accessible. PMID 23405887.

89. Lalwani, Gaurav (September 2013). "Tungsten disulfide nanotubes reinforced biodegradable polymers for bone tissue engineering". Acta Biomaterialia. 9 (9): 8365–8373. doi:10.1016/j.actbio.2013.05.018. PMC 3732565Freely accessible. PMID 23727293.

90. Gobin AM; O'Neal DP; Watkins DM; Halas NJ; Drezek RA; West JL (2005). "Near infrared laser-tissue welding using nanoshells as an exogenous absorber". Lasers Surg Med. 37 (2): 123–9. doi:10.1002/lsm.20206. PMID 16047329.

91. http://www.nanowerk.com/spotlight/spotid=19573.php

92. Nanomedicine, Volume IIA: Biocompatibility, by Robert A. Freitas Jr. 2003, ISBN 1-57059-700-6

93. Freitas, Robert A., Jr. (2005). "Current Status of Nanomedicine and Medical Nanorobotics" (PDF). Journal of Computational and Theoretical Nanoscience. 2 (4): 1–25. doi:10.1166/jctn.2005.001.

94. Nanofactory Collaboration

95. Kurzweil, Ray (2005). The Singularity Is Near. New York City: Viking Press. ISBN 978-0-670-03384-3. OCLC 57201348.

96. Richard P. Feynman (December 1959). "There's Plenty of Room at the Bottom". Retrieved March 2010. Check date values in: |access-date= (help)

CHAPTER 7

Mechanism and Mode of action

Chapter Contents

- **Introduction**
- **Drugs With Known Mechanisms of Action**
- **Mode of Action**

Mechanism of action describes the process by which a molecule, such as a drug, functions to produce a pharmacological effect. A drug's mechanism of action may refer to its effects on a biological readout such as cell growth, or its interaction and modulation of its direct biomolecular target, for example a protein or nucleic acid.

When bound, the drug can act as either an agonist or an antagonist. Agonist drugs activate the receptors they bind to, which either increases or decreases activity within the cell. Antagonist drugs, on the other hand, block the receptors so that natural agonists within the body cannot bind.

Most drugs bind to a specific type of receptor, and this term is called receptor selectivity. The ability of a drug to bind to a certain receptor is based on its unique chemical structure.

INTRODUCTION

In pharmacology, the term mechanism of action (MOA) refers to the specific biochemical interaction through which a drug substance produces its pharmacological effect. A mechanism of action usually includes mention of the specific molecular targets to which the drug binds, such as an enzyme or receptor. Receptor sites have specific affinities for drugs based on the chemical structure of the drug, as well as the specific action that occurs there. Drugs that do not bind to receptors produce their corresponding therapeutic effect by simply interacting with chemical or physical properties in the body. Common examples of drugs that work in this way are antacids and laxatives.

In comparison, a mode of action (MoA) describes functional or anatomical changes, at the cellular level, resulting from the exposure of a living organism to a substance.

DRUGS WITH KNOWN MECHANISMS OF ACTION

There are many drugs in which the mechanism of action is known. By knowing the interaction between a certain site of a drug and a receptor, other drugs can be formulated in a way that replicates this interaction, thus producing the same therapeutic effects. Indeed, this method is used to create new drugs.

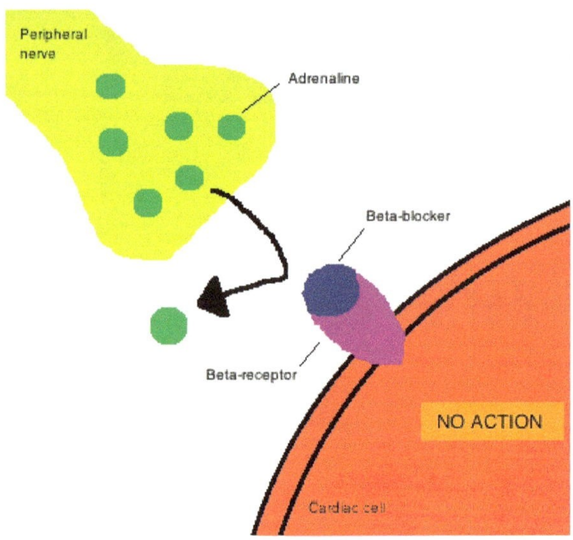

Mechanism of Action

Aspirin

The mechanism of action of aspirin involves irreversible inhibition of the enzyme cyclooxygenase; therefore suppressing the production of prostaglandins and thromboxanes, thus reducing pain and inflammation. This mechanism of action is specific to aspirin, and is not constant for all nonsteroidal anti-inflammatory drugs (NSAIDs). Rather, aspirin is the only NSAID that irreversibly inhibits COX-1.

Drugs with unknown mechanisms of action

Some drug mechanisms of action are still unknown. However, even though the mechanism of action of a certain drug is unknown, the drug still functions; it is just unknown or unclear how the drug interacts with receptors and produces its therapeutic effect.

- Acamprosate
- Armodafinil
- Antidepressants
- Cyclobenzaprine
- Demeclocycline
- Fabomotizole
- Lithium
- Meprobamate
- Methocarbamol
- Paracetamol
- Phenytoin
- PRL-8-53

Acamprosate

Acamprosate, sold under the brand name Campral, is a medication used along with counselling in the treatment of alcohol dependence.

Acamprosate is thought to stabilize the chemical balance in the brain that would otherwise be disrupted by alcohol withdrawal. Reports indicate that acamprosate works to best advantage in combination with psychosocial support and can help facilitate reduced consumption as well as full abstinence. Certain serious side effects include allergic reactions, abnormal heart rhythms, and low or high blood pressure, while less serious side effects include headaches, insomnia, and impotence. Diarrhea is the most common side-effect. Acamprosate should not be taken by people with kidney problems or allergies to the drug.

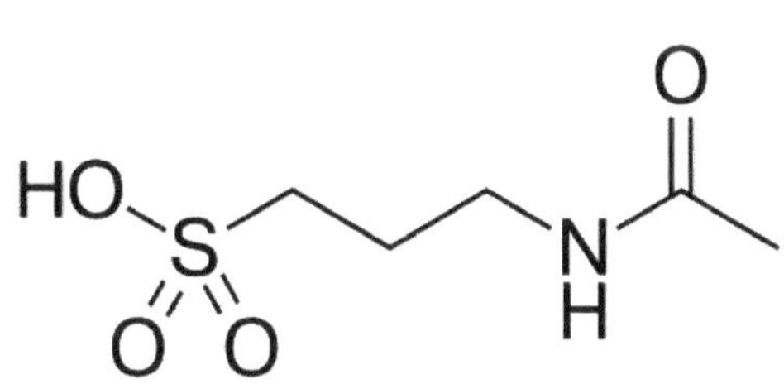

Acamprosate

Until it became a generic in the United States, Campral was manufactured and marketed in the United States by Forest Laboratories, while Merck KGaA markets it outside the US. It is sold as 333 mg white and odorless tablets of acamprosate calcium, which is the equivalent of 300 mg of acamprosate.

Medical Uses

Acamprosate is useful when used along with counselling in the treatment of alcohol dependence. Over three to twelve months it increases the number of people who do not drink at all and the number of days without alcohol. It appears to work as well as naltrexone.

Contraindications

Acamprosate is primarily removed by the kidneys and should not be given to people with severely impaired kidneys (creatinine clearance less than 30ml/min). A dose reduction is suggested in those with moderately impaired kidneys (creatinine clearance between 30ml/min and 50ml/min). It is also contraindicated in those who have a strong allergic reaction to acamprosate calcium or any of its components.

Interactions

Current studies have not shown any serious drug-drug interactions between acamprosate and alcohol, diazepam, imipramine, or disulfiram. One study found that giving acamprosate with naltrexone had no harmful effects and no clinically important effects on the pharmacokinetics of either drugs.

Pharmacology

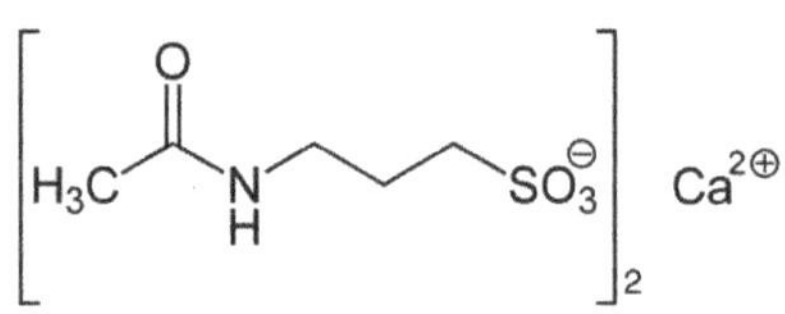

acamprosate calcium

The mechanism of action of acamprosate is unknown and controversial. At high concentrations, well above those that occur clinically (1–3 μM), reports of inhibition of glutamate receptor-activated responses (1 mM), enhancement of NMDA receptorfunction (300 μM), weak antagonization of the NMDA receptor, partial agonism of the polyamine site of the NMDA receptor, and possible inhibition of the mGluR1 and mGluR5 (10 μM) have all been published. However, no direct action of acamprosate at clinically-relevant concentrations has yet been reported. Moreover, a subsequent study found no action of acamprosate on the mGluR1 or mGluR5 at concentrations as high as 100 μM, nor at $GABA_A$ or glycine receptors or voltage-gated sodium channels.

GABA: Ethanol and benzodiazepines act on the central nervous system by binding to the $GABA_A$ receptor, increasing the effects of the inhibitory neurotransmitter GABA (i.e., it is a positive allosteric modulator). In chronic alcohol abuse, one of the main mechanisms of tolerance is attributed to $GABA_A$ receptors becoming downregulated (i.e.

becoming generally less sensitive to the inhibitory effect of the GABA system). When alcohol is no longer consumed, these down-regulated $GABA_A$ receptor complexes are so insensitive to GABA that the typical amount of GABA produced has little effect; compounded with the fact that GABA normally inhibits action potential formation, there are not as many receptors for GABA to bind to — meaning that sympathetic activation is unopposed, leading to sympathetic over-stimulation. Acamprosate's mechanism of action is supposed to be, at least partially, due to an enhancement effect on GABA receptors. It has been purported to open the chloride ion channel in a novel way as it does not require GABA as a cofactor, making it less liable for dependence than benzodiazepines. Acamprosate has been successfully used to control tinnitus, hyperacusis, ear pain and inner ear pressure during alcohol use due to spasms of the tensor tympani muscle.

NMDA: In addition, alcohol also inhibits the activity of *N*-methyl-D-aspartate receptors (NMDARs). Chronic alcohol consumption leads to the overproduction (upregulation) of these receptors. Thereafter, sudden alcohol abstinence causes the excessive numbers of NMDARs to be more active than normal and to contribute to the symptoms of delirium tremens and excitotoxic neuronal death. Withdrawal from alcohol induces a surge in release of excitatory neurotransmitters like glutamate, which activates NMDARs. Acamprosate reduces this glutamate surge. The drug also protects cultured cells from excitotoxicity induced by ethanol withdrawal and from glutamate exposure combined with ethanol withdrawal.

Calcium: In contrast to the aforementioned wide array of purported mechanisms of action, a 2013 profile animal study published in *Neuropsychopharmacology* suggests that acamprosate has by itself no psychotropic profile, no *N*-methyl-D-aspartate receptor or metabotropic glutamate receptor 5 activity, and that therapeutic effects are due to the active calcium moiety co-administered with the acamprosate salt form. These findings have not yet been reproduced.

Neuroprotective effects: In addition to its apparent ability to help patients refrain from drinking, some evidence suggests that acamprosate is neuroprotective (that is, it protects neurons from damage and death caused by the effects of alcohol withdrawal, and possibly other causes of neurotoxicity). For example, acamprosate has been found to protect cultured cells from damage induced by ischemia (inadequate blood flow). The drug also protected infant hamsters from brain damage induced by injections of the toxin ibotenic acid (which exacerbates excitotoxicity, the harmful over-activation of glutamate receptors).

One Brazilian study has shown that acamprosate may be an effective treatment for tinnitus.

Armodafinil

Armodafinil (trade name Nuvigil) is the enantiopure of the wakefulness-promoting agent, or *eugeroic*, modafinil(Provigil). It consists of just the (*R*)-(−)-enantiomer of the racemic modafinil. Armodafinil is produced by the pharmaceutical company Cephalon Inc. and was approved by the U.S. Food and Drug Administration (FDA) in June 2007.

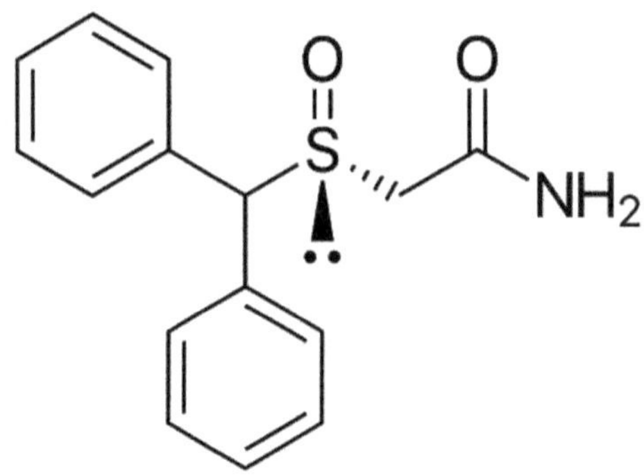

Armodafinil

Although they have similar half-lives, armodafinil reaches its peak concentration in the blood later after administration than modafinil does, which may make it more effective at improving wakefulness in patients with excessive daytime sleepiness.

Medical Uses

Armodafinil is currently FDA-approved to treat excessive daytime sleepiness associated with obstructive sleep apnea, narcolepsy, and shift work disorder. It is commonly used off-label to treat attention deficit hyperactivity disorder, chronic fatigue syndrome, and major depressive disorder. It has been shown to improve vigilance in air traffic controllers.

Sleep Disorders

Armodafinil is approved by the U.S. FDA for the treatment of narcolepsy and shift work sleep disorder, and as an adjuvant therapy for obstructive sleep apnea. For narcolepsy and obstructive sleep apnea, armodafinil is taken as a once daily 150 mg or 250 mg dose in the morning. For shift work sleep disorder, 150 mg of armodafinil are taken one hour prior to starting work. Slow dose titration is needed to mitigate some side effects.

Pharmacodynamics

The mechanism of action of armodafinil is unknown. Armodafinil (*R*-(−)-modafinil) has pharmacological properties almost identical to those of modafinil (a mixture of *R*-(−)- and (*S*)-(+)-modafinil). The (*R*)- and (*S*)-enantiomers have similar pharmacological action in animals. Armodafinil has wake-promoting actions similar to sympathomimetic agents including amphetamine and methylphenidate, although its pharmacologic profile is not identical to that of the sympathomimetic amines. Armodafinil is an indirect dopamine receptor agonist; it binds *in vitro* to the dopamine transporter (DAT) and inhibits dopamine reuptake. For modafinil, this activity has been associated *in vivo* with increased extracellular dopamine levels. In genetically engineered mice lacking the dopamine transporter, modafinil lacked wake-promoting activity, suggesting that this activity was DAT-dependent. However, the wake-promoting effects of modafinil, unlike those of amphetamine, were not antagonized by the dopamine receptor antagonist haloperidol in rats. In addition, alpha-methyl-p-tyrosine, an inhibitor of dopamine synthesis, blocks the action of amphetamine but does not block locomotor activity induced by modafinil.

In addition to its wake-promoting effects and ability to increase locomotor activity in animals, according to Nuvigil prescribing information from manufacturer Cephalon, armodafinil produces psychoactive and euphoric effects, alterations in mood, perception, thinking, and feelings typical of other central nervous system(CNS) stimulants in humans. Armodafinil, like racemic modafinil, may also possess reinforcing properties, as evidenced by its self-administration in monkeys previously trained to administer cocaine; armodafinil was also partially discriminated as stimulant-like. A Cephalon-founded study in which patients were administered modafinil, methylphenidate, and a placebo found that modafinil produces "psychoactive and euphoric effects and feelings consistent with [methylphenidate]."

Pharmacokinetics

Armodafinil exhibits linear time-independent kinetics following single and multiple oral dose administration. Increase in systemic exposure is proportional over the dose range of 50–400 mg. No time-dependent change in kinetics was observed through 12 weeks of dosing. Apparent steady state for armodafinil was reached within 7 days of dosing. At steady state, the systemic exposure for armodafinil is 1.8 times the exposure observed after a single dose. The concentration-time profiles of the (*R*)-(−)-enantiomer following a single dose of 50 mg Nuvigil or 100 mg Provigil (modafinil being a 1:1 mixture of (*R*)-(−)- and (*S*)-(−)- enantiomers) are nearly superimposable. However, the C_{max} of armodafinil at steady state was 37% higher following administration of 200 mg Nuvigil than the corresponding value of modafinil following administration of 200 mg Provigil due to the more rapid clearance of the (*S*)-(+)-enantiomer.

Absorption

Armodafinil is readily absorbed after oral administration. The absolute oral bioavailability was not determined due to the aqueous insolubility of armodafinil, which precluded intravenous administration. Peak plasma concentrations are attained at approximately 2 hours in the fasted state. Food effect on the overall bioavailability of armodafinil is considered minimal; however, time to reach peak concentration may be delayed 2–4 hours in the fed state. Since the delay in T_{max} is also associated with elevated plasma concentration later in time, food can potentially affect the onset and time course of pharmacologic action of armodafinil.

Cyclobenzaprine

Cyclobenzaprine, sold under the brand name Flexeril among others, is a muscle relaxer medication used to relieve skeletal muscle spasms and associated pain in acute musculoskeletal conditions. It is the best-studied drug for this application. It has also been used off-label for fibromyalgia treatment.

As of 2015 the cost for a typical course of medication in the United States is less than US$25.

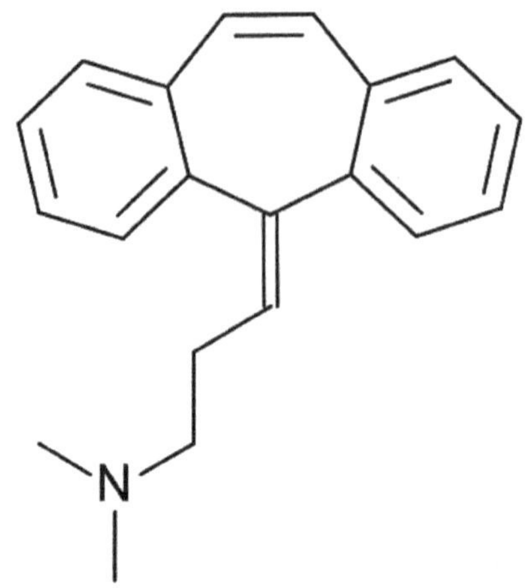

Cyclobenzaprine

Medical Use

After sustaining an injury, muscle spasms may occur to stabilize the affected body part and prevent further damage. They also generate pain. Cyclobenzaprine is used to treat such muscle spasms associated with acute, painful musculoskeletal conditions. It decreases pain in the first two weeks, peaking in the first few days, but has no proven benefit after two weeks. Since no benefit is proven beyond that, therapy should not be continued long-term. It is not useful for spasticity due to neurologic conditions such as cerebral palsy.

Cyclobenzaprine has also shown effectiveness in the treatment of fibromyalgia symptoms, with a report of 4.8 patients needing treatment for each (1) patient reporting pain reduction (but no change in fatigue or tender points). It may also be used along with other treatments for tetanus.

Side Effects

Meta-analysis studies have found significantly increased rates of drowsiness (38% of patients), dry mouth (24%), dizziness (10%), and adverse events of any kind in patients taking cyclobenzaprine versus placebo. Drowsiness and dry mouth appear to intensify with increasing dose.

The sedative effects of cyclobenzaprine are likely due to its antagonistic effect on histamine, serotonin, and muscarinic receptors. Agitation is a common side effect observed especially in the elderly. In general, the National Committee for Quality Assurance recommends avoiding the use of cyclobenzaprine in the elderly because of the potential for more severe side effects. Treatment protocols and support should follow the same as for any structurally related tricyclic, such as tricyclic antidepressants.

Some experts believe that cyclobenzaprine should be avoided in elderly patients because it can cause confusion, delirium, and cognitive impairment.

Overdose

The most common effects of overdose are drowsiness and tachycardia. Rare but potentially critical complications are cardiac arrest, abnormal heart rhythms, severe low blood pressure, seizures, and neuroleptic malignant syndrome.Life-threatening overdose is rare, however, as the median lethal dose is about 338 milligrams/kilogram in mice and 425 mg/kg in rats. The potential harm is increased when central nervous system depressants and antidepressants are also used; deliberate overdose often includes alcohol among other drugs.

Interactions

Cyclobenzaprine has major contraindications with monoamine oxidase inhibitors (MAOIs). At least one study also found increased risk of serotonin syndrome when cyclobenzaprine was taken with the serotonergic drugs duloxetine or phenelzine.

These substances may interact with cyclobenzaprine:

- Alcohol;
- Central nervous system depressants (e.g. opioids, benzodiazepines, nonbenzodiazepines, phenothiazines, carbamates, barbiturates);
- Tricyclic antidepressants may increase the chance of side effects and
- Monoamine oxidase inhibitors taken within two weeks of cyclobenzaprine may result in serious, life-threatening side effects.

If co-administered with opioids, the dose of one or both medicines should be reduced accordingly. The patient should be monitored for excessive sedation.

Comparison to Other Medications

Cyclobenzaprine has been found to be not inferior to tizanidine, orphenadrine, and carisoprodol in the treatment of acute lower back pain, although none has been proven to be effective for long-term use (beyond two weeks of treatment). No differences in pain or spasm scores were noted among these agents, nor when compared to benzodiazepines. However, nonbenzodiazepine (including cyclobenzaprine) treatment was found to have a lower risk of medication abuse and continuation of use against medical advice. Side effects such as sedation and ataxia are also less pronounced with nonbenzodiazepine antispasmodics.

In a study on the treatment of musculoskeletal pain treatment with cyclobenzaprine alone or in combination with ibuprofen, no significant differences in pain scores were noted among the three treatment groups. Peak benefit was found to occur on day seven of the treatment for all groups.

Formulations

By mouth, cyclobenzaprine is marketed as Apo-Cyclobenzaprin, Fexmid and Novo-Cycloprine. Flexeril was discontinued.It is available in generic form. A once-a-day, extended-release formulation, Amrix, is available. Cyclobenzaprine is also used by compounding pharmacies in topical creams.

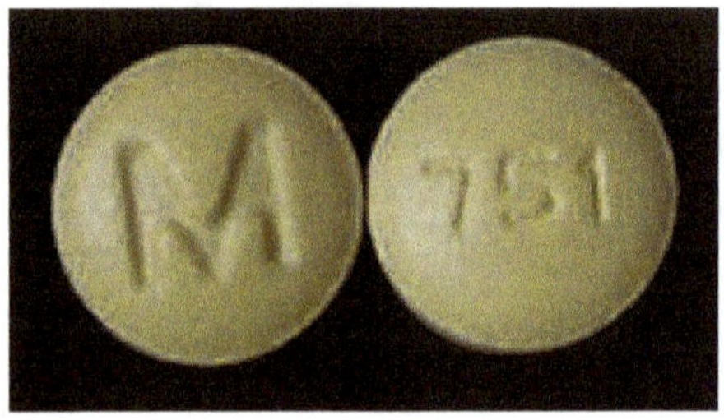

Cyclobenzaprine 10mg

Cyclobenzaprine is regulated in the U.S. for prescription use only. Though it does not fall within most governmental guidelines as a controlled substance, possession of it without a valid or current prescription may be illegal, depending upon various state and local laws.

Demeclocycline

Demeclocycline (INN, BAN, USAN) (brand names Declomycin, Declostatin, Ledermycin, Bioterciclin, Deganol, Deteclo), also known under the brand names Detravis, Meciclin, Mexocine, Clortetrin, is a semisynthetictetracycline antibiotic which was derived from a strain of *Streptomyces aureofaciens*.

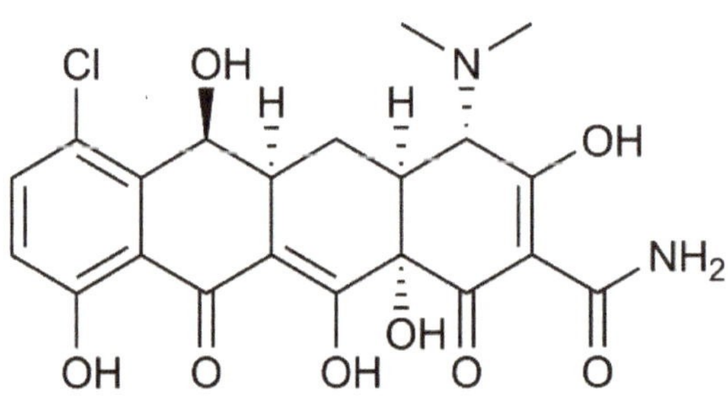

Demeclocycline

Uses

It is officially indicated for the treatment of various types of bacterial infections. It is used as an antibiotic in the treatment of Lyme disease, acne, and bronchitis. Resistance, though, is gradually becoming more common, and demeclocycline is now rarely used for infections.

It is widely used (though off-label in many countries) in the treatment of hyponatremia (low blood sodium concentration) due to the syndrome of inappropriate antidiuretic hormone (SIADH) when fluid restriction alone has been ineffective.Physiologically, this works by reducing the responsiveness of the collecting tubule cells to ADH.

The use in SIADH actually relies on a side effect; demeclocycline induces nephrogenic diabetes insipidus (dehydration due to the inability to concentrate urine). The use of demeclocycline in SIADH was first reported in 1975, and, in 1978, a larger study found it to be more effective and better tolerated than lithium carbonate, the only available treatment at the time. Demeclocycline has since been the drug of choice for treating SIADH, although it may be superseded as vasopressin receptor antagonists, such as tolvaptan, become available.

Contraindications

Like other tetracyclines, demeclocycline is contraindicated in children and pregnant or nursing women. All members of this class interfere with bone development and may discolor teeth.

Side Effects and Interactions

These are similar to those of other tetracyclines. Skin reactions with sunlight have been reported. Demeclocycline is unique in that it is the only tetracycline known to cause nephrogenic diabetes insipidus.

Tetracyclines bind to cations, such as calcium, iron (when given orally), and magnesium, rendering them insoluble and inabsorbable for the gastrointestinal tract. Demeclocycline should not be taken with food (particularly milk and other dairy products) or antacids.

Mechanism of Action

As with related tetracycline antibiotics, demeclocycline acts by binding to the 30S ribosomal subunit to inhibit binding of aminoacyl tRNA which impairs protein synthesis by bacteria. It is bacteriostatic (it impairs bacterial growth, but does not kill bacteria directly).

Demeclocycline inhibits the renal action of antidiuretic hormone by interfering with the intracellular second messenger cascade (specifically, inhibiting adenylyl cyclase activation) after the hormone binds to vasopressin V_2 receptors in the kidney. Exactly how demeclocycline does this has yet to be elucidated, however.

Fabomotizole

Fabomotizole (INN) (brand name Afobazole) is an anxiolytic drug launched in Russia in the early 2000's. It produces anxiolytic and neuroprotective effects without any sedative or muscle relaxant actions. Its mechanism of action remains poorly defined however, with GABAergic, NGF- and BDNF-release-promoting, MT1 receptor agonism, MT3 receptor antagonism, and sigma agonism suggested as potential mechanisms. Fabomotizole was shown to inhibit MAO-A reversibly and there might be also some involvement with serotonin receptors. Clinical trials have shown fabomotizole to be well tolerated and reasonably effective for the treatment of anxiety.

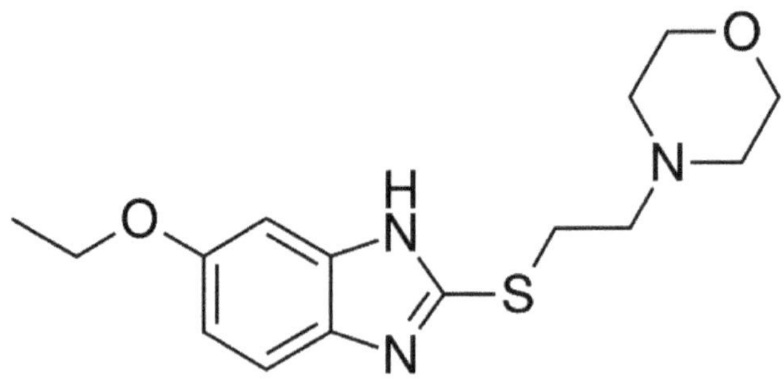

Fabomotizole

Experiments of mice have shown antimutagenic and antiteratogenic properties.

Fabomotizole has found little clinical use outside Russia and has not been evaluated by the FDA.

Lithium (Medication)

Lithium compounds, also known as lithium salts, are primarily used as a psychiatric medication. This includes in the treatment of major depressive disorder that does not improve following the use of other antidepressants and bipolar disorder. In these disorders, it reduces the risk of suicide. Lithium is given orally by mouth.

Common side effects include increased urination, shakiness of the hands, and increased thirst. Serious side effects include hypothyroidism, diabetes insipidus, and lithium toxicity. Blood level monitoring is recommended to decrease the risk of potential toxicity. If levels become too high, diarrhea, vomiting, poor coordination, sleepiness, and ringing in the ears may occur. If used during pregnancy, lithium can cause problems for the baby. It appears to be safe to use while breastfeeding. Lithium salts are classified as mood stabilizers. How they work is not specifically known.

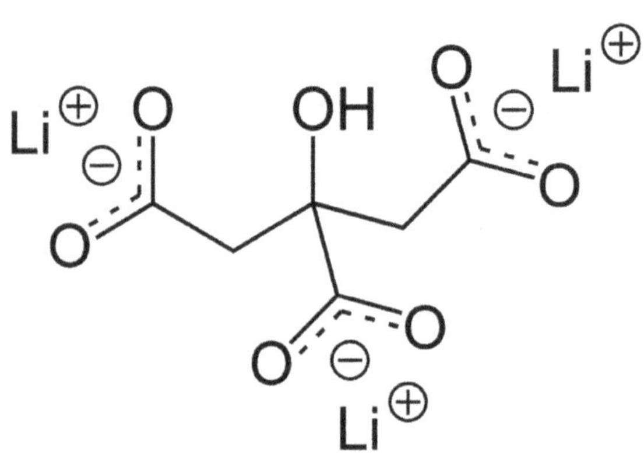

Lithium

In the 1800s, lithium was used in people who had gout, epilepsy, and cancer. Its use in the treatment of mental disorder began in 1948 by John Cade in Australia. It is on the World Health Organization's List of Essential Medicines, the most important medications needed in a basic health system. It is available as a generic medication. The wholesale cost in the developing world in 2014 was between 0.12 and 0.20 USD per day. In the United States at usual doses it costs about 0.90 to 1.20 USD per day.

Medical Uses

Lithium is used primarily for bipolar disorder. It is sometimes used when other treatments are not effective in a number of other conditions, including major depression, schizophrenia, and some psychiatric disorders in children. In mood disorders, of which bipolar is one, it decreases the risk of suicide. This benefit is not seen with other medications.

Bipolar Disorder

Lithium carbonate treatment was previously considered to be unsuitable for children; however, more recent studies show its effectiveness for treatment of early-onset bipolar disorder in children as young as eight. The required dosage is slightly less than the toxic level, requiring close monitoring of blood levels of lithium carbonate during treatment. A limited amount of evidence suggests lithium carbonate may contribute to treatment of substance abuse for some people with bipolar disorder.

Suicide

High levels of naturally occurring lithium in drinking water have been associated with lower rates of suicide.

Monitoring

Those who use lithium should receive regular serum level tests and should monitor thyroid and kidney function for abnormalities, as it interferes with the regulation of sodium and water levels in the body, and can cause dehydration. Dehydration, which is compounded by heat, can result in increasing lithium levels. The dehydration is due to lithium inhibition of the action of antidiuretic hormone, which normally enables the kidney to reabsorb water from urine. This causes an inability to concentrate urine, leading to consequent loss of body water and thirst.

Lithium concentrations in whole blood, plasma, serum or urine may be measured using instrumental techniques as a guide to therapy, to confirm the diagnosis in potential poisoning victims or to assist in the forensic investigation in a case of fatal overdosage. Serum lithium concentrations are usually in the 0.5–1.3 mmol/l range in well-controlled people, but may increase to 1.8–2.5 mmol/l in those who accumulate the drug over time and to 3–10 mmol/l in acute overdose.

Lithium salts have a narrow therapeutic/toxic ratio, so should not be prescribed unless facilities for monitoring plasma concentrations are available. Doses are adjusted to achieve plasma concentrations of 0.4 to 1.2 mmol Li^{+}/l (lower end of the range for maintenance therapy and the elderly, higher end for children) on samples taken 12 hours after the preceding dose.

Interactions

Lithium concentrations are known to be increased with concurrent use of diuretics — especially loop diuretics (such as furosemide) and thiazides — and non-steroidal anti-inflammatory drugs (NSAIDs) such as ibuprofen. Lithium concentrations can also be increased with concurrent use of ACE inhibitors such as captopril, enalapril, and lisinopril.

Lithium is mainly removed from the body through glomerular function, but some is then reabsorbed together with sodium through the proximal tubule. Its levels are therefore sensitive to water and electrolyte balance. Diuretics act by lowering water and sodium levels; this causes more reabsorption of lithium in the proximal tubules so that the removal of lithium from the body is less, leading to increased levels of lithium. ACE inhibitors have also been shown in a retrospective case-control study to increase lithium concentrations. This is likely due to constriction of the afferent arteriole of the glomerulus, resulting in decreased glomerular filtration rate and clearance. Another possible mechanism is that ACE inhibitors can lead to a decrease in sodium and water. This will increase lithium reabsorption and its concentrations in the body.

There are also drugs that can increase the clearance of lithium from the body, which can result in decreased lithium levels in the blood. These drugs include theophylline, caffeine, and acetazolamide. Additionally, increasing dietary sodium intake may also reduce lithium levels by prompting the kidneys to excrete more lithium.

Lithium is also known to be a potential precipitant of serotonin syndrome in people concurrently on serotonergic medications such as antidepressants, buspirone and certain opioids such as pethidine (meperidine), tramadol, oxycodone, fentanyl and others. Lithium co-treatment is also a risk factor for neuroleptic malignant syndrome in people on antipsychotics and other antidopaminergic medications.

High doses of haloperidol, fluphenazine, or flupenthixol may be hazardous when used with lithium; irreversible toxic encephalopathy has been reported. Indeed these and other antipsychotics have been associated with increased risk of lithium neurotoxicity, even with low therapeutic lithium doses.

Overdose

Lithium toxicity may occur on an acute basis, in persons taking excessive amounts either accidentally or intentionally, or on a chronic basis, in people who accumulate high levels during ongoing therapy. The manifestations include nausea, emesis, diarrhea, asthenia, ataxia, confusion, lethargy, polyuria, seizures and coma. Other toxic effects of lithium include coarse tremor, muscle twitching, convulsions and renal failure. People who survive a poisoning episode may develop persistent neurotoxicity. Several authors have described a "Syndrome of Irreversible Lithium-Effected Neurotoxicity" (SILENT), associated with episodes of acute lithium toxicity or long-term treatment within the appropriate dosage range. Symptoms are said to include cerebellar dysfunction.

Overdosage, usually with plasma concentrations over 1.5 mmol Li^+/l, may be fatal, and toxic effects include tremor, ataxia, dysarthria, nystagmus, renal impairment, confusion, and convulsions. If these potentially hazardous signs occur, treatment should be stopped, plasma lithium concentrations redetermined, and steps taken to reverse lithium toxicity.

Lithium toxicity is compounded by sodium depletion. Concurrent use of diuretics that inhibit the uptake of sodium by the distal tubule (e.g. thiazides) is hazardous and should be avoided because this can cause increased resorption of lithium in the proximal convoluted tubule, leading to elevated, potentially toxic levels. In mild cases, withdrawal of lithium and administration of generous amounts of sodium and fluid will reverse the toxicity. Plasma concentrations in excess of 2.5 mmol Li^+/l are usually associated with serious toxicity requiring emergency treatment. When toxic concentrations are reached, there may be a delay of one or two days before maximum toxicity occurs.

In long-term use, therapeutic concentrations of lithium have been thought to cause histological and functional changes in the kidney. The significance of such changes is not clear, but is of sufficient concern to discourage long-term use of lithium unless it is definitely indicated. Doctors may change a bipolar patient's medication from lithium to another mood-stabilizing drug, such as valproate (Depakote), if problems with the kidneys arise. An important potential consequence of long-term lithium use is the development of renal diabetes insipidus (inability to concentrate urine). Patients should therefore be maintained on lithium treatment after three to five years only if, on assessment, benefit persists. Conventional and sustained-release tablets are available. Preparations vary widely in bioavailability, and a change in the formulation used requires the same precautions as initiation of treatment. There are few reasons to prefer any one simple salt of lithium; the carbonate has been the more widely used, but the citrate is also available.

Mechanism of Action

The specific biochemical mechanism of lithium action in stabilizing mood is unknown.

Upon ingestion, lithium becomes widely distributed in the central nervous system and interacts with a number of neurotransmitters and receptors, decreasing norepinephrine release and increasing serotonin synthesis.

Unlike many other psychoactive drugs, Li^+ typically produces no obvious psychotropic effects (such as euphoria) in normal individuals at therapeutic concentrations. Lithium may also increase the release of serotonin by neurons in the brain. In vitro studies performed on serotonergic neurons from rat raphe nuclei have shown that when these neurons are treated with lithium, serotonin release is enhanced during a depolarization compared to no lithium treatment and the same depolarization.

Several authors proposed that pAp-phosphatase could be one of the therapeutic targets of lithium. This hypothesis was supported by the low Ki of lithium for human pAp-phosphatase compatible within the range of therapeutic concentrations of lithium in the plasma of people (0.8–1 mM). Importantly, the Ki of human pAp-phosphatase is ten times lower than that of GSK3β (glycogen synthase kinase 3β). Inhibition of pAp-phosphatase by lithium leads to increased levels of pAp (3′-5′ phosphoadenosine phosphate), which was shown to inhibit PARP-1

Another mechanism proposed in 2007 is that lithium may interact with nitric oxide (NO) signaling pathway in the central nervous system, which plays a crucial role in the neural plasticity. The NO system could be involved in the antidepressant effect of lithium in the Porsolt forced swimming test in mice. It was also reported that NMDA receptor blockage augments antidepressant-like effects of lithium in the mouse forced swimming test, indicating the possible involvement of NMDA receptor/NO signaling in the action of lithium in this animal model of learned helplessness.

Lithium possesses neuroprotective properties by preventing apoptosis and increasing cell longevity.

Oxidative metabolism: Evidence suggests that mitochondrial dysfunction is present in patients with bipolar disorder. Oxidative stress and reduced levels of anti-oxidants (such as glutathione) lead to cell death. Lithium may protect against oxidative stress by up-regulating complex I and II of the mitochondrial electron transport chain.

Dopamine and G-protein coupling: During mania, there is an increase in neurotransmission of dopamine that causes a secondary homeostatic down-regulation, resulting in decreased neurotransmission of dopamine, which can cause depression. Additionally, the post-synaptic actions of dopamine are mediated through G-protein coupled receptors. Once dopamine is coupled to the G-protein receptors, it stimulates other secondary messenger systems that modulate neurotransmission. Studies found that in autopsies (which do not necessarily reflect living people), people with bipolar disorder had increased G-protein coupling compared to people without bipolar disorder. Lithium treatment alters the function of certain subunits of the dopamine associated G-protein, which may be part of its mechanism of action.

Glutamate and NMDA receptors: Glutamate levels are observed to be elevated during mania. Lithium is thought to provide long-term mood stabilization and have anti-manic properties by modulating glutamate levels. It is proposed that lithium competes with magnesium for binding to NMDA glutamate receptor, increasing the availability of glutamate in post-synaptic neurons. The NMDA receptor is also affected by other neurotransmitters such as serotonin and dopamine. Effects observed appear exclusive to lithium and have not been observed by other monovalent ions such as rubidium and caesium.

GABA receptors: GABA is an inhibitory neurotransmitter that plays an important role in regulating dopamine and glutamate neurotransmission. It was found that patients with bipolar disorder had lower GABA levels, which results in excitotoxicity and can cause apoptosis (cell loss). Lithium counteracts these degrading processes by decreasing pro-apoptotic proteins and stimulating release of neuroprotective proteins.

Cyclic AMP secondary messengers: The cyclic AMP secondary messenger system is shown to be modulated by lithium. Lithium was found to increase the basal levels of cyclic AMP but impair receptor coupled stimulation of cyclic AMP production. It is hypothesized that the dual effects of lithium are due the inhibition of G-proteins that then mediate cyclic AMP production. Over a long period of lithium treatment, cyclic AMP and adenylate cyclase levels are further changed by gene transcription factors.

Inositol depletion hypothesis: Lithium treatment has been found to inhibit the enzyme inositol monophosphatase, involved in degrading inositol monophosphate to inositol required in PIP_2synthesis. This leads to lower levels of inositol triphosphate, created by decomposition of PIP_2. This effect has been suggested to be further enhanced with an inositol triphosphate reuptake inhibitor. Inositol disruptions have been linked to memory impairment and depression. It is known with good certainty that signals from the receptors coupled to the phosphoinositide signal transduction is effected by lithium. myo-inositol is also regulated by the high affinity sodium mI transport system (SMIT). Lithium is hypothesized to inhibit mI entering the cells and mitigating the function of SMIT. Reductions of cellular levels of myo-inositol results in the inhibition of the phosphoinositide cycle

Intracellular calcium: In 2014, it was proposed that lithium treatment works by affecting calcium signaling by blocking excitotoxic processes such as antagonizing NMDA receptors and inhibiting inositol monophosphatase (IMPase).

Meprobamate

Meprobamate — marketed as *Miltown* by Wallace Laboratories and *Equanil* by Wyeth, among others — is a carbamate derivative used as an anxiolytic drug. It was the best-selling minor tranquilizer for a time, but has largely been replaced by the benzodiazepines due to their wider therapeutic index (lower risk of toxicity at therapeutically prescribed doses) and lower incidence of serious side effects.

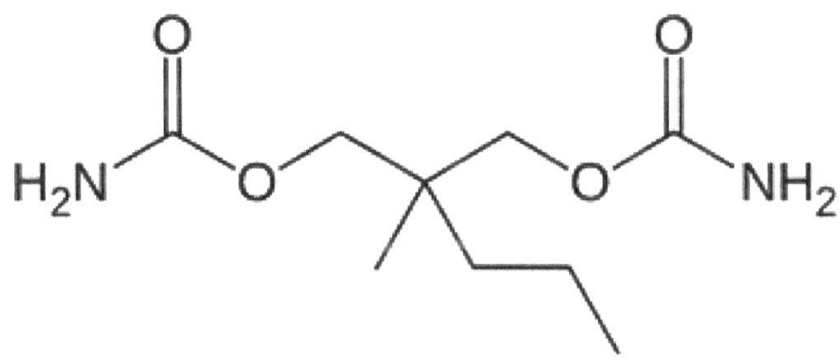

Meprobamate

Pharmacology

Although it was marketed as being safer, meprobamate has most of the pharmacological effects and dangers of the barbiturates and acts at the barbiturate binding site (though it is less sedating at effective doses). It is reported to have some anticonvulsant properties against absence seizures, but can exacerbate generalized tonic-clonic seizures.

Meprobamate's mechanism of action is not completely known. It has been shown in animal studies to have effects at multiple sites in the central nervous system, including the thalamus and limbic system. Meprobamate binds to $GABA_A$ receptors which interrupts neuronal communication in the reticular formation and spinal cord, causing sedation and altered perception of pain. It has been shown that meprobamate has the ability to activate currents even in the absence of GABA. This relatively unique property makes meprobamate exceptionally dangerous when used in combination with other GABA-mediated drugs (including alcohol). It is also a potent adenosine reuptake inhibitor (AdoRI), which is most likely responsible for its lesser degree of sedation compared to barbiturates. Related drugs include carisoprodol and tybamate (prodrugs of meprobamate), felbamate, mebutamate, and methocarbamol.

Indications

Meprobamate is licensed for the short-term relief of anxiety, although it is not known whether the purported anti-anxiety effects of meprobamate are separable from its sedative effects. Its effectiveness as a selective agent for the treatment of anxiety has not been proven in humans, and is not used as often as the benzodiazepines for this purpose.

Meprobamate is available in 200 mg and 400 mg tablets for oral administration. Meprobamate is also a component of the combination drug Equagesic(discontinued in the UK in 2002) acting as a muscle relaxant.

Meprobamate, like barbiturates, possesses an analgesic/anesthetic potential. It is also found as a component of the combination analgesic "Stopayne" capsules (along with paracetamol (acetaminophen), caffeine, and codeine phosphate).

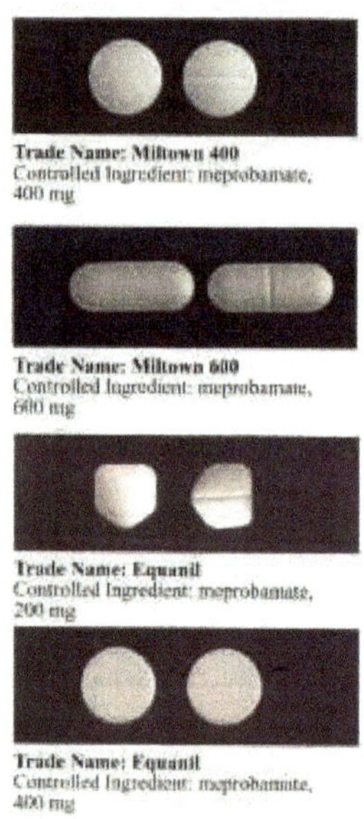

Overdose

Symptoms of meprobamate overdose include: drowsiness, sluggishness, unresponsiveness, or coma; loss of muscle control; severe impairment or cessation of breathing; or shock. Death has been reported with ingestion of as little as 12 g of meprobamate and survival with as much as 40 g. In an overdose, meprobamate tablets may form a gastric bezoar, requiring physical removal of the undissolved mass of tablets through an endoscope;

therefore, administration of activated charcoal should be considered even after 4 or more hours or if levels are rising.

Preparations which contain paracetamol may also induce severe liver toxicity resulting from paracetamol poisoning. The exact form of the preparation used should be identified immediately if possible, as patients who have also overdosed on paracetamol can reduce/avoid permanent liver damage with the administration of acetylcysteine.

Meprobamate overdosage is still a continuing problem.

Health issues

Meprobamate is a Schedule IV drug (US) (S5 in South Africa) under the Convention on Psychotropic Substances. With protracted use it can cause physical dependence and a potentially life-threatening abstinence syndrome similar to that of barbiturates and alcohol (delerium tremens). For this reason, discontinuation is often achieved through an extended regimen of slowly decreasing doses over a period of weeks, or even months. Alternatively, the patient may be switched to a longer-acting gabaminergic agent such as diazepam (in a manner similar to the use of methadone therapy for opiate addiction) before attempting de-titration.

An acute cerebral edema caused by a reaction to Equagesic, a combination of aspirin and meprobamate, is believed to have caused the death of Bruce Lee.

"In the January 2008 issue of Drug Safety Update, a Stop press article announced the recent European review of carisoprodol for which the Committee for Medicinal Products for Human Use (CHMP) concluded that the risks of treatment outweigh the benefits. This review was triggered by concerns from the Norwegian Medical Agency that carisoprodol (converted to meprobamate after administration) was associated with increased risk of abuse, addiction, intoxication, and psychomotor impairment." February 2008.

European Medicines Agency recommended suspension of marketing authorisations for meprobamate-containing medicines in the European Union in January 2012.

Synthesis

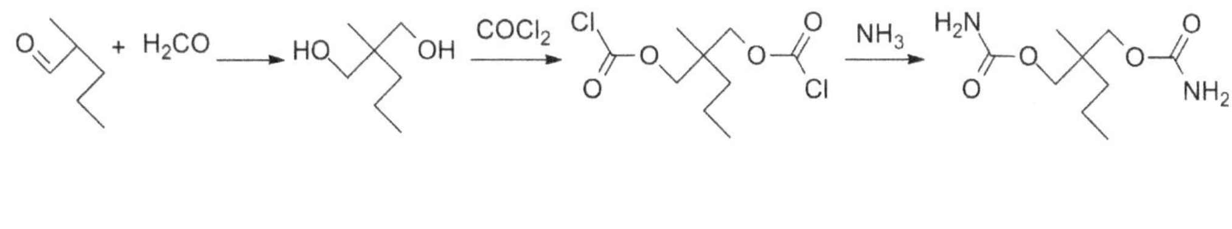

Meprobamate synthesis:

Meprobamate, 2-methyl-2-propyl-1,3-propandiol dicarbamate is synthesized by the reaction of 2-methylvaleraldehyde with two molecules of formaldehyde and the subsequent transformation of the resulting 2-methyl-2-propylpropan-1,3-diol into the dicarbamate via successive reactions with phosgene and ammonia.

Methocarbamol

Methocarbamol is a central muscle relaxant used to treat skeletal muscle spasms. Under the trade name Robaxin, it is marketed by Actient Pharmaceuticals in the United States and Pfizer in Canada. The mechanism of action of methocarbamol is currently unknown, but may involve the inhibition of carbonic anhydrase. The muscle relaxant effects of methocarbamol are largely attributed to central depressant effects; however, peripheral effects of methocarbamol to prolong muscle refractory period have also been reported. As of 2015 the cost for a typical month of medication in the United States is less than 25 USD.

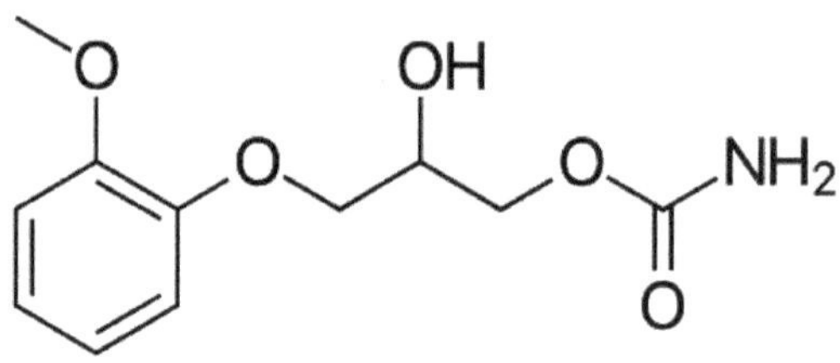

Methocarbamol

Side-Effects

Potential side-effects include: drowsiness, dizziness, clumsiness (ataxia), upset stomach, flushing, blurred vision, and fever. Both tachycardia (fast heart rate) and bradycardia (slow heart rate) have been reported; these can be serious. Other serious side-effects include the development of a severe skin rash or itching, fainting, jaundice, persistent nausea/vomiting, stomach/abdominal pain, mental/mood changes, trouble urinating, and signs of infection. If taken in large amounts at once or more than directed or as prescribed, dysphoria or suicidal thoughts may occur. In addition, methocarbamol may cause urine to turn black, blue, or green. However, this effect is harmless.

Methocarbamol has a high therapeutic index, i.e., a wide range of safe and effective dosages. Consumer (OTC) doses are in the range 3–6 g per day, while clinical doses can be as high as 24 g per day for severe conditions such as tetanus.

Because of the potential for side-effects, this drug is considered to be a high-risk medication for the elderly.

Abuse potential: Unlike other carbamates such as meprobamate and its prodrug carisoprodol, methocarbamol has greatly reduced abuse potential. Studies comparing it to the benzodiazepine lorazepam and the antihistamine diphenhydramine, along with placebo, find that methocarbamol produces increased "liking" responses and some sedative-like effects, however, at higher doses dysphoria is reported. It is considered to have an abuse profile similar to, but weaker than, lorazepam.

Metabolism

Methocarbamol is the carbamate of guaifenesin, but does not produce guaifenesin as a metabolite, because the carbamate bond is not hydrolyzed metabolically; metabolism is by Phase I ring hydroxylation and *O*-demethylation, followed by Phase II conjugation. All the major metabolites are unhydrolyzed carbamates.

Marketing

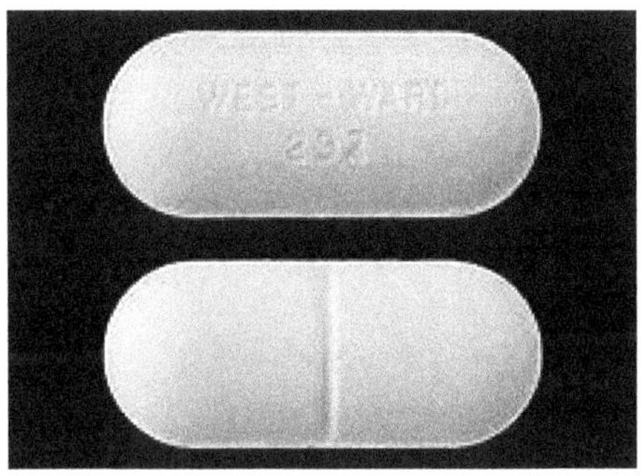

Generic Methocarbamol 750mg Oral Tablet.

Methocarbamol is marketed under different names when presented in combination with other active ingredients. In combination with acetaminophen (Paracetamol), under trade names Robaxacet and Tylenol Body Pain Night, whereas Robax Platinum is the trade name for a formulation of methocarbamol and ibuprofen. A combination of methocarbamol and aspirin is marketed as Robaxisal, however in Spain the tradename Robaxisal is used for the Paracetamol combination instead of Robaxacet.

Paracetamol

Paracetamol, also known as acetaminophen or APAP, is a medication used to treat pain and fever. It is typically used for mild to moderate pain. There is poor evidence for fever relief in children. It is often sold in combination with other ingredients such as in many cold medications. In combination with opioid pain medication, paracetamol is used for more severe pain such as cancer pain and after surgery. It is typically used either by mouth or rectally but is also available intravenously. Effects last between two and four hours.

Paracetamol is generally safe at recommended doses. Serious skin rashes may rarely occur, and too high a dose can result in liver failure. It appears to be safe during pregnancy and when breastfeeding. In those with liver disease, it may still be used, but lower doses should be taken. Paracetamol is classified as a mild analgesic. It does not have significant anti-inflammatory activity and how it works is not entirely clear.

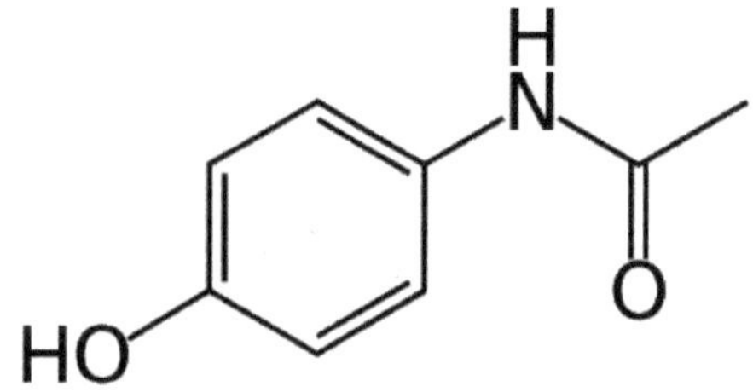

Paracetamol

Paracetamol was discovered in 1877. It is the most commonly used medication for pain and fever in both the United States and Europe. It is on the WHO Model List of Essential Medicines, the most important medications needed in a basic health system. Paracetamol is available as a generic medication with trade names including *Tylenol* and *Panadol* among others. The wholesale price in the developing world is less than 0.01 USD per dose. In the United States it costs about 0.04 USD per dose.

Medical uses

Fever: Paracetamol is used for reducing fever in people of all ages. The World Health Organization (WHO) recommends that paracetamol be used to treat fever in children only if their temperature is greater than 38.5 °C (101.3 °F). The efficacy of paracetamol by itself in children with fevers has been questioned and a meta-analysis showed that it is less effective than ibuprofen.

Pain: Paracetamol is used for the relief of mild to moderate pain. The use of the intravenous form for pain of sudden onset in people in the emergency department is supported by limited evidence.

Osteoarthritis: The American College of Rheumatology recommends paracetamol as one of several treatment options for people with arthritis pain of the hip, hand, or knee that does not improve with exercise and weight loss. A 2015 review, however, found it provided only a small benefit in osteoarthritis.

Paracetamol has relatively little anti-inflammatory activity, unlike other common analgesics such as the NSAIDs aspirin and ibuprofen, but ibuprofen and paracetamol have similar effects in the treatment of headache. Paracetamol can relieve pain in mild arthritis, but has no effect on the underlying inflammation, redness, and swelling of the joint. It has analgesic properties comparable to those of aspirin, while its anti-inflammatory effects are weaker. It is better tolerated than aspirin due to concerns about bleeding with aspirin.

Low back pain: Based on a systematic review, paracetamol is recommended by the American College of Physicians and the American Pain Society as a first-line treatment for low back pain. However, other systematic reviews concluded that evidence for its efficacy is lacking.

Headaches: A joint statement of the German, Austrian, and Swiss headache societies and the German Society of Neurology recommends the use of paracetamol in combination with caffeine as one of several first line therapies for treatment of tension or migraine headache. In the treatment of acute migraine, it is superior to placebo, with 39% of people experiencing pain relief at 1 hour compared to 20% in the control group.

Postoperative pain: Paracetamol combined with NSAIDs may be more effective for treating postoperative pain than either paracetamol alone or NSAIDs alone.

Dental use: NSAIDs such as ibuprofen, naproxen, diclofenac are more effective than paracetamol for controlling dental pain or pain arising from dental procedures; combinations of NSAIDs and paracetamol are more effective than either alone. Paracetamol is particularly useful when NSAIDs are contraindicated due to hypersensitivity or history of gastrointestinal ulceration or bleeding. It can also be used in combination with NSAIDs when these are ineffective in controlling dental pain alone. The Cochrane review of preoperative analgesics for additional pain relief in children and adolescents shows no evidence of benefit in taking paracetamol before dental treatment to help reduce pain after treatment for procedures under local anaesthetic, however the quality of evidence is low.

Other: The efficacy of paracetamol when used in combination with weak opioids (such as codeine) improved for approximately 50% of people but with increases in the number experiencing side effects. Combination drugs of paracetamol and strong opioids like morphine improve analgesic effect.

The combination of paracetamol with caffeine is superior to paracetamol alone for the treatment of common pain conditions including dental pain, postpartum pain, and headache.

Adverse Effects

Healthy adults taking regular doses of up to 4,000 mg a day show little evidence of toxicity (although some researchers disagree). They are more likely to have abnormal liver function tests, but the significance of this is uncertain.

Liver damage: Acute overdoses of paracetamol can cause potentially fatal liver damage. In 2011, US Food and Drug Administration launched a public education program to help consumers avoid overdose, warning: "Acetaminophen can cause serious liver damage if more than directed is used." In a 2011 Safety Warning the FDA immediately required manufacturers to update labels of all prescription combination acetaminophen products to warn of the potential risk for severe liver injury and required that such combinations contain no more than 325 mg of acetaminophen. FDA has likewise requested prescribers to limit combination opioids to 325 mg of acetaminophen. Such overdoses are frequently related to high-dose recreational use of prescription opioids, as these opioids are most often combined with acetaminophen. The overdose risk may be heightened by frequent consumption of alcohol.

Paracetamol toxicity is the foremost cause of acute liver failure in the Western world and accounts for most drug overdoses in the United States, the United Kingdom, Australia, and New Zealand. According to the FDA, in the United States there were "56,000 emergency room visits, 26,000 hospitalizations, and 458 deaths per year related to acetaminophen-associated overdoses during the 1990s. Within these estimates, unintentional acetaminophen overdose accounted for nearly 25 percent of the emergency department visits, 10 percent of the hospitalizations, and 25 percent of the deaths."

Paracetamol is metabolised by the liver and is hepatotoxic; side effects are multiplied when combined with alcoholic drinks, and are very likely in chronic alcoholicsor patients with liver damage. Some studies have suggested the possibility of a moderately increased risk of upper gastrointestinal complications such as stomach bleeding when high doses are taken chronically. Kidney damage is seen in rare cases, most commonly in overdose.

Skin reactions: On August 2, 2013, the U.S. Food and Drug Administration (FDA) issued a new warning about paracetamol. It stated that the drug could cause rare and possibly fatal skin reactions such as Stevens–Johnson syndrome and toxic epidermal necrolysis. Prescription-strength products will be required to carry a warning label about skin reactions, and the FDA has urged manufacturers to do the same with over-the-counter products.

Asthma: There is an association between paracetamol use and asthma, but the evidence suggests that this likely reflects confounders rather than a causal role. A 2014 review found that among children the association disappeared when respiratory infections were taken into account.

As of 2014, the American Academy of Pediatrics and the National Institute for Health and Care Excellence (NICE) continue to recommend paracetamol for pain and discomfort in children, but some experts have recommended that paracetamol use by children with asthma or at risk for asthma should be avoided.

Other factors

In contrast to aspirin, paracetamol does not prevent blood from clotting (it is not an antithrombotic), and thus may be used in patients where failure of blood coagulation is a concern; and it does not cause gastric irritation. However, paracetamol does not help reduce inflammation, while aspirin does. Compared to ibuprofen—whose side effects may include diarrhea, vomiting and abdominal pain—paracetamol has fewer adverse gastrointestinal effects. Unlike aspirin, paracetamol is generally considered safe for children, as it is not associated with a risk of Reye's syndrome in children with viral illnesses. If taken recreationally with opioids, there is weak evidence suggesting that it may cause hearing loss.

Overdose: Untreated paracetamol overdose results in a lengthy, painful illness. Signs and symptoms of paracetamol toxicity may initially be absent or non-specific symptoms. The first symptoms of overdose usually begin several hours after ingestion, with nausea, vomiting, sweating, and pain as acute liver failure starts. People who take overdoses of paracetamol do not fall asleep or lose consciousness, although most people who attempt suicide with paracetamol wrongly believe that they will be rendered unconscious by the drug. The process of dying from an overdose takes from 3–5 days to 4–6 weeks.

Paracetamol hepatotoxicity is by far the most common cause of acute liver failure in both the United States and the United Kingdom. Paracetamol overdose results in more calls to poison control centers in the US than overdose of any other pharmacological substance. Toxicity of paracetamol is believed to be due to its quinone metabolite.

Untreated overdose can lead to liver failure and death within days. Treatment is aimed at removing the paracetamol from the body and replacing glutathione.Activated charcoal can be used to decrease absorption of paracetamol if the patient presents for treatment soon after the overdose. While the antidote, acetylcysteine (also called N-acetylcysteine or NAC), acts as a precursor for glutathione, helping the body regenerate enough to prevent or at least decrease the possible damage to the liver, a liver transplant is often required if damage to the liver becomes severe. NAC was usually given following a treatment nomogram (one for patients with risk factors, and one for those without) but the use of the nomogram is no longer recommended as evidence to support the use of risk factors was poor and inconsistent, and many of the risk factors are imprecise and difficult to determine with sufficient certainty in clinical practice. NAC also helps in neutralizing the imidoquinone metabolite of paracetamol. Kidney failure is also a possible side effect.

Until 2004, tablets were available (brand-name in the UK Paradote) that combined paracetamol with an antidote (methionine) to protect the liver in case of an overdose. One theoretical, but rarely if ever used, option in the United States is to request a compounding pharmacy to make a similar drug mix for at-risk patients.

In June 2009, a U.S. Food and Drug Administration (FDA) advisory committee recommended that new restrictions be placed on paracetamol usage in the United States to help protect people from the potential toxic effects. The maximum dosage at any given time would be decreased from 1000 mg to 650 mg, while combinations of paracetamol and opioid analgesics would be prohibited. Committee members were particularly concerned by the fact that the present maximum dosages of paracetamol had been shown to produce alterations in hepatic function.

In January 2011, the FDA asked manufacturers of prescription combination products containing paracetamol to limit the amount of paracetamol to no more than 325 mg per tablet or capsule and began requiring manufacturers to update the labels of all prescription combination paracetamol products to warn of the potential risk of severe liver damage. Manufacturers had three years to limit the amount of paracetamol in their prescription drug products to 325 mg per dosage unit. In November 2011, the Medicines and Healthcare products Regulatory Agency revised UK dosing of liquid paracetamol for children.

*Pregnancy:*Experimental studies in animals and cohort studies in humans indicate no detectable increase in congenital malformations associated with paracetamol use during pregnancy. Additionally, paracetamol does not affect the closure of the fetal ductus arteriosus as NSAIDs can.

Paracetamol use by the mother during pregnancy is associated with an increased risk of childhood asthma. It is also associated with an increase in ADHD but it is unclear whether the relationship is causal. A 2015 review states that paracetamol remains a first-line recommended medication for pain and fever during pregnancy, despite these concerns.

Cancer: Some studies have found an association between paracetamol and a slight increase in kidney cancer, but no effect on bladder cancer risk.

Mechanism of Action

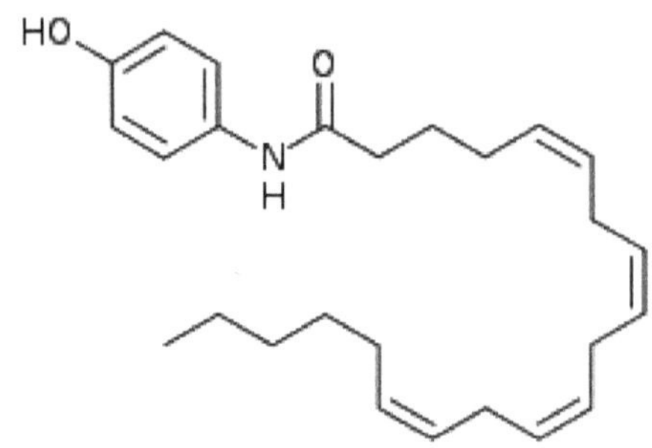

AM404 – Metabolite of paracetamol

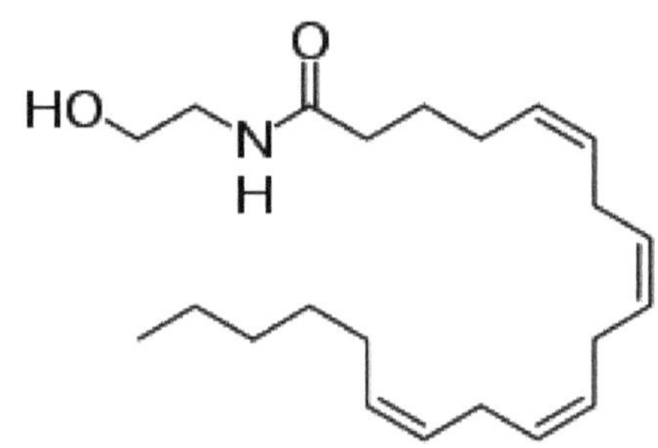

Anandamide – Endogenous cannabinoid

inhibition of cyclooxygenase (COX), and recent findings suggest that it is highly selective for COX-2. Because of its selectivity for COX-2, it does not significantly inhibit the production of the pro-clotting thromboxanes. While it has analgesic and antipyretic properties comparable to those of aspirin or other NSAIDs, its peripheral anti-inflammatory activity is usually limited by several factors, one of which is the high level of peroxides present in inflammatory lesions.

An article in Nature Communications from researchers in London, UK and Lund, Sweden in November 2011 has found a hint to the analgesic mechanism of paracetamol, being that the metabolites of paracetamol (e.g., NAPQI), act on TRPA1-receptors in the spinal cord to suppress the signal transduction from the superficial layers of the dorsal horn, to alleviate pain.

This conclusion has been contested in a new hypothesis paper on how paracetamol might act. The author concedes that NAPQI is the active metabolite but that this reactive compound should react not only with the thiol in TRPA1 but also with any other suitably available nucleophile that it happens to encounter. It is suggested that thiol groups in cysteine proteases, e.g. the proteases that take part in the processing of procytokines, such as those generating IL-1β and IL-6, might be the targets giving rise to overall analgesic effects.

The COX family of enzymes are responsible for the metabolism of arachidonic acid to prostaglandin H_2, an unstable molecule that is, in turn, converted to numerous other pro-inflammatory compounds. Classical anti-inflammatories such as the NSAIDs block this step. Only when appropriately oxidised is the COX enzyme highly active. Paracetamol reduces the oxidised form of the COX enzyme, preventing it from forming pro-inflammatory chemicals. This leads to a reduced amount of *prostaglandin E2* in the CNS, thus lowering the hypothalamic set-point in the thermoregulatory centre.

Aspirin is known to inhibit the cyclooxygenase (COX) family of enzymes and, because paracetamol's action is partially similar to aspirin's, much research has focused on whether paracetamol also inhibits COX. It is now clear that paracetamol acts via at least two pathways.

The exact mechanisms by which COX is inhibited in various circumstances are still a subject of discussion. Because of differences in the activity of paracetamol, aspirin, and other NSAIDs, it has been postulated that further COX variants may exist. One theory holds that paracetamol works by inhibiting the COX-3 isoform—a COX-1 splice variant—of the COX family of enzymes. When expressed in dogs, this enzyme shares a strong similarity to the other COX enzymes, produces pro-inflammatory chemicals, and is selectively inhibited by paracetamol. However, some research has suggested that, in humans and mice, the COX-3 enzyme is without inflammatory action and paracetamol's blockage of it is not significant in its functioning in humans.

Another possibility is that paracetamol blocks cyclooxygenase (as in aspirin), but that, in an inflammatory environment where the concentration of peroxides is high, the high oxidation state of paracetamol prevents its actions. This idea would mean that paracetamol has no direct effect at the site of inflammation, but instead acts in the CNS where the environment is not oxidative, to reduce temperature, etc.

Paracetamol also modulates the endogenous cannabinoid system. Paracetamol is metabolised to AM404, a compound with several actions; what is most important is that it inhibits the reuptake of the endogenous cannabinoid/vanilloid anandamide by neurons. Anandamide reuptake lowers synaptic levels of anandamide and results in more activation of the main pain receptor (nociceptor) of the body, the TRPV1 (older name: vanilloid receptor). By inhibiting anandamide reuptake, levels in the synapse remain high and are able to desensitise the TRPV1 receptor much like capsaicin. Furthermore, AM404 inhibits sodium channels, as do the anesthetics lidocaine and procaine. Both of these actions by themselves have been shown to reduce pain, and are a possible mechanism for paracetamol. It has been demonstrated that when cannabinoid receptors are blocked with synthetic antagonists, paracetamol's analgesic effects are prevented, suggesting its pain-relieving action involves the endogenous cannabinoid system. Spinal TRPA1 receptors have also been demonstrated to mediate antinociceptive effects of paracetamol and Δ9-tetrahydrocannabinol in mice.

Increase of social behavior in mice dosed with paracetamol (which corresponds to a reduction of social rejection response in humans) does not appear to be due to cannabinoid receptor type 1 activity. It may result from serotonin receptor agonism.

Pharmacokinetics

After being taken by mouth it is rapidly absorbed by the GI tract (although absorption through the stomach is negligible);its volume of distribution is roughly 50 L. The concentration in serum after a typical dose of paracetamol usually peaks below 30 μg/ml, which equals 200 μmol/L. After 4 hours the concentration is usually less than 10 μg/mL, which equals 66 μmol/L.

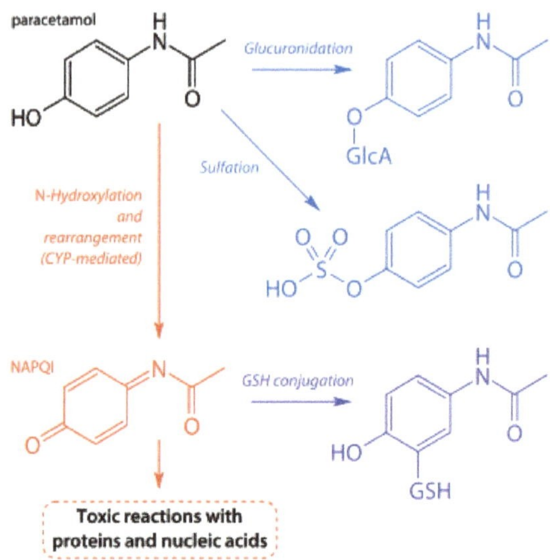

Main pathways of paracetamol metabolism. Pathways shown in blue and purple lead to non-toxic metabolites; the pathway in red leads to toxic NAPQI.

Paracetamol is metabolised primarily in the liver, into toxic and non-toxic products. Three metabolic pathways are notable:

- Glucuronidation (45-55%), by UGT1A1 and UGT1A6;
- Sulfation (sulfate conjugation) (20–30%) by SULT1A1;
- *N*-hydroxylation and dehydration, then glutathione conjugation, (less than 15%). The hepatic cytochrome P450 enzyme system metabolises paracetamol, forming a minor yet significant alkylating metabolite known as NAPQI (*N*-acetyl-*p*-benzoquinone imine) (also known as *N*-acetylimidoquinone). NAPQI is then irreversibly conjugated with the sulfhydryl groups of glutathione.

All three pathways yield final products that are inactive, non-toxic, and eventually excreted by the kidneys. In the third pathway, however, the intermediate product NAPQI is toxic. NAPQI is primarily responsible for the toxic effects of paracetamol; this constitutes an example of toxication. Production of NAPQI is due primarily to two isoenzymes of cytochrome P450: CYP2E1 and CYP3A4. At usual doses, NAPQI is quickly detoxified by conjugation with glutathione.

Chemistry

Chemical properties: Paracetamol consists of a benzene ring core, substituted by one hydroxyl group and the nitrogen atom of an amide group in the *para* (1,4) pattern. The amide group is acetamide (ethanamide). It is an extensively conjugated system, as the lone pair on the hydroxyl oxygen, the benzene pi cloud, the nitrogen lone pair, the p orbital on the carbonyl carbon, and the lone pair on the carbonyl oxygen are all conjugated. The presence of two activating groups also make the benzene ring highly reactive toward electrophilic aromatic substitution. As the substituents are *ortho, para*-directing and *para* with respect to each other, all positions on the ring are more or less equally activated. The conjugation also greatly reduces the basicity of the oxygens and the nitrogen, while making the hydroxyl acidic through delocalisation of charge developed on the phenoxideanion.

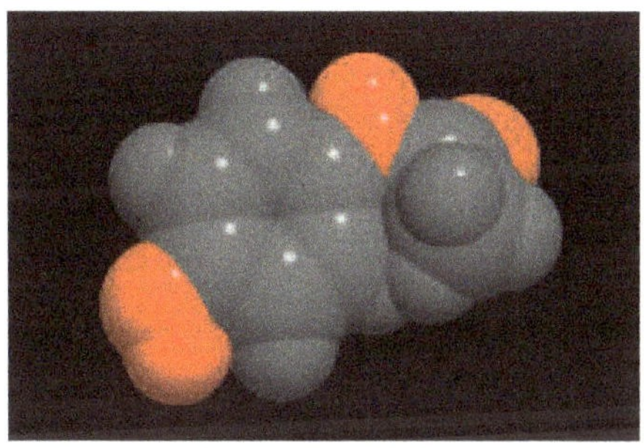

Paracetamol molecule polar surface area

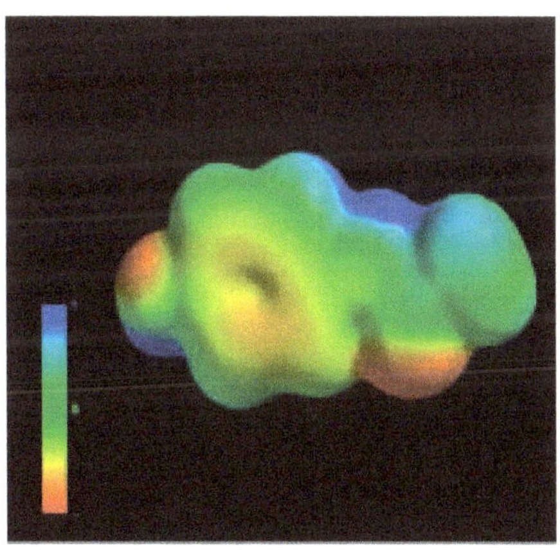

Paracetamol electron map electrostatic surface area

Paracetamol is part of the class of drugs known as "aniline analgesics"; it is the only such drug still in use today. It is not considered an NSAID because it does not exhibit significant anti-inflammatory activity (it is a weak COX inhibitor).This is despite the evidence that paracetamol and NSAIDs have some similar pharmacological activity.

Synthesis

Original (Boots) method: The original method for production involves the nitration of phenol with sodium nitrate gives a mixture of two isomers, from which the wanted 4-nitrophenol (bp 279 °C) can easily be separated by steam distillation. In this electrophilic aromatic substitution reaction, phenol's oxygen is strongly activating, thus the reaction requires only mild conditions as compared to nitration of benzene itself. The nitro group is then reduced to an amine, giving 4-aminophenol. Finally, the amine is acetylated with acetic anhydride. Industrially direct hydrogenation is used, but in the laboratory scale sodium borohydride serves.

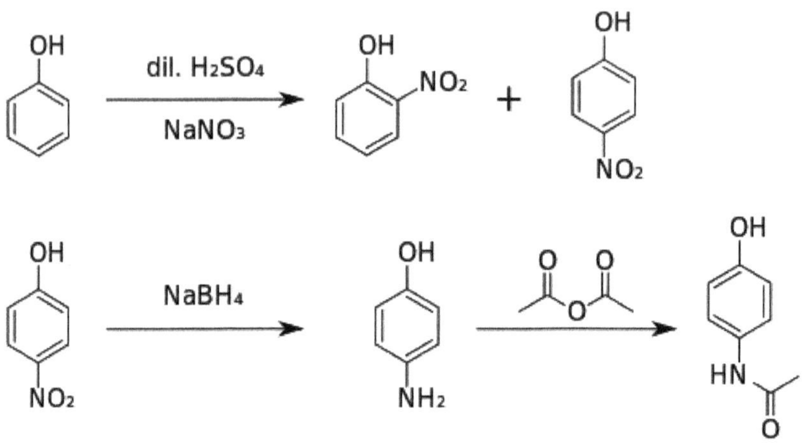

Green(er) synthesis: An alternative industrial synthesis developed by Hoechst–Celanese involves direct acylation of phenol with acetic anhydride catalyzed by HF, conversion of the ketone to a ketoxime with hydroxylamine, followed by the acid-catalyzed Beckmann rearrangement to give the amide.

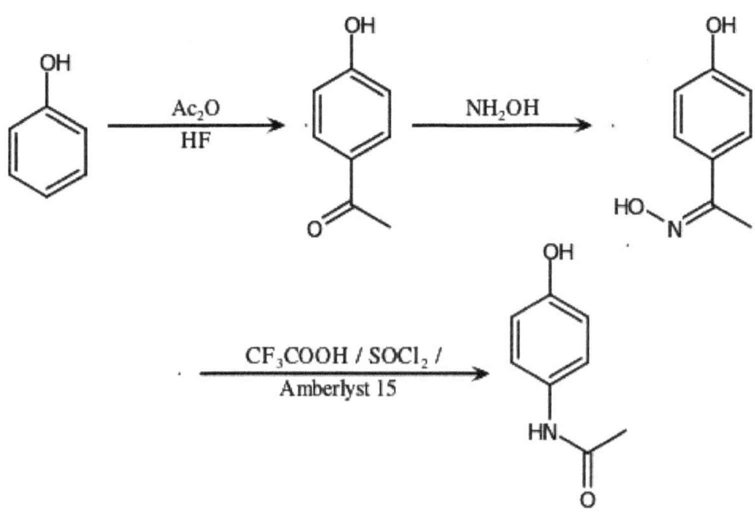

Direct synthesis: More recently (2014) a "one-pot" synthesis from hydroquinone has been described before the Royal Society of Chemistry. The process may be summarized as follows:

Hydroquinone, ammonium acetate, and acetic acid were mixed in an argon atmosphere and heated slowly to 230 °C. The mixture was stirred at this temperature for 15 hours. After cooling the acetic acid was evaporated and the precipitate was filtered, washed with water and dried to give paracetamol as a white solid.

The authors go on to claim an 88% yield and 99% purity.

Reactions: 4-Aminophenol may be obtained by the amide hydrolysis of paracetamol. *4*-Aminophenol prepared this way, and related to the commercially available Metol, has been used as a developer in photography by hobbyists. This reaction is also used to determine paracetamol in urine samples: After hydrolysis with hydrochloric acid, *4*-aminophenol reacts in ammonia solution with a phenol derivate, e.g. salicylic acid, to form an indophenol dye under oxidization by air.

Phenytoin

Phenytoin, sold under the brand name Dilantin among others, is an anti-seizure medication. It is useful for the prevention of tonic-clonic seizures, partial seizures, but not absence seizures. The intravenous form is used for status epilepticus that does not improve with benzodiazepines. It may also be used for certain heart arrhythmias or neuropathic pain. It can be taken intravenously or by mouth. The intravenous form generally begins working within 30 minutes and is effective for 24 hours. Blood levels can be measured to determine the proper dose. Common side effects include nausea, stomach pain, loss of appetite, poor coordination, increased hair growth, and enlargement of the gums. Potentially serious side effects include sleepiness, self harm, liver problems, bone marrow suppression, low blood pressure, and toxic epidermal necrolysis. There is evidence that use during pregnancy results in abnormalities in the baby. It appears to be safe to use when breastfeeding. Alcohol may interfere with the medication's effects.

Phenytoin was first made in 1908 by the German chemist Heinrich Biltz and found useful for seizures in 1936. It is on the World Health Organization's List of Essential Medicines, the most important medications needed in a basic health system. Phenytoin is available as a generic medication and usually not too expensive. The wholesale cost in the developing world is between US$0.003 and US$0.15 per dose. A month of treatment is about US$30 in the United States.

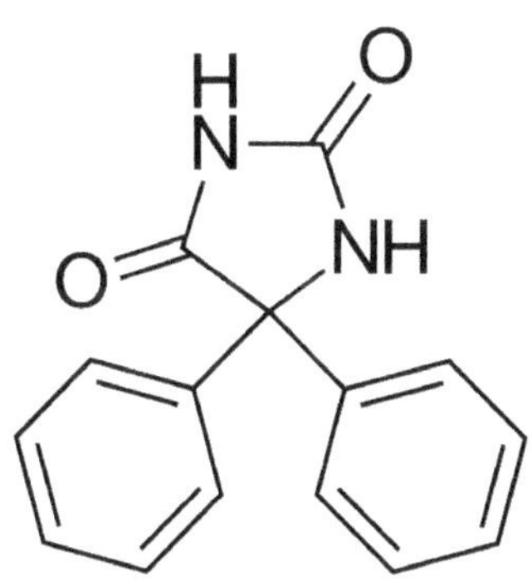

Phenytoin

Medical uses

Seizures

- Tonic-clonic seizures: Mainly used in the prophylactic management of tonic-clonic seizures with complex symptomatology (psychomotor seizures). A period of 5–10 days may be required to achieve anticonvulsant effects.
- Focal seizures: Mainly used to protect against the development of focal seizures with complex symptomatology (psychomotor and temporal lobe seizures). Also effective in controlling partial seizures with autonomic symptoms.
- Absence seizures: Not used in treatment of pure absence seizures due to risk for increasing frequency of seizures. However, can be used in combination with other anticonvulsants during combined absence and tonic-clonic seizures.
- Seizures during surgery: Used as prevention and treatment of seizures occurring during and after neurosurgery.
- Status epilepticus: Considered after failed treatment using a benzodiazepine due to slow onset of action.

Other

- Abnormal heart rhythms: may be used in the treatment of ventricular tachycardia and sudden episodes of atrial tachycardia after other antiarrhythmic medications or cardioversion has failed. It is a class 1b antiarrhythmic.
- Digoxin toxicity: IV formulation is drug of choice for arrhythmias caused by cardiac glycoside toxicity.
- Trigeminal neuralgia: Second choice drug to carbamazepine.

Special considerations

- Monitoring plasma concentrations: Narrow therapeutic index. Anticonvulsant effect: 10–20 μg/mL; Antiarrhythmic effect: 10–20 μg/mL
- Avoid giving intramuscular formulation unless necessary due to skin cell death and local tissue destruction.
- Elderly: May show earlier signs of toxicity.
- Obese: Use ideal body weight for dosing calculations.
- Pregnancy: Pregnancy Category D due to risk of fetal hydantoin syndrome and fetal bleeding. However, optimal seizure control is very important during pregnancy so drug may be continued if benefits outweigh the risks. Due to decreased drug concentrations during pregnancy, dose of phenytoin may need to be increased if only option for seizure control.
- Breast feeding: The manufacturer does not recommend breast feeding because low concentrations of phenytoin are excreted in breast milk.
- Liver disease: Do not use oral loading dose. Consider using decreased maintenance dose.
- Kidney disease: Do not use oral loading dose. Can begin with standard maintenance dose and adjust as needed.

- IV use is contraindicated in patients with sinus bradycardia, SA block, second- or third-degree AV block, Stokes-Adams syndrome, or have known hypersensitivity to phenytoin or any ingredient in the respective formulation or to other hydantoins.

Side Effects

Common side effects include nausea, stomach pain, loss of appetite, poor coordination, increased hair growth, and enlargement of the gums. Potentially serious side effects include sleepiness, self harm, liver problems, bone marrow suppression, low blood pressure, and toxic epidermal necrolysis. There is evidence that use during pregnancy results in abnormalities in the baby. It appears to be okay during breastfeeding. Alcohol may interfere with the medication's effects.

Heart and blood vessels: Severe low blood pressure and abnormal heart rhythms can be seen with rapid infusion of IV phenytoin. IV infusion should not exceed 50 mg/min in adults or 1–3 mg/kg/min (or 50 mg/min, whichever is slower) in children. Heart monitoring should occur during and after IV infusion. Due to these risks, oral phenytoin should be used if possible.

Neurological: At therapeutic doses, phenytoin may produce nystagmus on lateral gaze. At toxic doses, patients experience vertical nystagmus, double vision, sedation, slurred speech, cerebellar ataxia, and tremor. If phenytoin is stopped abruptly, this may result in increased seizure frequency, including status epilepticus.

Phenytoin may accumulate in the cerebral cortex over long periods of time which can cause atrophy of the cerebellum. The degree of atrophy is related to the duration of phenytoin treatment and is not related to dosage of the medication.

Abrupt discontinuation of phenytoin can precipitate status epilepticus.

Phenytoin is known to be a causal factor in the development of peripheral neuropathy.

Blood: It has been suggested that phenytoin causes a reduction in folic acid levels, predisposing patients to megaloblastic anemia. Folate is presented in foods as polyglutamate, which is then converted into monoglutamates by intestinal conjugase. Phenytoin acts by inhibiting this enzyme, thereby causing folate deficiency.Other side effects may include: agranulocytosis, aplastic anemia, decreased white blood cell count, and a low platelet count.

Pregnancy: Phenytoin is a known teratogen. The syndrome consists of craniofacial anomalies (broad nasal bridge, cleft lip and palate, smaller than normal head) and a mild form of mental retardation (average IQ=71). This syndrome resembles the well-described Fetal Alcohol Syndrome and has also been called the "fetal hydantoin syndrome". Some recommend avoiding polytherapy and maintaining the minimal dose possible during pregnancy, but acknowledge that current data do not provide clear answers. Data now being collected by the Epilepsy and Antiepileptic Drug Pregnancy Registry may one day answer this question definitively.

Cancer: There is no good evidence that phenytoin is a human carcinogen.

Mouth: Phenytoin has been associated with drug-induced gingival enlargement (overgrowth of the gums), probably due to above-mentioned folate deficiency; indeed, evidence from a randomized controlled trial suggests that folic acid supplementation can prevent gingival enlargement in children who take phenytoin. Plasma concentrations needed to induce gingival lesions have not been clearly defined. Effects consist of the following: bleeding upon probing, increased gingival exudate, pronounced gingival inflammatory response to plaque levels, associated in some instances with bone loss but without tooth detachment.

Skin: Hypertrichosis, Stevens-Johnson syndrome, purple glove syndrome, rash, exfoliative dermatitis, itching, excessive hairiness, and coarsening of facial features can be seen in those taking phenytoin.

Phenytoin therapy has been linked to the life-threatening skin reactions Stevens–Johnson syndrome (SJS) and toxic epidermal necrolysis (TEN). These conditions are significantly more common in patients with a particular HLA-B allele, HLA-B*1502. This allele occurs almost exclusively in patients with ancestry across broad areas of Asia, including South Asian Indians.

Phenytoin is primarily metabolized to its inactive form by the enzyme CYP2C9. Variations within the CYP2C9 gene that result in decreased enzymatic activity have been associated with increased phenytoin concentrations, as well as reports of drug toxicities due to these increased concentrations. The U.S. Food and Drug Administration (FDA) notes on the phenytoin drug label that since strong evidence exists linking HLA-B*1502 with the risk of developing SJS or TEN in patients taking carbamazepine, consideration should be given to avoiding phenytoin as an alternative to carbamazepine in patients carrying this allele.

*Immune System:*Phenytoin has been known to cause drug-induced lupus.

Phenytoin is also associated with induction of reversible IgA deficiency.

Psychological: Phenytoin may increase risk of suicidal thoughts or behavior. People on phenytoin should be monitored for any changes in mood, the development or worsening depression, and/or any thoughts or behavior of suicide.

Bones: Chronic phenytoin use has been associated with decreased bone density and increased bone fractures. Phenytoin induces metabolizing enzymes in the liver. This leads to increased metabolism of vitamin D, thus decreased vitamin D levels. Vitamin D deficiency, as well as low calcium and phosphate in the blood cause decreased bone mineral density.

Interactions

Phenytoin is an inducer of the CYP3A4 and CYP2C19 families of the P450 enzyme responsible for the liver's degradation of various drugs.

A 1981 study by the National Institutes of Health showed that antacids administered concomitantly with phenytoin "altered not only the extent of absorption but also appeared to alter the rate of absorption. Antacids administered in a peptic ulcer regimen may decrease the AUC of a single dose of phenytoin. Patients should be cautioned against concomitant use of antacids and phenytoin."

Warfarin (Coumadin) and trimethoprim increase serum phenytoin levels and prolong the serum half-life of phenytoin by inhibiting its metabolism. Consider using other options if possible.

Mechanism of Action

Phenytoin is believed to protect against seizures by causing voltage-dependent block of voltage gated sodium channels.This blocks sustained high frequency repetitive firing of action potentials. This is accomplished by reducing the amplitude of sodium-dependent action potentials through enhancing steady state inactivation. Sodium channels exist in three main conformations: the resting state, the open state, and the inactive state.

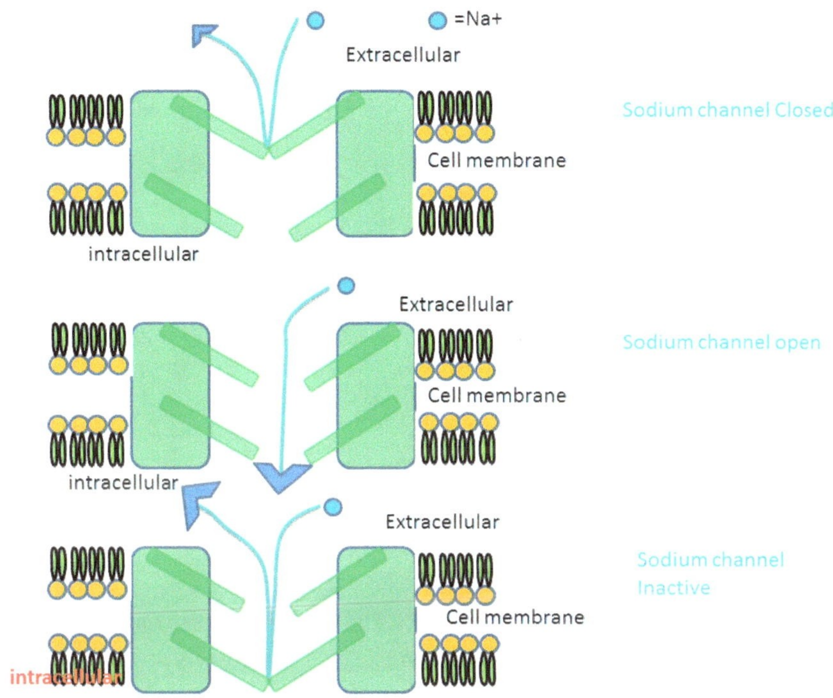

The mechanism of action of phenytoin sodium. Sodium channels are: 1) Closed 2) Open 3) Inactive (phenytoin effect)

Phenytoin binds preferentially to the inactive form of the sodium channel. Because it takes time for the bound drug to dissociate from the inactive channel, there is a time dependent block of the channel. Since the fraction of inactive channels is increased by membrane depolarization as well as by repetitive firing, the binding to the inactive state by phenytoin sodium can produce voltage-dependent, use-dependent and time-dependent block of sodium-dependent action potentials.

The primary site of action appears to be the motor cortex where spread of seizure activity is inhibited. Possibly by promoting sodium efflux from neurons, phenytoin tends to stabilize the threshold against hyperexcitability caused by excessive stimulation or environmental changes capable of reducing membrane sodium gradient. This includes the reduction of post-tetanic potentiation at synapses which prevents cortical seizure foci from detonating adjacent cortical areas. Phenytoin reduces the maximal activity of brain stem centers responsible for the tonic phase of generalized tonic-clonic seizures.

Pharmacokinetics

Phenytoin elimination kinetics show mixed-order behaviour at therapeutic concentrations. A small increase in dose may lead to a large increase in drug concentration as elimination becomes saturated. The time to reach steady state is often longer than 2 weeks.

PRL-8-53

PRL-8-53 is a nootropic research chemical derived from benzoic acid and phenylmethylamine (Benzylamine) that has been shown to act as a hypermnesic drug in humans; it was first synthesized by medical chemistry professor Nikolaus Hansl at Creighton University in the 1970s as part of his work on amino ethyl meta benzoic acid esters.

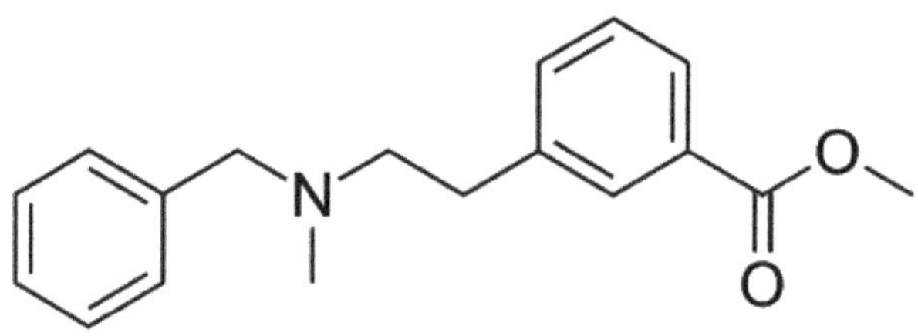

PRL-8-53

Nootropic Effects

A single study in humans was reported in 1978. The double-blind trial of PRL-8-53 in 47 healthy volunteers measured its effects on a variety of cognitive measures. 5 mg of the drug was administered orally 2–2.5 hours before the study tasks. Overall improvements in recollection differed based on how many words were recalled under placebo, with the poor performers (six words or fewer) experiencing a 87.5-105% increase in recollection and the high performers (eight or more words) a 7.9-14% increase which failed to reach statistical significance; when controlling for subjects over the age of 30 only, a 108-152% increase was noted.. No side effects were reported during the trial.

Mechanism of Action

The exact mechanism of action of PRL-8-53 remains unknown. Doses up to 200 mg/kg are not observed to have stimulant properties, and a dosage of 20 mg/kg does not potentiate the effects of dextroamphetamine in rats. It displays possible cholinergic properties, and potentiates dopamine while partially inhibiting serotonin. PRL-8-53 reverses the catatonic and ptotic effects of reserpine.

Toxicity

PRL-8-53 is relatively non-toxic, with an oral LD_{50} in mice of 860 mg/kg, giving the drug a high therapeutic index. Doses above 8 mg/kg have brief hypotensiveeffects in the canine. High doses depress motor activity in the rat and mouse, with the ED_{50} for a 50% reduction in motor activity of mice at 160 mg/kg. PRL-8-53 displays spasmolytic effects.

Synonyms

Methyl 3-(2-(benzylmethylamino)ethyl)benzoate hydrochloride

3-(2-benzylmethylaminoethyl) benzoic acid methyl ester hydrochloride

3-(2-(Methyl(phenylmethyl)amino)ethyl)benzoic acid methyl ester hydrochloride

Versus Mode of Action

In some literature articles, the term mechanism of action and mode of action (MoA) are used interchangeably and typically referring to the way in which the drug interacts and produces a medical effect. However, in actuality, a mode of action describes functional or anatomical changes, at the cellular level, resulting from the exposure of a living organism to a substance. This differs from a mechanism of action, as it is a more specific term that focuses on the interaction between the drug itself and an enzyme or receptor and its particular form of interaction, whether through inhibition, activation, agonism, or antagonism. Furthermore, the term mechanism of action is the main term that is primarily used in pharmacology, whereas mode of action will more often appear in the field of microbiology or certain aspects of biology.

Methods of Determination

Microscopy-Based Methods

Bioactive compounds induce phenotypic changes in target cells, changes that are observable by microscopy, and which can give insight into the mechanism of action of the compound. With antibacterial agents, for example, the conversion of target cells to spheroplasts can be an indication that peptidoglycan synthesis is being targeted, and filamentation of target cells can be an indication that FtsZ or DNA is being targeted. In the case of anticancer agents, bleb formation can be an indication that the compound is disrupting the plasma membrane. A current limitation of this approach is the time required to manually generate and interpret data, but advances in automated microscopy and image analysis software may help resolve this.

Direct Biochemical Methods

Direct biochemical methods include methods in which a protein or a small molecule, such as a drug candidate, is labeled and is traced throughout the body. This proves to be the most direct approach to find target protein that will bind to small targets of interest, such as a basic representation of a drug outline, in order to identify the pharmacophore of the drug. Due to the physical interactions between the labeled molecule and a protein, biochemical methods can be used to determine the toxicity, efficacy, and the mechanism of action of the drug.

Computation Inference Methods

Typically, computation inference methods are primarily used to predict protein targets for small molecule drugs based on computer based pattern recognition.However, this method could also be used for finding new targets for existing or newly developed drugs. By identifying the pharmacophore of the drug molecule, the profiling method of pattern recognition can be carried out where a new target is identified. This provides an insight at a possible mechanism of action, as it is known what certain functional components of the drug are responsible for interacting with a certain area on a protein, thus, leading to a therapeutic effect.

MODE OF ACTION

A mode of action (MoA) describes a functional or anatomical change, at the cellular level, resulting from the exposure of a living organism to a substance. In comparison, a mechanism of action (MOA) describes such changes at the molecular level.

A mode of action is important in classifying chemicals as it represents an intermediate level of complexity in between molecular mechanisms and physiological outcomes, especially when the exact molecular target has not yet been elucidated or is subject to debate. A mechanism of action of a chemical could be "binding to DNA" while its broader mode of action would be "transcriptional regulation". However, there is no clear consensus and the term mode of action is also often used, especially in the study of pesticides, to describe molecular mechanisms such as action on specific nuclear receptors or enzymes.

REFERENCES

1. Spratto, George R.; Adrienne L. Woods (2010). Delmar Nurse's Drug Handbook. Cengage Learning. ISBN 978-1-4390-5616-5.
2. Grant RL, Combs AB, Acosta D (2010) "Experimental Models for the Investigation of Toxicological Mechanisms". In McQueen CA. Comprehensive Toxicology (2nd ed.). Oxford: Elsevier. p. 204. ISBN 978-0-08-046884-6.
3. L. Tóth, L. Muszbek, I. Komaromi "Mechanism of the irreversible inhibition of human cyclooxygenase-1 by aspirin as predicted by QM/MM calculations", J Mol Graph Model. 2013 Mar;40: pp.99-109
4. Sharma, S.; Sharma, S. C. (1997-10-01). "An update on eicosanoids and inhibitors of cyclooxygenase enzyme systems". Indian Journal of Experimental Biology. 35 (10): 1025–1031. ISSN 0019-5189. PMID 9475035.
5. "Mechanisms and mode of dioxin action" (PDF). US EPA. Retrieved 11 June 2012.
6. Fetz, V.; Prochnow, H.; Brönstrup, M.; Sasse, F. (2016). "Target identification by image analysis". Natural Product Reports. 33 (5): 655–667. doi:10.1039/c5np00113g. PMID 26777141.
7. Cushnie, T.P.; O'Driscoll, N.H.; Lamb, A.J. (2016). "Morphological and ultrastructural changes in bacterial cells as an indicator of antibacterial mechanism

of action". Cellular and Molecular Life Sciences. doi:10.1007/s00018-016-2302-2. PMID 27392605.

8. Dubovskii, P.V.; Vassilevski, A.A.; Kozlov, S.A.; Feofanov, A.V.; Grishin, E.V.; Efremov, R.G. (2015). "Latarcins: versatile spider venom peptides". Cellular and Molecular Life Sciences. 72 (23): 4501–4522. doi:10.1007/s00018-015-2016-x. PMID 26286896.
9. c Schenone, Monica; Dančík, Vlado; Wagner, Bridget K.; Clemons, Paul A. (2013-04-01). "Target identification and mechanism of action in chemical biology and drug discovery". Nature Chemical Biology. 9 (4): 232–240. doi:10.1038/nchembio.1199. ISSN 1552-4450.
10. "Campral Description" (PDF). Archived (PDF) from the original on 2006-03-18. Retrieved 2006-04-02.
11. Plosker, GL (July 2015). "Acamprosate: A Review of Its Use in Alcohol Dependence.". Drugs. 75 (11): 1255–68. doi:10.1007/s40265-015-0423-9. PMID 26084940.
12. Williams, SH. (2005). "Medications for treating alcohol dependence". American Family Physician. 72 (9): 1775–1780. PMID 16300039.
13. Mason, BJ (2001). "Treatment of alcohol-dependent outpatients with acamprosate: a clinical review.". The Journal of Clinical Psychiatry. 62 Suppl 20: 42–8. PMID 11584875.
14. Nutt, DJ (2014). "Doing it by numbers: A simple approach to reducing the harms of alcohol". JOURNAL OF PSYCHOPHARMACOLOGY. 28: 3–7. doi:10.1177/0269881113512038. PMID 24399337.
15. "Acamprosate". drugs.com. 2005-03-25. Archived from the original on 22 December 2006. Retrieved 2007-01-08.
16. Wilde, MI; Wagstaff, AJ (June 1997). "Acamprosate. A review of its pharmacology and clinical potential in the management of alcohol dependence after detoxification". Drugs. 53 (6): 1038–53. doi:10.2165/00003495-199753060-00008. PMID 9179530.
17. "Acamprosate Oral - Who should not take this medication?". WebMD.com. Retrieved 2007-01-08.
18. c Saivin, S; Hulot, T; Chabac, S; Potgieter, A; Durbin, P; Houin, G (Nov 1998). "Clinical Pharmacokinetics of Acamprosate". Clinical Pharmacokinetics. 35 (5): 331–345. doi:10.2165/00003088-199835050-00001. PMID 9839087.
19. "Campral Prescribing Information" (PDF). Forest Pharmaceuticals. 2004. Retrieved 28 October 2014.
20. Mason, BJ; Goodman, AM; Dixon, RM; Hameed, MH; Hulot, T; Wesnes, K; Hunter, JA; Boyeson, MG (Oct 2002). "A pharmacokinetic and pharmacodynamic drug interaction study of acamprosate and naltrexone". Neuropsychopharmacology. 27 (4): 596–606. doi:10.1016/s0893-133x(02)00368-8. PMID 12377396.
21. Reilly, Matthew T.; Lobo, Ingrid A.; McCracken, Lindsay M.; Borghese, Cecilia M.; Gong, Diane; Horishita, Takafumi; Adron Harris, R. (2008).

"Effects of Acamprosate on Neuronal Receptors and Ion Channels Expressed inXenopusOocytes". Alcoholism: Clinical and Experimental Research. 32 (2): 188–196. doi:10.1111/j.1530-0277.2007.00569.x. ISSN 0145-6008.

22. Tsai, G; Coyle, JT (1998). "The role of glutamatergic neurotransmission in the pathophysiology of alcoholism". Annual Review of Medicine. 49: 173–84. doi:10.1146/annurev.med.49.1.173. PMID 9509257.
23. Tsai, GE; Ragan, P; Chang, R; Chen, S; Linnoila, VM; Coyle, JT (1998). "Increased glutamatergic neurotransmission and oxidative stress after alcohol withdrawal". The American Journal of Psychiatry. 155 (6): 726–32. PMID 9619143.
24. De Witte, P; Littleton, J; Parot, P; Koob, G (2005). "Neuroprotective and abstinence-promoting effects of acamprosate: elucidating the mechanism of action". CNS Drugs. 19 (6): 517–37. doi:10.2165/00023210-200519060-00004. PMID 15963001.
25. Mayer, S; Harris, BR; Gibson, DA; Blanchard, JA; Prendergast, MA; Holley, RC; Littleton, J (2002). "Acamprosate, MK-801, and ifenprodil inhibit neurotoxicity and calcium entry induced by ethanol withdrawal in organotypic slice cultures from neonatal rat hippocampus". Alcoholism: Clinical and Experimental Research. 26 (10): 1468–78. doi:10.1097/01.ALC.0000033261.14548.D2. PMID 12394279.
26. Al Qatari, M; Khan, S; Harris, B; Littleton, J (2001). "Acamprosate is neuroprotective against glutamate-induced excitotoxicity when enhanced by ethanol withdrawal in neocortical cultures of fetal rat brain". Alcoholism: Clinical and Experimental Research. 25 (9): 1276–83. doi:10.1111/j.1530-0277.2001.tb02348.x. PMID 11584146.
27. Spanagel R, Vengeliene V, Jandeleit B, Fischer WN, Grindstaff K, Zhang X, Gallop MA, Krstew EV, Lawrence AJ, Kiefer F (March 2014). "Acamprosate produces its anti-relapse effects via calcium.". Neuropsychopharmacology. 39 (4): 783–791. doi:10.1038/npp.2013.264. PMID 24081303.
28. Mann K, Kiefer F, Spanagel R, Littleton J (July 2008). "Acamprosate: recent findings and future research directions". Alcohol. Clin. Exp. Res. 32 (7): 1105–10. doi:10.1111/j.1530-0277.2008.00690.x. PMID 18540918.
29. Engelhard, K; Werner C; Lu H; Mollenberg O; Zieglgansberger W; Kochs E (2006). "The neuroprotective effect of the glutamate antagonist acamprosate following experimental cerebral ischemia. A study with the lipid peroxidase inhibitor u-101033e". Anaesthesist. 49 (9): 816–821. PMID 11076270.
30. Adde-Michel, C; Hennebert O; Laudenbach V; Marret S; Leroux P (2005). "Effect of acamprosate on neonatal excitotoxic cortical lesions in in utero alcohol-exposed hamsters". Neuroscience Letters. 374 (2): 109–112. doi:10.1016/j.neulet.2004.10.037. PMID 15644274.
31. Azevedo AA, Figueiredo RR (2005). "Tinnitus treatment with acamprosate: double-blind study". Braz J Otorhinolaryngol. 71 (5): 618–23. doi:10.1590/S0034-72992005000500012. PMID 16612523.

32. "FDA Approves New Drug for Treatment of Alcoholism". FDA Talk Paper. Food and Drug Administration. 2004-07-29. Archived from the original on 2008-01-17. Retrieved 2009-08-15.

CHAPTER 8

Drug Class

Chapter Contents

- **Introduction**
- **Chemical Class**
- **Therapeutic Class**
- **Amalgamated Classes**

A drug may be classified by the chemical type of the active ingredient or by the way it is used to treat a particular condition. Each drug can be classified into one or more drug classes. A drug class is a group of drugs that have something in common. They are similar in some way, but they are not identical.

Drugs can be in a class with other drugs because;

- The drugs are related by their chemical structure;
- The drugs work in the same way and
- The drugs are used for the same purpose.

INTRODUCTION

A drug class is a set of medications that have similar chemical structures, the same mechanism of action (i.e., bind to the same biological target), a related mode of action, and/or are used to treat the same disease.

In several dominant drug classification systems, these four types of classifications form a hierarchy. For example, the fibrates are a chemical class of drugs (amphipathic carboxylic acids) that share the same mechanism of action (PPAR agonist), mode of action (reducing blood triglycerides), and are used to prevent and to treat the same disease (atherosclerosis). Conversely not all PPAR agonists are fibrates, not all triglyceride lowering agents are PPAR agonists, and not all drugs that are used to treat atherosclerosis are triglyceride lowering agents. The most widely used drug classification system is the Anatomical Therapeutic Chemical Classification System (ATC). The Systematized Nomenclature of Medicine (SNOMED) also includes a section devoted to drug classification.

CHEMICAL CLASS

Examples of drug classes that are based on chemical structures include:

- β-lactam antibiotic
- Benzodiazepine
- Cardiac glycoside
- Fibrate
- Thiazide diuretic

β-Lactam Antibiotic

β-lactam antibiotics (beta-lactam antibiotics) are a class of broad-spectrum antibiotics, consisting of all antibiotic agents that contain a β-lactam ring in their molecular structures. This includes penicillin derivatives (penams), cephalosporins (cephems), monobactams, and carbapenems. Most β-lactam antibiotics work by inhibiting cell wall biosynthesis in the bacterial organism and are the most widely used group of antibiotics. Until 2003, when measured by sales, more than half of all commercially available antibiotics in use were β-lactam compounds.

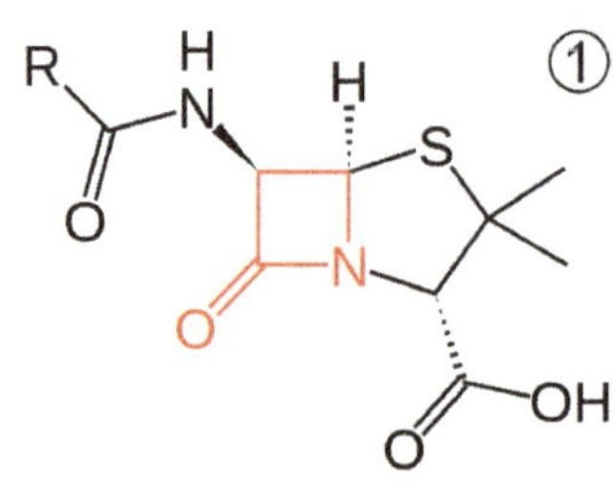

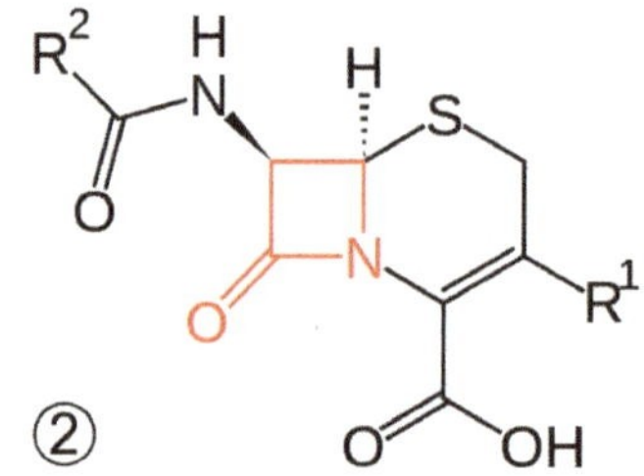

Core structure of penicillins (top) and cephalosporins (bottom). β-lactam ring in red.

Bacteria often develop resistance to β-lactam antibiotics by synthesizing a β-lactamase, an enzyme that attacks the β-lactam ring. To overcome this resistance, β-lactam antibiotics are often given with β-lactamase inhibitors such as clavulanic acid.

Medical Use

β-lactam antibiotics are indicated for the prophylaxis and treatment of bacterial infections caused by susceptible organisms. At first, β-lactam antibiotics were mainly active only against Gram-positive bacteria, yet the recent development of broad-spectrum β-lactam antibiotics active against various Gram-negative organisms has increased their usefulness.

Adverse Effects

Adverse Drug Reactions

Common adverse drug reactions for the β-lactam antibiotics include diarrhea, nausea, rash, urticaria, superinfection (including candidiasis).

Infrequent adverse effects include fever, vomiting, erythema, dermatitis, angioedema, pseudomembranous colitis.

Pain and inflammation at the injection site is also common for parenterally administered β-lactam antibiotics.

Allergy/Hypersensitivity

Immunologically mediated adverse reactions to any β-lactam antibiotic may occur in up to 10% of patients receiving that agent (a small fraction of which are truly IgE-mediated allergic reactions, see amoxicillin rash). Anaphylaxis will occur in approximately 0.01% of patients. There is perhaps a 5%-10% cross-sensitivity between penicillin-derivatives, cephalosporins, and carbapenems; but this figure has been challenged by various investigators.

Nevertheless, the risk of cross-reactivity is sufficient to warrant the contraindication of all β-lactam antibiotics in patients with a history of severe allergic reactions (urticaria, anaphylaxis, interstitial nephritis) to any β-lactam antibiotic.

A Jarisch-Herxheimer reaction may occur after initial treatment of a spirochetal infection such as syphilis with a β-lactam antibiotic.

Mode of Action

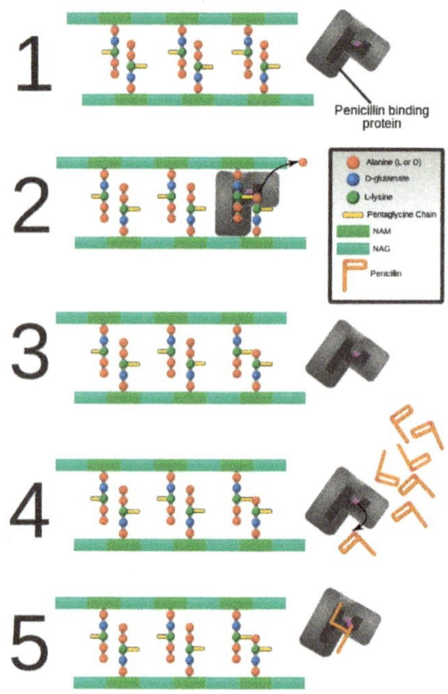

Penicillin and most other β-lactam antibiotics act by inhibiting penicillin-binding proteins, which normally catalyze cross-linking of bacterial cell walls.

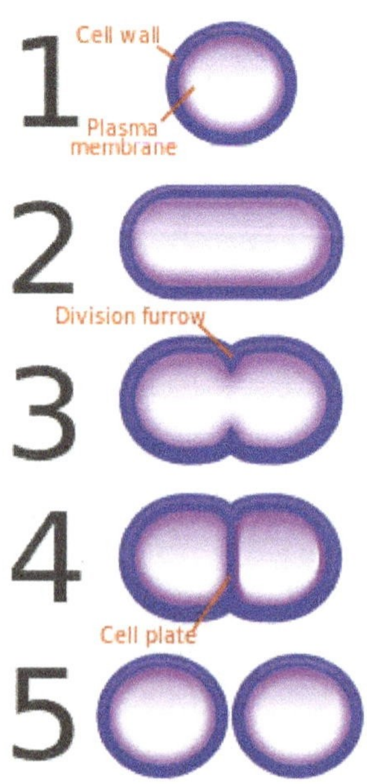

In the absence of β-lactam antibiotics, the bacterial cell wall plays an important role in bacterial reproduction.

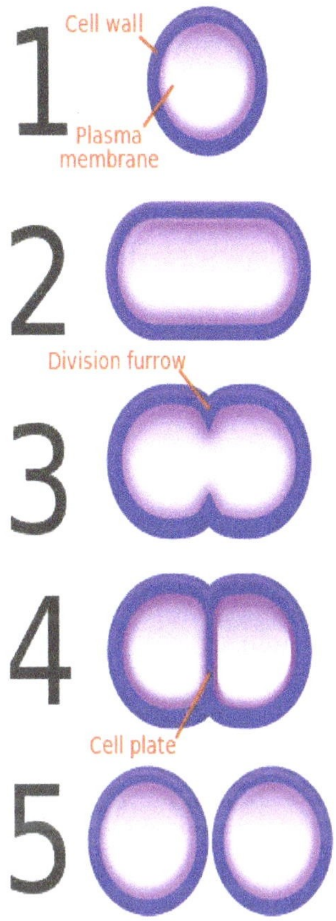

Adding β-lactam antibiotics to the cell medium while bacteria are dividing will cause them to shed their cell walls and fail to divide, forming large, fragile spheroplasts.

β-lactam antibiotics are bacteriocidal, and act by inhibiting the synthesis of the peptidoglycan layer of bacterial cell walls. The peptidoglycan layer is important for cell wall structural integrity, especially in Gram-positive organisms, being the outermost and primary component of the wall. The final transpeptidation step in the synthesis of the peptidoglycan is facilitated by DD-transpeptidases which are penicillin-binding proteins (PBPs). PBPs vary in their affinity for binding penicillin or other β-lactam antibiotics. The amount of PBPs varies among bacterial species.

β-lactam antibiotics are analogues of d-alanyl-d-alanine—the terminal amino acid residues on the precursor NAM/NAG-peptide subunits of the nascent peptidoglycan layer. The structural similarity between β-lactam antibiotics and d-alanyl-d-alanine facilitates their binding to the active site of PBPs. The β-lactam nucleus of the molecule irreversibly binds to (acylates) the Ser_{403} residue of the PBP active site. This irreversible inhibition of the PBPs prevents the final crosslinking (transpeptidation) of the nascent peptidoglycan layer, disrupting cell wall synthesis.

β-lactam antibiotics block not only the division of bacteria, including cyanobacteria, but also the division of cyanelles, the photosynthetic organelles of the glaucophytes, and the division of chloroplasts of bryophytes. In contrast, they have no effect on the plastids of the highly developed vascular plants. This is supporting the endosymbiotic theory and indicates an evolution of plastid division in land plants.

Under normal circumstances, peptidoglycan precursors signal a reorganization of the bacterial cell wall and, as a consequence, trigger the activation of autolytic cell wall hydrolases. Inhibition of cross-linkage by β-lactams causes a build-up of peptidoglycan precursors, which triggers the digestion of existing peptidoglycan by autolytic hydrolases without the production of new peptidoglycan. As a result, the bactericidal action of β-lactam antibiotics is further enhanced.

Potency

Two structural features of β-lactam antibiotics have been correlated with their antibiotic potency. The first is known as "Woodward's parameter", h, and is the height (in angstroms) of the pyramid formed by the nitrogen atom of the β-lactam as the apex and the three adjacent carbon atoms as the base. The second is called "Cohen's parameter", c, and is the distance between the carbon atom of the carboxylate and the oxygen atom of the β-lactam carbonyl. This distance is thought to correspond to the distance between the carboxylate-binding site and the oxyanion hole of the PBP enzyme. The best antibiotics are those with higher h values (more reactive to hydrolysis) and lower c values (better binding to PBPs).

Modes of Resistance

By definition, all β-lactam antibiotics have a β-lactam ring in their structure. The effectiveness of these antibiotics relies on their ability to reach the PBP intact and their ability to bind to the PBP. Hence, there are two main modes of bacterial resistance to β-lactams:

Enzymatic Hydrolysis of the β-Lactam Ring

If the bacterium produces the enzyme β-lactamase or the enzyme penicillinase, the enzyme will hydrolyse the β-lactam ring of the antibiotic, rendering the antibiotic ineffective. (An example of such an enzyme is NDM-1, discovered in 2009.) The genes encoding these enzymes may be inherently present on the bacterial chromosome or may be acquired via plasmid transfer (plasmid mediated resistance), and β-lactamase gene expression may be induced by exposure to β-lactams.

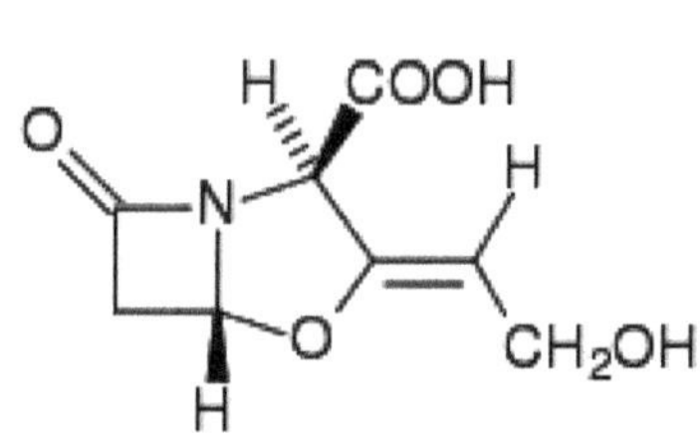

Clavulanic acid

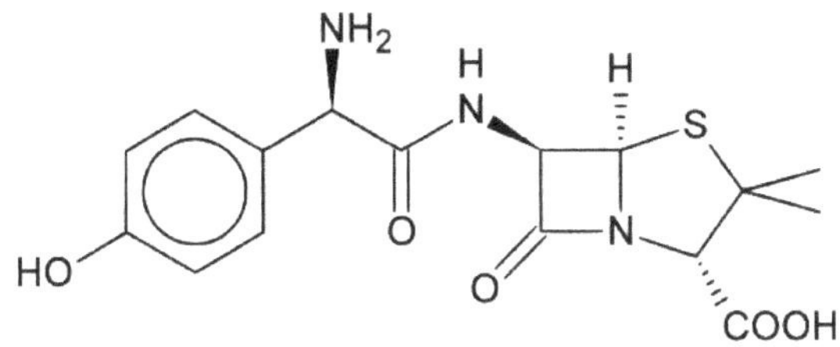

Amoxicillin

The production of a β-lactamase by a bacterium does not necessarily rule out all treatment options with β-lactam antibiotics. In some instances, β-lactam antibiotics may be co-administered with a β-lactamase inhibitor. For example, Augmentin (FGP) is made of amoxicillin (a β-lactam antibiotic) and clavulanic acid (a β-lactamase inhibitor). The clavulanic acid is designed to overwhelm all β-lactamase enzymes, and effectively serve as an antagonist so that the amoxicillin is not affected by the β-lactamase enzymes.

Other β-Lactamase inhibitors such as boronic acids are being studied in which they irreversibly bind to the active site of β-lactamases. This is a benefit over clavulonic acid and similar beta-lactam competitors, because they cannot be hydrolysed, and therefore rendered useless. Extensive research is currently being done to develop tailored boronic acids to target different isozymes of beta-lactamases.

However, in all cases where infection with β-lactamase-producing bacteria is suspected, the choice of a suitable β-lactam antibiotic should be carefully considered prior to treatment. In particular, choosing appropriate β-lactam antibiotic therapy is of utmost importance against organisms which harbor some level of β-lactamase expression. In this case, failure to use the most appropriate β-lactam antibiotic therapy at the onset of treatment could result in selection for bacteria with higher levels of β-lactamase expression, thereby making further efforts with other β-lactam antibiotics more difficult.

Possession of Altered Penicillin-Binding Proteins

As a response to increased efficacy of β-lactams, some bacteria have changed the proteins to which β-lactam antibiotics bind. β-lactams cannot bind as effectively to these altered PBPs, and, as a result, the β-lactams are less effective at disrupting cell wall synthesis. Notable examples of this mode of resistance include methicillin-resistant *Staphylococcus aureus* (MRSA) and penicillin-resistant *Streptococcus pneumoniae*. Altered PBPs do not necessarily rule out all treatment options with β-lactam antibiotics.

Nomenclature

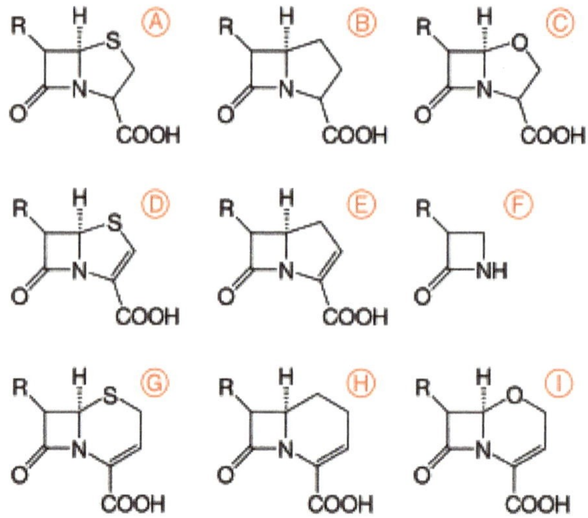

The β-lactam core structures. **(A)** A penam. **(B)** A carbapenam. **(C)** An oxapenam. **(D)** A penem. **(E)** A carbapenem. **(F)** A monobactam. **(G)** A cephem. **(H)** A carbacephem. **(I)** An oxacephem.

β-Lactams are classified according to their core ring structures.

- β-Lactams fused to saturated five-membered rings:
    - β-Lactams containing thiazolidine rings are named penams.
    - β-Lactams containing pyrrolidine rings are named carbapenams.
    - β-Lactams fused to oxazolidine rings are named oxapenams or clavams.
- β-Lactams fused to unsaturated five-membered rings:
    - β-Lactams containing 2,3-dihydrothiazole rings are named penems.
    - β-Lactams containing 2,3-dihydro-1H-pyrrole rings are named carbapenems.
- β-Lactams fused to unsaturated six-membered rings:
    - β-Lactams containing 3,6-dihydro-2H-1,3-thiazine rings are named cephems.
    - β-Lactams containing 1,2,3,4-tetrahydropyridine rings are named carbacephems.
    - β-Lactams containing 3,6-dihydro-2H-1,3-oxazine rings are named oxacephems.
- β-Lactams not fused to any other ring are named monobactams.

By convention, the bicyclic β-lactams are numbered starting with the position occupied by sulfur in the penams and cephems, regardless of which atom it is in a given class. That is, position 1 is always adjacent to the β-carbon of β-lactam ring. The numbering continues clockwise from position one until the β-carbon of β-lactam is reached, at which point numbering continues counterclockwise around the lactam ring to number the remaining to carbons. For example, the nitrogen atom of all bicyclic β-lactams fused to five-membered rings is labelled position 4, as it is in penams, while in cephems, the nitrogen is position 5.

The numbering of monolactams follows that of the IUPAC; the nitrogen atom is position 1, the carbonyl carbon is 2, the α-carbon is 3, and the β-carbon 4.

Biosynthesis

To date, two distinct methods of biosynthesizing the β-lactam core of this family of antibiotics have been discovered. The first pathway discovered was that of the penams and cephems. This path begins with a nonribosomal peptide synthetase (NRPS), ACV synthetase (ACVS), which generates the linear tripeptide δ-(L-α-aminoadipyl)-L-cysteine-D-valine (ACV). ACV is oxidatively cyclized (two cyclizations by a single enzyme) to bicyclic intermediate isopenicillin N by isopenicillin N synthase (IPNS) to form the penam core structure. Various transamidations lead to the different natural penicillins.

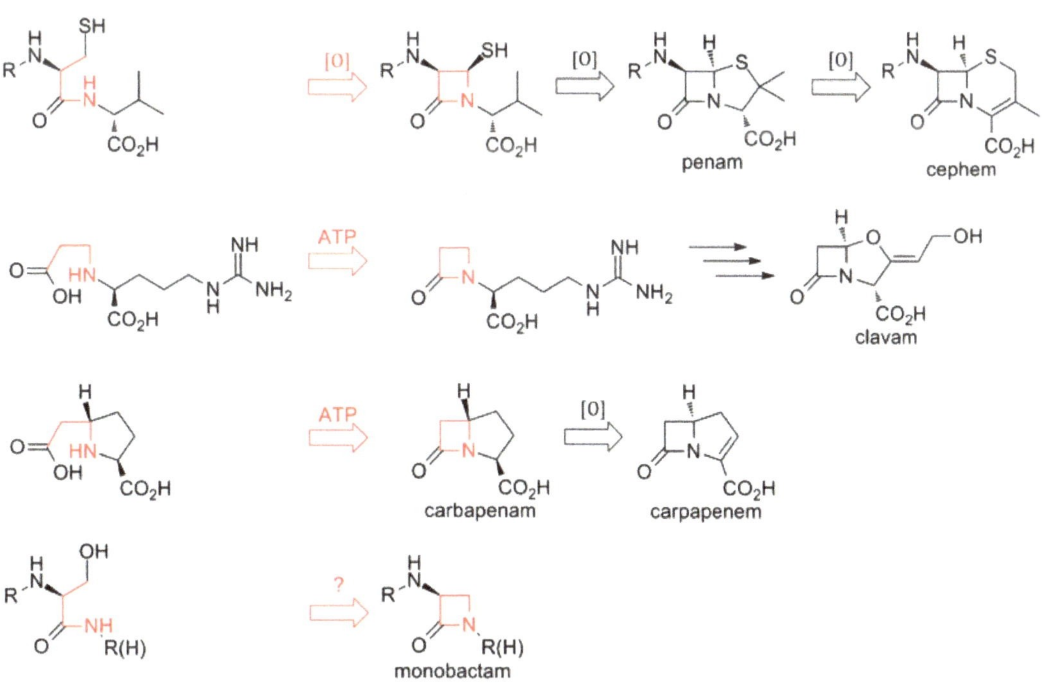

This figure outlines the different methods of β-lactam closure among the various classes of β-lactam compounds. Penams and cephems are cyclized oxidatively (first row); clavams and carbapenems are closed by ATP-utilizing amidation (second and third row); and some monobactams may be closed by a third method (fourth row).

The biosynthesis of cephems branch off at isopenicillin N by an oxidative ring expansion to the cephem core. As with the penams, the variety of cephalosporins and cephamycins come from different transamidations, as is the case for the penicillins.

While the ring closure in penams and cephems is between positions 1 and 4 of the β-lactam and is oxidative, the clavams and carbapenems have their rings closed by two-electron processes between positions 1 and 2 of the ring. β-lactam synthetases are responsible for these cyclizations, and the carboxylate of the open-ring substrates is activated by ATP. In clavams, the β-lactam is formed prior to the second ring; in carbapenems, the β-lactam ring is closed second in sequence.

The biosynthesis of the β-lactam ring of tabtoxin mirrors that of the clavams and carbapenems. The closure of the lactam ring in the other monobactams, such as sulfazecin and the nocardicins, may involve a third mechanism involving inversion of configuration at the β-carbon.

Benzodiazepine

Benzodiazepines (BZD, BZs), sometimes called "benzos", are a class of psychoactive drugs whose core chemical structure is the fusion of a benzene ring and a diazepine ring. The first such drug, chlordiazepoxide (Librium), was discovered accidentally by Leo Sternbach in 1955, and made available in 1960 by Hoffmann–La Roche, which, since 1963, has also marketed the benzodiazepine diazepam (Valium). In 1977 benzodiazepines were globally the most prescribed medications.

Benzodiazepines enhance the effect of the neurotransmitter gamma-aminobutyric acid (GABA) at the $GABA_A$ receptor, resulting in sedative, hypnotic (sleep-inducing), anxiolytic (anti-anxiety), anticonvulsant, and muscle relaxant properties. High doses of many shorter-acting benzodiazepines may also cause anterograde amnesia and dissociation. These properties make benzodiazepines useful in treating anxiety, insomnia, agitation, seizures, muscle spasms, alcohol withdrawal and as a premedication for medical or dental procedures. Benzodiazepines are categorized as either short-, intermediate-, or long-acting. Short- and intermediate-acting benzodiazepines are preferred for the treatment of insomnia; longer-acting benzodiazepines are recommended for the treatment of anxiety.

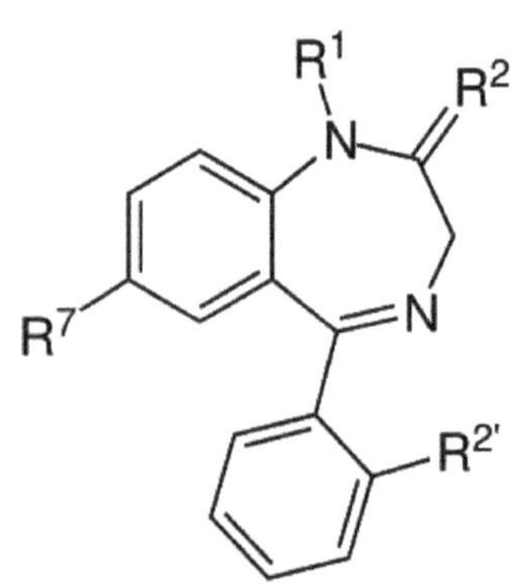

The core structure of benzodiazepines. "R" labels denote common locations of side chains, which give different benzodiazepines their unique properties.

Benzodiazepines are generally viewed as safe and effective for short-term use, although cognitive impairment and paradoxical effects such as aggression or behavioral disinhibition occasionally occur. A minority of people can have paradoxical reactions such as worsened agitation or panic. Long-term use is controversial because of concerns about adverse psychological and physical effects, decreasing effectiveness, and physical dependence and withdrawal. As a result of adverse effects associated with the long-term use of benzodiazepines, withdrawal from benzodiazepines, in general, leads to improved physical and mental health. The elderly are at an increased risk of suffering from both short- and long-term adverse effects, and as a result, all benzodiazepines are listed in the Beers List of inappropriate medications for older adults.

There is controversy concerning the safety of benzodiazepines in pregnancy. While they are not major teratogens, uncertainty remains as to whether they cause cleft palate in a small number of babies and whether neurobehavioural effects occur as a result of prenatal exposure; they are known to cause withdrawal symptoms in the newborn. Benzodiazepines can be taken in overdoses and can cause dangerous deep unconsciousness. However, they are less toxic than their predecessors, the barbiturates, and death rarely results when a benzodiazepine is the only drug taken. When combined with other central nervous system (CNS) depressants such as ethanol and opioids, the potential for toxicity and fatal overdose increases. Benzodiazepines are commonly misused and taken in combination with other drugs of abuse.

Medical Uses

Benzodiazepines possess sedative, hypnotic, anxiolytic, anticonvulsant, muscle relaxant, and amnesic actions, which are useful in a variety of indications such as alcohol dependence, seizures, anxiety disorders, panic, agitation, and insomnia. Most are administered orally; however, they can also be given intravenously, intramuscularly, or rectally. In general, benzodiazepines are well-tolerated and are safè and effective drugs in the short term for a wide range of conditions.

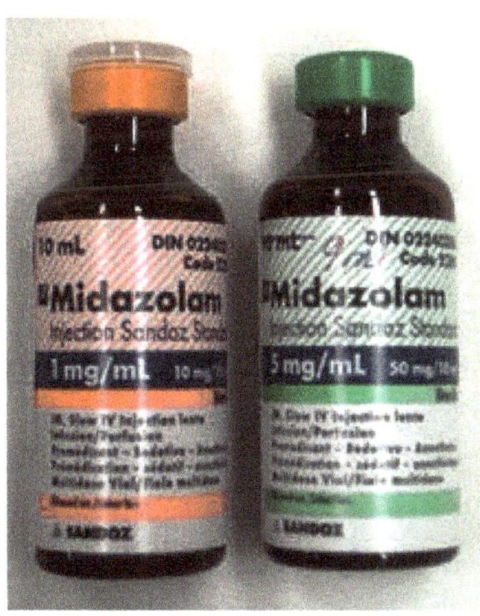

Midazolam 1 & 5 mg/mL injections(US)

Tolerance can develop to their effects and there is also a risk of dependence, and upon discontinuation a withdrawal syndrome may occur. These factors, combined with other possible secondary effects after prolonged use such as psychomotor, cognitive, or memory impairments, limit their long-term applicability. The effects of long-term use or misuse include the tendency to cause or worsen cognitive deficits, depression, and anxiety. The College of Physicians and Surgeons of British Columbia recommends discontinuing the usage of benzodiazepines in those on opioids and those who have used them long term.

Panic Disorder

Because of their effectiveness, tolerability, and rapid onset of anxiolytic action, benzodiazepines are frequently used for the treatment of anxiety associated with panic disorder. However, there is disagreement among expert bodies regarding the long-term use of benzodiazepines for panic disorder. The views range from those that hold that benzodiazepines are not effective long-term and that they should be reserved for treatment-resistant cases to that they are as effective in the long term as selective serotonin reuptake inhibitors.

The American Psychiatric Association (APA) guidelines note that, in general, benzodiazepines are well tolerated, and their use for the initial treatment for panic disorder is strongly supported by numerous controlled trials. APA states that there is insufficient evidence to recommend any of the established panic disorder treatments over another. The choice of treatment between benzodiazepines, SSRIs, serotonin–norepinephrine reuptake inhibitors, tricyclic antidepressants, and psychotherapy should be based on the patient's history, preference, and other individual characteristics. Selective serotonin reuptake inhibitors are likely to be the best choice of pharmacotherapy for many patients with panic disorder, but benzodiazepines are also often used, and some studies suggest that these medications are still used with greater frequency than the SSRIs. One advantage of benzodiazepines is that they alleviate the anxiety symptoms much faster than antidepressants, and therefore may be preferred in patients for whom rapid symptom control is critical. However, this advantage is offset by the possibility of developing benzodiazepine dependence. APA does not recommend benzodiazepines for persons with depressive symptoms or a recent history of substance abuse. The APA guidelines state that, in general, pharmacotherapy of panic disorder should be continued for at least a year, and that clinical experience support continuing benzodiazepine treatment to prevent recurrence. Although major concerns about benzodiazepine tolerance and withdrawal have been raised, there is no evidence for significant dose escalation in patients using benzodiazepines long-term. For many such patients stable doses of benzodiazepines retain their efficacy over several years.

Guidelines issued by the UK-based National Institute for Health and Clinical Excellence (NICE), carried out a systematic review using different methodology and came to a different conclusion. They questioned the accuracy of studies that were not placebo-controlled. And, based on the findings of placebo-controlled studies, they do not recommend use of benzodiazepines beyond two to four weeks, as tolerance and physical dependence develop rapidly, with withdrawal symptoms including rebound anxiety occurring after six weeks or more of use. Nevertheless, benzodiazepines continue to be prescribed for the long-term treatment of anxiety disorders, although specific antidepressants and psychological therapies are recommended as the first-line treatment options with the anticonvulsant drug pregabalin indicated as a second- or third-line treatment and suitable for long-term use. NICE stated that long-term use of benzodiazepines for panic disorder with or without agoraphobia is an unlicensed indication, does not have long-term efficacy, and is, therefore, not recommended by clinical guidelines. Psychological therapies such as cognitive behavioural therapy are recommended as a first-line therapy for panic disorder; benzodiazepine use has been found to interfere with therapeutic gains from these therapies.

Benzodiazepines are usually administered orally; however, very occasionally lorazepam or diazepam may be given intravenously for the treatment of panic attacks.

Generalized Anxiety Disorder

Benzodiazepines have robust efficacy in the short-term management of generalized anxiety disorder (GAD), but were not shown to be effective in producing long-term improvement overall. According to National Institute for Health and Clinical Excellence (NICE), benzodiazepines can be used in the immediate management of GAD, if necessary. However, they should not usually be given for longer than 2–4 weeks. The only medications NICE recommends for the longer term management of GAD are antidepressants.

Likewise, Canadian Psychiatric Association (CPA) recommends benzodiazepines alprazolam, bromazepam, lorazepam, and diazepam only as a second-line choice, if the treatment with two different antidepressants was unsuccessful. Although they are second-line agents, benzodiazepines can be used for a limited time to relieve severe anxiety and agitation. CPA guidelines note that after 4–6 weeks the effect of benzodiazepines may decrease to the level of placebo, and that benzodiazepines are less effective than antidepressants in alleviating ruminative worry, the core symptom of GAD. However, in some cases, a prolonged treatment with benzodiazepines as the add-on to an antidepressant may be justified.

A 2015 review found a larger effect with medications than talk therapy. Medications with benefit include serotonin-noradrenaline reuptake inhibitors, benzodiazepines, and selective serotonin reuptake inhibitors.

Insomnia

Benzodiazepines can be useful for short-term treatment of insomnia. Their use beyond 2 to 4 weeks is not recommended due to the risk of dependence. It is preferred that benzodiazepines be taken intermittently and at the lowest effective dose. They improve sleep-related problems by shortening the time spent in bed before falling asleep, prolonging the sleep time, and, in general, reducing wakefulness. However, they worsen sleep quality by increasing light sleep and decreasing deep sleep. Other drawbacks of hypnotics, including benzodiazepines, are possible tolerance to their effects, rebound insomnia, and reduced slow-wave sleep and a withdrawal period typified by rebound insomnia and a prolonged period of anxiety and agitation.

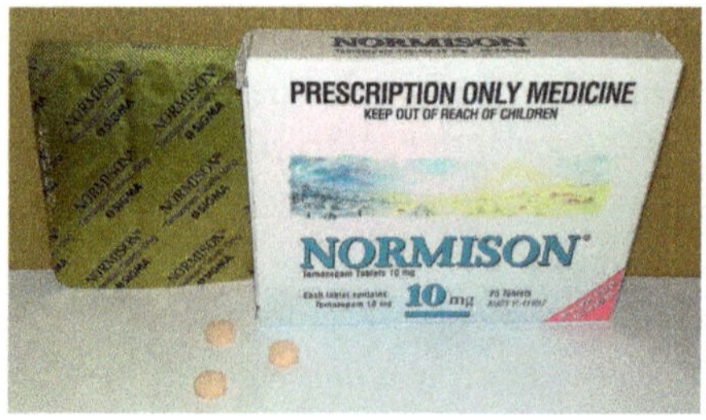

Temazepam (Normison) 10 mg tablets

The list of benzodiazepines approved for the treatment of insomnia is fairly similar among most countries, but which benzodiazepines are officially designated as first-line hypnotics prescribed for the treatment of insomnia can vary distinctly between countries. Longer-acting benzodiazepines such as nitrazepam and diazepam have residual effects that may persist into the next day and are, in general, not recommended.

Since the release of nonbenzodiazepines in 1992 in response to safety concerns, individuals with insomnia and other sleep disorders have increasingly been prescribed nonbenzodiazepines (2.3% in 1993 to 13.7% of Americans in 2010), less often prescribed benzodiazepines (23.5% in 1993 to 10.8% in 2010). It is not clear as to whether the new nonbenzodiazepine hypnotics (Z-drugs) are better than the short-acting benzodiazepines. The efficacy of these two groups of medications is similar. According to the US Agency for Healthcare Research and Quality, indirect comparison indicates that side-effects from benzodiazepines may be about twice as frequent as from nonbenzodiazepines. Some experts suggest using nonbenzodiazepines preferentially as a first-line long-term treatment of insomnia. However, the UK National Institute for Health and Clinical Excellence did not find any convincing evidence in favor of Z-drugs. NICE review pointed out that short-acting Z-drugs were inappropriately compared in clinical trials with long-acting benzodiazepines. There have been no trials comparing short-acting Z-drugs with appropriate doses of short-acting benzodiazepines. Based on this, NICE recommended choosing the hypnotic based on cost and the patient's preference.

Older adults should not use benzodiazepines to treat insomnia unless other treatments have failed to be effective. When benzodiazepines are used, patients, their caretakers, and their physician should discuss the increased risk of harms, including evidence which shows twice the incidence of traffic collisions among driving patients as well as falls and hip fracture for all older patients.

Seizures

Prolonged convulsive epileptic seizures are a medical emergency that can usually be dealt with effectively by administering fast-acting benzodiazepines, which are potent anticonvulsants. In a hospital environment, intravenous clonazepam, lorazepam, and diazepam are first-line choices, clonazepam due to its stronger and more potent anticonvulsant action, diazepam due to its faster onset and lorazepam for its longer duration of action.

In the community, intravenous administration is not practical and so rectal diazepam or (more recently) buccal midazolam are used, with a preference for midazolam as its administration is easier and more socially acceptable.

When benzodiazepines were first introduced, they were enthusiastically adopted for treating all forms of epilepsy. However, drowsiness and tolerance become problems with continued use and none are now considered first-line choices for long-term epilepsy therapy. Clobazam is widely used by specialist epilepsy clinics worldwide and clonazepam is popular in the Netherlands, Belgium and France. Clobazam was approved for use in the United States in 2011. In the UK, both clobazam and clonazepam are second-line choices for treating many forms of epilepsy. Clobazam also has a useful role for very short-term seizure prophylaxisand in catamenial epilepsy. Discontinuation after long-term use in epilepsy requires additional caution because of the risks of rebound seizures. Therefore, the dose is slowly tapered over a period of up to six months or longer.

Alcohol Withdrawal

Chlordiazepoxide is the most commonly used benzodiazepine for alcohol detoxification, but diazepam may be used as an alternative. Both are used in the detoxification of individuals who are motivated to stop drinking, and are prescribed for a short period of time to reduce the risks of developing tolerance and dependence to the benzodiazepine medication itself. The benzodiazepines with a longer half-life make detoxification more tolerable, and dangerous (and potentially lethal) alcohol withdrawal effects are less likely to occur. On the other hand, short-acting benzodiazepines may lead to breakthrough seizures, and are, therefore, not recommended for detoxification in an outpatient setting. Oxazepam and lorazepam are often used in patients at risk of drug accumulation, in particular, the elderly and those with cirrhosis, because they are metabolized differently from other benzodiazepines, through conjugation. Benzodiazepines are the preferred choice in the management of alcohol withdrawal syndrome, in particular, for the prevention and treatment of the dangerous complication of seizures and in subduing severe delirium. Lorazepam is the only benzodiazepine with predictable intramuscular absorption and it is the most effective in preventing and controlling acute seizures.

Anxiety

Benzodiazepines are sometimes used in the treatment of acute anxiety, as they bring about rapid and marked or moderate relief of symptoms in most individuals; however, they are not recommended beyond 2–4 weeks of use due to risks of tolerance and dependence and a lack of long-term effectiveness. As for insomnia, they may also be used on an irregular/"as-needed" basis, such as in cases where said anxiety is at its worst. Compared to other pharmacological treatments, benzodiazepines are twice as likely to lead to a relapse of the underlying condition upon discontinuation. Psychological therapies and other pharmacological therapies are recommended for the long-term treatment of generalized anxiety disorder. Antidepressants have higher remission rates and are, in general, safe and effective in the short and long term.

Other Indications

Benzodiazepines are often prescribed for a wide range of conditions:

- They can be very useful in intensive care to sedate patients receiving mechanical ventilation or those in extreme distress. Caution is exercised in this situation due to the occasional occurrence of respiratory depression, and it is recommended that benzodiazepine overdose treatment facilities should be available.
- Benzodiazepines are effective as medication given a couple of hours before surgery to relieve anxiety. They also produce amnesia, which can be useful, as patients will not be able to remember any unpleasantness from the procedure. They are also used in patients with dental phobia as well as some ophthalmic procedures like refractive surgery; although such use is controversial and only recommended for those who are very anxious. Midazolam is the most commonly prescribed for this use because of its strong sedative actions and fast recovery time, as well as its water solubility, which reduces pain upon injection. Diazepam and lorazepam are sometimes used. Lorazepam has particularly marked amnesic properties that may make it more effective when amnesia is the desired effect.
- Benzodiazepines are well known for their strong muscle-relaxing properties and can be useful in the treatment of muscle spasms, although tolerance often develops to their muscle relaxant effects. Baclofen or tizanidine are sometimes used as an alternative to benzodiazepines. Tizanidine has been found to have superior tolerability compared to diazepam and baclofen.
- Benzodiazepines are also used to treat the acute panic caused by hallucinogen intoxication. Benzodiazepines are also used to calm the acutely agitated individual and can, if required, be given via an intramuscular injection. They can sometimes be effective in the short-term treatment of psychiatric emergencies such as acute psychosis as in schizophrenia or mania, bringing about rapid tranquillization and sedation until the effects of lithium or neuroleptics(antipsychotics) take effect. Lorazepam is most commonly used but clonazepam is sometimes prescribed for acute psychosis or mania; their long-term use is not recommended due to risks of dependence. Further research investigating the use of benzodiazepines alone and in combination with antipsychotic medications for treating acute psychosis is warranted.
- Clonazepam, a benzodiazepine is used to treat many forms of parasomnia. Rapid eye movement behavior disorder responds well to low doses of clonazepam. Restless legs syndrome can be treated using clonazepam as a third line treatment option as the use of clonazepam is still investigational.
- Benzodiazepines are sometimes used for obsessive–compulsive disorder (OCD), although they are generally believed to be ineffective for this indication; effectiveness was, however, found in one small study. Benzodiazepines can be considered as a treatment option in treatment resistant cases.
- Antipsychotics are generally a first-line treatment for delirium; however, when delirium is caused by alcohol or sedative hypnotic withdrawal, benzodiazepines are a first-line treatment.

- There is some evidence that low doses of benzodiazepines reduce adverse effects of electroconvulsive therapy.

Contraindications

Because of their muscle relaxant action, benzodiazepines may cause respiratory depression in susceptible individuals. For that reason, they are contraindicated in people with myasthenia gravis, sleep apnea, bronchitis, and COPD. Caution is required when benzodiazepines are used in people with personality disorders or intellectual disability because of frequent paradoxical reactions. In major depression, they may precipitate suicidal tendencies and are sometimes used for suicidal overdoses. Individuals with a history of alcohol, opioid and barbiturate abuse should avoid benzodiazepines, as there is a risk of life-threatening interactions with these drugs.

Pregnancy

In the United States, the Food and Drug Administration has categorized benzodiazepines into either category D or X meaning potential for harm in the unborn has been demonstrated.

Exposure to benzodiazepines during pregnancy has been associated with a slightly increased (from 0.06 to 0.07%) risk of cleft palate in newborns, a controversial conclusion as some studies find no association between benzodiazepines and cleft palate. Their use by expectant mothers shortly before the delivery may result in a floppy infant syndrome, with the newborns suffering from hypotonia, hypothermia, lethargy, and breathing and feeding difficulties. Cases of neonatal withdrawal syndrome have been described in infants chronically exposed to benzodiazepines in utero. This syndrome may be hard to recognize, as it starts several days after delivery, for example, as late as 21 days for chlordiazepoxide. The symptoms include tremors, hypertonia, hyperreflexia, hyperactivity, and vomiting and may last for up to three to six months. Tapering down the dose during pregnancy may lessen its severity. If used in pregnancy, those benzodiazepines with a better and longer safety record, such as diazepam or chlordiazepoxide, are recommended over potentially more harmful benzodiazepines, such as temazepam or triazolam. Using the lowest effective dose for the shortest period of time minimizes the risks to the unborn child.

Elderly

The benefits of benzodiazepines are least and the risks are greatest in the elderly. The elderly are at an increased risk of dependence and are more sensitive to the adverse effects such as memory problems, daytime sedation, impaired motor coordination, and increased risk of motor vehicle accidents and falls, and an increased risk of hip fractures. The long-term effects of benzodiazepines and benzodiazepine dependence in the elderly can resemble dementia, depression, or anxiety syndromes, and progressively worsens over time. Adverse effects on cognition can be mistaken for the effects of old age. The benefits of withdrawal include improved cognition, alertness, mobility, reduced risk incontinence, and a reduced risk of falls and fractures. The success of gradual-tapering benzodiazepines is as great in the elderly as in younger people. Benzodiazepines should be prescribed to the elderly only with caution and only for a short period at low doses.

Short to intermediate-acting benzodiazepines are preferred in the elderly such as oxazepam and temazepam. The high potency benzodiazepines alprazolam and triazolam and long-acting benzodiazepines are not recommended in the elderly due to increased adverse effects. Nonbenzodiazepines such as zaleplon and zolpidem and low doses of sedating antidepressants are sometimes used as alternatives to benzodiazepines. Long-term use of benzodiazepines has been associated with increased risk of cognitive impairment, but its relationship with dementia remains inconclusive. The association of a past history of benzodiazepine use and cognitive decline is unclear, with some studies reporting a lower risk of cognitive decline in former users, some finding no association and some indicating an increased risk of cognitive decline. Benzodiazepines are sometimes prescribed to treat behavioral symptoms of dementia. However, like antidepressants, they have little evidence of effectiveness, although antipsychotics have shown some benefit. Cognitive impairing effects of benzodiazepines that occur frequently in the elderly can also worsen dementia.

Adverse Effects

The most common side-effects of benzodiazepines are related to their sedating and muscle-relaxing action. They include drowsiness, dizziness, and decreased alertness and concentration. Lack of coordination may result in falls and injuries, in particular, in the elderly. Another result is impairment of driving skills and increased likelihood of road traffic accidents. Decreased libido and erection problems are a common side effect. Depression and disinhibition may emerge. Hypotension and suppressed breathing (hypoventilation) may be encountered with intravenous use. Less common side effects include nausea and changes in appetite, blurred vision, confusion, euphoria, depersonalization and nightmares. Cases of liver toxicity have been described but are very rare.

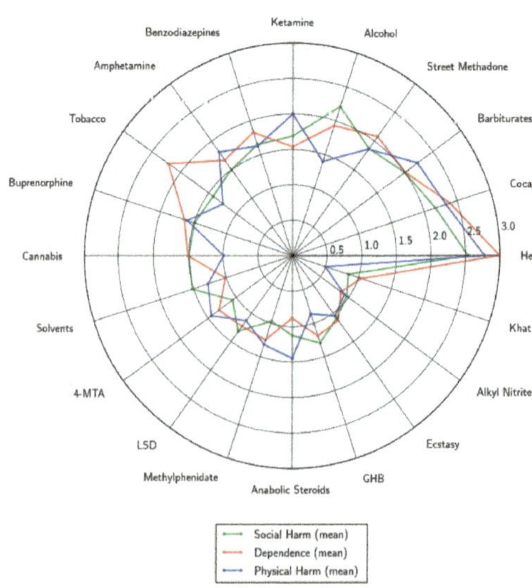

Addiction experts in psychiatry, chemistry, pharmacology, forensic science, epidemiology, and the police and legal services engaged in delphic analysis regarding 20 popular recreational drugs. Benzodiazepines were ranked 7th in dependence, physical harm, and social harm.

The long-term effects of benzodiazepine use can include cognitive impairment as well as affective and behavioural problems. Feelings of turmoil, difficulty in thinking constructively, loss of sex-drive, agoraphobia and social phobia, increasing anxiety and depression, loss of interest in leisure pursuits and interests, and an inability to experience or express feelings can also occur. Not everyone, however, experiences problems with long-term use. Additionally an altered perception of self, environment and relationships may occur.

Cognitive Effects

The short-term use of benzodiazepines adversely affects multiple areas of cognition, the most notable one being that it interferes with the formation and consolidation of memories of new material and may induce complete anterograde amnesia. However, researchers hold contrary opinions regarding the effects of long-term administration. One view is that many of the short-term effects continue into the long-term and may even worsen, and are not resolved after stopping benzodiazepine usage. Another view maintains that cognitive deficits in chronic benzodiazepine users occur only for a short period after the dose, or that the anxiety disorder is the cause of these deficits.

While the definitive studies are lacking, the former view received support from a 2004 meta-analysis of 13 small studies This meta-analysis found that long-term use of benzodiazepines was associated with moderate to large adverse effects on all areas of cognition, with visuospatial memory being the most commonly detected impairment. Some of the other impairments reported were decreased IQ, visiomotor coordination, information processing, verbal learning and concentration. The authors of the meta-analysis and a later reviewer noted that the applicability of this meta-analysis is limited because the subjects were taken mostly from withdrawal clinics; the coexisting drug, alcohol use, and psychiatric disorders were not defined; and several of the included studies conducted the cognitive measurements during the withdrawal period.

Paradoxical Effects

Paradoxical reactions, such as increased seizures in epileptics, aggression, violence, impulsivity, irritability and suicidal behavior sometimes occur. These reactions have been explained as consequences of disinhibition and the subsequent loss of control over socially unacceptable behavior. Paradoxical reactions are rare in the general population, with an incidence rate below 1% and similar to placebo. However, they occur with greater frequency in recreational abusers, individuals with borderline personality disorder, children, and patients on high-dosage regimes. In these groups, impulse control problems are perhaps the most important risk factor for disinhibition; learning disabilities and neurological disorders are also significant risks. Most reports of disinhibition involve high doses of high-potency benzodiazepines. Paradoxical effects may also appear after chronic use of benzodiazepines.

Long-Term Worsening of Psychiatric Symptoms

While benzodizapines may have short-term benefits for anxiety, sleep and agitation in some patients, long-term (i.e., greater than 2–4 weeks) use can result in a worsening of the very symptoms the medications are meant to treat. Potential explanations include exacerbating cognitive problems that are already common in anxiety disorders, causing or worsening depression and suicidality, disrupting sleep architecture by inhibiting deep stage sleep, withdrawal symptoms or rebound symptoms in between doses mimicking or exacerbating underlying anxiety or sleep disorders, inhibiting the benefits of psychotherapy by inhibiting memory consolidation and reducing fear extinction, and reducing coping with trauma/stress and increasing vulnerability to future stress. Anxiety, insomnia and irritability may be temporarily exacerbated during withdrawal, but psychiatric symptoms after discontinuation are usually less than even while taking benzodiazepines. Fortunately, for those with benzodiazepine-induced problems, functioning significantly improves within 1 year of discontinuation.

Reinforcement Disorders

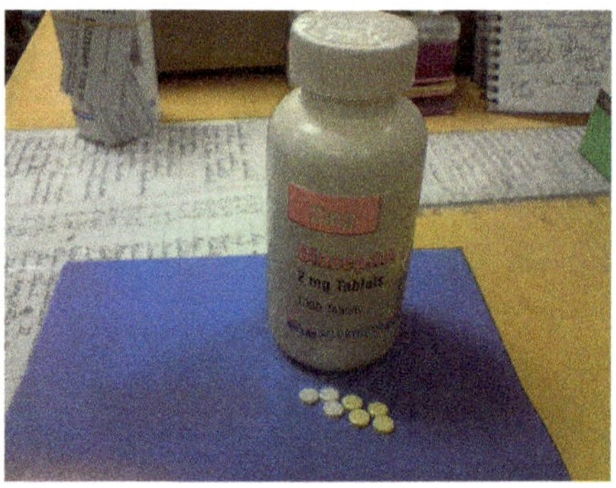

Diazepam 2 mg and 5 mg diazepam tablets, which are commonly used in the treatment of benzodiazepine withdrawal.

Tolerance

The main problem of the chronic use of benzodiazepines is the development of tolerance and dependence. Tolerance manifests itself as diminished pharmacological effect and develops relatively quickly to the sedative, hypnotic, anticonvulsant, and muscle relaxant actions of benzodiazepines. Tolerance to anti-anxiety effects develops more slowly with little evidence of continued effectiveness beyond four to six months of continued use. In general, tolerance to the amnesic effects does not occur. However, controversy exists as to tolerance to the anxiolytic effects with some evidence that benzodiazepines retain efficacy and opposing evidence from a systematic review of the literature that tolerance frequently occurs and some evidence that anxiety may worsen with long-term use. The question of tolerance to the amnesic effects of benzodiazepines is, likewise, unclear. Some evidence suggests that partial tolerance does develop, and that, "memory impairment is limited to a narrow window within 90 minutes after each dose".

A major disadvantage of benzodiazepines that tolerance to therapeutic effects develops relatively quickly while many adverse effects persist. Tolerance develops to hypnotic and myorelexant effects within days to weeks, and to anticonvulsant and anxiolytic effects within weeks to months. Therefore, benzodiazepines are unlikely to be effective long-term treatments for sleep and anxiety. While BZD therapeutic effects disappear with tolerance, depression and impulsivity with high suicidal risk commonly persist. Several studies have confirmed that long-term benzodiazepines are not significantly different from placebo for sleep or anxiety. This may explain why patients commonly increase doses over time and many eventually take more than one type of benzodiazepine after the first loses effectiveness. Additionally, because tolerance to benzodiazepine sedating effects develops more quickly than does tolerance to brainstem depressant effects, those taking more benzodiazepines to achieve desired effects may suffer sudden respiratory depression, hypotension or death. Most patients with anxiety disorders and PTSD have symptoms which persist for at least several months, making tolerance to therapeutic effects a distinct problem for them and necessitating the need for more effective long-term treatment (e.g., psychotherapy, serotonergic antidepressants).

Withdrawal Symptoms and Management

Discontinuation of benzodiazepines or abrupt reduction of the dose, even after a relatively short course of treatment (three to four weeks), may result in two groups of symptoms—rebound and withdrawal. Rebound symptoms are the return of the symptoms for which the patient was treated but worse than before. Withdrawal symptoms are the new symptoms that occur when the benzodiazepine is stopped. They are the main sign of physical dependence.

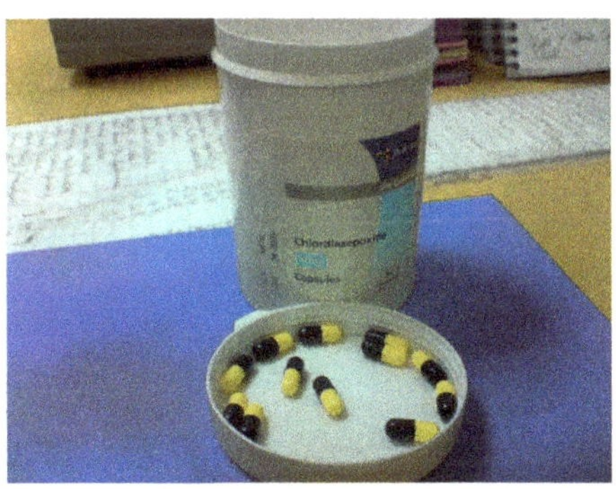

Chlordiazepoxide 5 mg capsules, which are sometimes used as an alternative to diazepam for benzodiazepine withdrawal. Like diazepam it has a long elimination half-life and long-acting active metabolites.

The most frequent symptoms of withdrawal from benzodiazepines are insomnia, gastric problems, tremors, agitation, fearfulness, and muscle spasms. The less frequent effects are irritability, sweating, depersonalization, derealization, hypersensitivity to stimuli, depression, suicidal behavior, psychosis, seizures, and delirium tremens. Severe symptoms usually occur as a result of abrupt or over-rapid withdrawal. Abrupt withdrawal can be dangerous, therefore a gradual reduction regimen is recommended.

Symptoms may also occur during a gradual dosage reduction, but are typically less severe and may persist as part of a protracted withdrawal syndrome for months after cessation of benzodiazepines. Approximately 10% of patients will experience a notable protracted withdrawal syndrome, which can persist for many months or in some cases a year or longer. Protracted symptoms tend to resemble those seen during the first couple of months of withdrawal but usually are of a sub-acute level of severity. Such symptoms do gradually lessen over time, eventually disappearing altogether.

Benzodiazepines have a reputation with patients and doctors for causing a severe and traumatic withdrawal; however, this is in large part due to the withdrawal process being poorly managed. Over-rapid withdrawal from benzodiazepines increases the severity of the withdrawal syndrome and increases the failure rate. A slow and gradual withdrawal customized to the individual and, if indicated, psychological support is the most effective way of managing the withdrawal. Opinion as to the time needed to complete withdrawal ranges from four weeks to several years. A goal of less than six months has been suggested, but due to factors such as dosage and type of benzodiazepine, reasons for prescription, lifestyle, personality, environmental stresses, and amount of available support, a year or more may be needed to withdraw.

Withdrawal is best managed by transferring the physically dependent patient to an equivalent dose of diazepam because it has the longest half-life of all of the benzodiazepines, is metabolized into long-acting active metabolites and is available in low-potency tablets, which can be quartered for smaller doses. A further benefit is that it is available in liquid form, which allows for even smaller reductions. Chlordiazepoxide, which also has a long half-life and long-acting active metabolites, can be used as an alternative.

Nonbenzodiazepines are contraindicated during benzodiazepine withdrawal as they are cross tolerant with benzodiazepines and can induce dependence. Alcohol is also cross tolerant with benzodiazepines and more toxic and thus caution is needed to avoid replacing one dependence with another. During withdrawal, fluoroquinolone-based antibiotics are best avoided if possible; they displace benzodiazepines from their binding site and reduce GABA function and, thus, may aggravate withdrawal symptoms. Antipsychotics are not recommended for benzodiazepine withdrawal (or other CNS depressant withdrawal states) especially clozapine, olanzapine or low potency phenothiazines e.g. chlorpromazine as they lower the seizure threshold and can worsen withdrawal effects; if used extreme caution is required.

Withdrawal from long term benzodiazepines is beneficial for most individuals. Withdrawal of benzodiazepines from long-term users, in general, leads to improved physical and mental health particularly in the elderly; although some long term users report continued benefit from taking benzodiazepines, this may be the result of suppression of withdrawal effects.

Overdose

Although benzodiazepines are much safer in overdose than their predecessors, the barbiturates, they can still cause problems in overdose. Taken alone, they rarely cause severe complications in overdose; statistics in England showed that benzodiazepines were responsible for 3.8% of all deaths by poisoning from a single drug. However, combining these drugs with alcohol, opiates or tricyclic antidepressants markedly raises the toxicity. The elderly are more sensitive to the side effects of benzodiazepines, and poisoning may even occur from their long-term use. The various benzodiazepines differ in their toxicity; temazepam appears to be most toxic in overdose and when used with other drugs. The symptoms of a benzodiazepine overdose may include; drowsiness, slurred speech, nystagmus, hypotension, ataxia, coma, respiratory depression, and cardiorespiratory arrest.

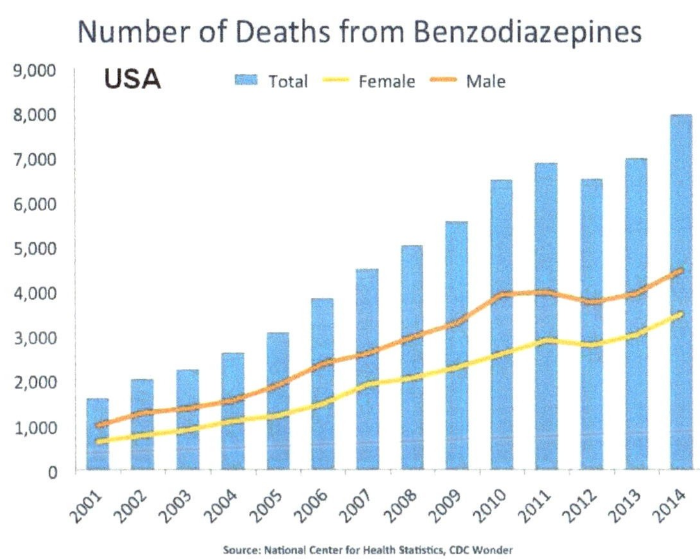

Timeline of number of yearly U.S. overdose deaths involving benzodiazepines.

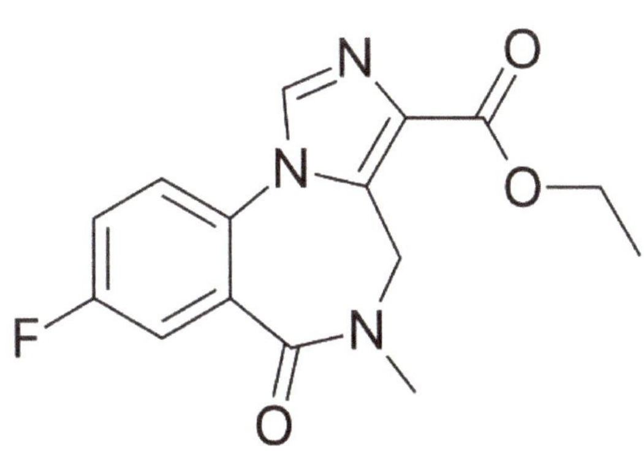

The use of flumazenil is controversial following benzodiazepine overdose.

A reversal agent for benzodiazepines exists, flumazenil (Anexate). Its use as an antidote is not routinely recommended because of the high risk of resedation and seizures. In a double-blind, placebo-controlled trial of 326 patients, 4 patients suffered serious adverse events and 61% became resedated following the use of flumazenil. Numerous contraindications to its use exist. It is contraindicated in patients with a history of long-term use of benzodiazepines, those having ingested a substance that lowers the seizure threshold or may cause an arrhythmia, and in those with abnormal vital signs. One study found that only 10% of the patient population presenting with a benzodiazepine overdose are suitable candidates for treatment with flumazenil.

Interactions

Individual benzodiazepines may have different interactions with certain drugs. Depending on their metabolism pathway, benzodiazepines can be divided roughly into two groups. The largest group consists of those that are metabolized by cytochrome P450 (CYP450) enzymes and possess significant potential for interactions with other drugs. The other group comprises those that are metabolized through glucuronidation, such as lorazepam, oxazepam, and temazepam, and, in general, have few drug interactions.

Many drugs, including oral contraceptives, some antibiotics, antidepressants, and antifungal agents, inhibit cytochrome enzymes in the liver. They reduce the rate of elimination of the benzodiazepines that are metabolized by CYP450, leading to possibly excessive drug accumulation and increased side-effects. In contrast, drugs that induce cytochrome P450 enzymes, such as St John's wort, the antibiotic rifampicin, and the anticonvulsantscarbamazepine and phenytoin, accelerate elimination of many benzodiazepines and decrease their action. Taking benzodiazepines with alcohol, opioids and other central nervous system depressants potentiates their action. This often results in increased sedation, impaired motor coordination, suppressed breathing, and other adverse effects that have potential to be lethal. Antacids can slow down absorption of some benzodiazepines; however, this effect is marginal and inconsistent.

Recreational Use

Benzodiazepines are considered to be major drugs of abuse. Benzodiazepine abuse is mostly limited to individuals who abuse other drugs, i.e., poly-drug abusers. On the international scene, benzodiazepines are categorized as Schedule IV controlled drugs by the INCB, apart from flunitrazepam which is a Schedule III drug under the Convention on Psychotropic Substances. Some variation in drug scheduling exists in individual countries; for example, in the United Kingdom, midazolam and temazepam are Schedule III controlled drugs.

British law requires temazepam (but *not* midazolam) to be stored in safe custody. Safe custody requirements ensures that pharmacists and doctors holding stock of temazepam must store it in securely fixed double-locked steel safety cabinets and maintain a written register, which must be bound and contain separate entries for temazepam and must be written in ink with no use of correction fluid (although a written register is not required for temazepam in the United Kingdom). Disposal of expired stock must be witnessed by a designated inspector (either a local drug-enforcement police officer or official from health authority). Benzodiazepine abuse ranges from occasional binges on large doses, to chronic and compulsive drug abuse of high doses.

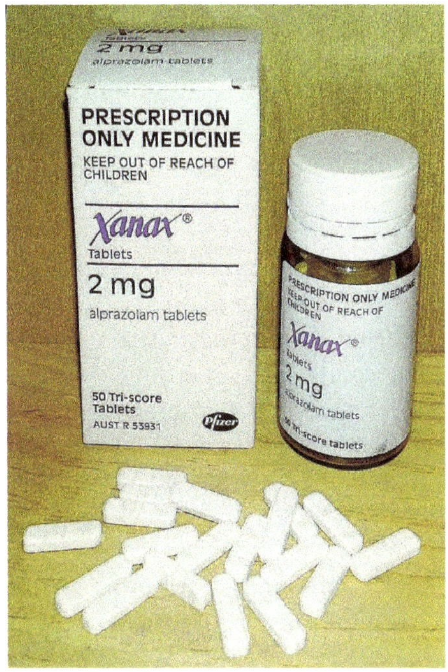

Xanax (alprazolam) 2 mg tri-score tablets

Benzodiazepines are used recreationally and by problematic drug misusers. Mortality is higher among poly-drug misusers that also use benzodiazepines. Heavy alcohol use also increases mortality among poly-drug users. Dependence and tolerance, often coupled with dosage escalation, to benzodiazepines can develop rapidly among drug misusers; withdrawal syndrome may appear after as little as three weeks of continuous use. Long-term use has the potential to cause both physical and psychological dependence and severe withdrawal symptoms such as depression, anxiety (often to the point of panic attacks), and agoraphobia. Benzodiazepines and, in particular, temazepam are sometimes used intravenously, which, if done incorrectly or in an unsterile manner, can lead to medical complications including abscesses, cellulitis, thrombophlebitis, arterial puncture, deep vein thrombosis, and gangrene. Sharing syringes and needles for this purpose also brings up the possibility of transmission of hepatitis, HIV, and other diseases. Benzodiazepines are also misused intranasally, which may have additional health consequences. Once benzodiazepine dependence has been established, a clinician usually converts the patient to an equivalent dose of diazepam before beginning a gradual reduction program.

A 1999–2005 Australian police survey of detainees reported preliminary findings that self-reported users of benzodiazepines were less likely than non-user detainees to work full-time and more likely to receive government benefits, use methamphetamine or heroin, and be arrested or imprisoned. Benzodiazepines are sometimes used for criminal purposes; they serve to incapacitate a victim in cases of drug assisted rape or robbery.

Overall, anecdotal evidence suggests that temazepam may be the most psychologically habit-forming (addictive) benzodiazepine. Temazepam abuse reached epidemic proportions in some parts of the world, in particular, in Europe and Australia, and is a major drug of abuse in many Southeast Asian countries. This led authorities of various countries to place temazepam under a more restrictive legal status. Some countries, such as Sweden, banned the drug outright. Temazepam also has certain pharmacokinetic properties of absorption, distribution, elimination, and clearance that make it more apt to abuse compared to many other benzodiazepines.

Veterinary Use

Benzodiazepines are used in veterinary practice in the treatment of various disorders and conditions. As in humans, they are used in the first-line management of seizures, status epilepticus, and tetanus, and as maintenance therapy in epilepsy (in particular, in cats). They are widely used in small and large animals (including horses, swine, cattle and exotic and wild animals) for their anxiolytic and sedative effects, as pre-medication before surgery, for induction of anesthesia and as adjuncts to anesthesia.

Cardiac Glycoside

Cardiac glycosides are organic compounds containing a glycoside (sugar) that act on the contractile force of the cardiac muscle. Because of their potency in disrupting the function of the heart, most are extremely toxic. These glycosides are found as secondary metabolites in several plants, and in some insects, such as the milkweed butterflies, that consume the plants.

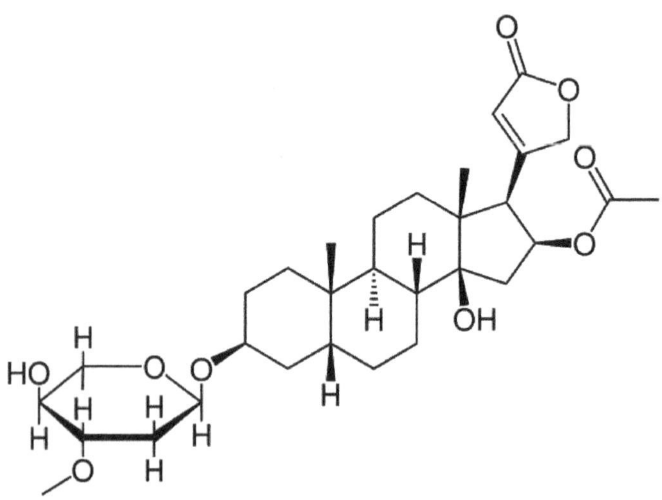

Example of the chemical structure of oleandrin, a potent toxic cardiac glycoside extracted from the Oleander bush.

Chemically, the aglycone [non-sugar] part of cardiac glycoside is a steroidal moiety.

Uses

From ancient times, humans have used cardiac-glycoside-containing plants and their crude extracts as arrow coatings, homicidal or suicidal aids, rat poisons, heart tonics, diuretics and emetics. In modern times, purified extracts or synthetic analogues of a few have been adapted for the treatment of congestive heart failure and cardiac arrhythmia.

Therapeutic uses of cardiac glycosides primarily involve the treatment of cardiac failure. Their utility results from an increased cardiac output by increasing the force of contraction. By increasing intracellular calcium as described below, cardiac glycosides increase calcium-induced calcium release and thus contraction. They also delay depolarization thus decreasing heart rate.

Bufalin, ouabain and digoxin are a few toxic cardiac glycosides. Digoxin from the foxglove plant is used clinically, whereas bufalin and ouabain are used only experimentally due to their extremely high potency.

Fibrate

In pharmacology, the fibrates are a class of amphipathic carboxylic acids. They are used for a range of metabolicdisorders, mainly hypercholesterolemia (high cholesterol), and are therefore hypolipidemic agents.

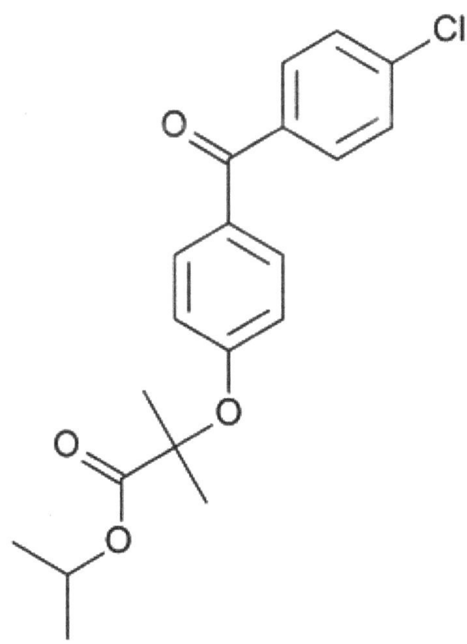

Fenofibrate, one of the most popular fibrates

Indications

Fibrates are used in accessory therapy in many forms of hypercholesterolemia, usually in combination with statins. Clinical trials do support their use as monotherapy agents. Fibrates reduce the number of non-fatal heart attacks, but do not improve all-cause mortality and are therefore indicated only in those not tolerant to statins.

Although less effective in lowering LDL levels, the ability of fibrates to increase HDL and lower triglyceride levels seems to reduce insulin resistance when the dyslipidemia is associated with other features of the metabolic syndrome (hypertension and diabetes mellitus type 2). They are therefore used in many hyperlipidemias. Due to a rare paradoxical decrease in HDL-C seen in some patients on fenofibrate, as per US FDA label change, it is recommended that the HDL-C levels be checked within the first few months after initiation of fibrate therapy. If a severely depressed HDL-C level is detected, fibrate therapy should be withdrawn, and the HDL-C level monitored until it has returned to baseline.

Side Effects

Most fibrates can cause mild stomach upset and myopathy (muscle pain with CPK elevations). Since fibrates increase the cholesterol content of bile, they increase the risk for gallstones.

In combination with statin drugs, fibrates cause an increased risk of rhabdomyolysis, idiosyncratic destruction of muscle tissue, leading to renal failure. A powerful statin drug, cerivastatin (Lipobay), was withdrawn because of this complication. The less lipophilic statins are less prone to cause this reaction, and are probably safer when combined with fibrates.

Drug toxicity includes acute kidney injury.

Thiazide

Thiazide is a type of molecule and a class of diuretics often used to treat hypertension (high blood pressure) and edema (such as that caused by heart failure, liver failure, or kidney failure).

The thiazides and thiazide-like diuretics reduce the risk of death, stroke, heart attack, and heart failure due to hypertension. The class was discovered and developed at Merck and Co. in the 1950's and the first approved drug of this class, chlorothiazide, was marketed under the trade name Diuril beginning in 1958. In most countries, the thiazides are the cheapest antihypertensive drugs available.

Medical Uses

Hypertension

Regarding effectiveness in the treatment of hypertension, a systematic review by the Cochrane Collaboration found:

- Chlorthalidone reduces systolic and diastolic blood pressure by 12.0/4 mmHg and the reduction is not dose related when tested at a range of doses from 12.5 mg to 75 mg/day.

- Hydrochlorothiazide's effect is dose related and at a maximum dose of 50 mg/day, the reduction is 11 mmHg/5 mmHg.

Thiazides and thiazide-like diuretics have been in constant use since their introduction in 1958. They "have remained a cornerstone in the management of hypertension for more than half a century since their introduction Very few agents used for the treatment of any disease can boast such staying power, which is a testament both to the efficacy and safety of these compounds.

Several clinical practice guidelines address the use of thiazides. They are the recommended first-line treatment in the US (JNC VII) guidelines for hypertension and a recommended treatment in the European (ESC/ESH) guidelines. However, the recent 2011 UK National Institute for Health and Clinical Excellence (NICE) guideline on the management of primary hypertension in adults (CG127) recommend calcium channel blockers (CCBs) as first line agents in hypertension and advise that thiazide-like diuretics should only be used first line if CCBs are not suitable or if the patient has oedema or has a high risk of developing heart failure. Thiazides have also been replaced by angiotensin converting enzyme (ACE) inhibitors in Australia due to their propensity to increase risk of diabetes mellitus type 2.

The mechanism of action of thiazides in lowering blood pressure in the long term is not fully understood. When administered acutely thiazides lower blood pressure by causing diuresis, a fall in plasma volume and a reduction in cardiac output. However, after chronic use thiazides cause a reduction in blood pressure by lowering peripheral resistance (i.e. vasodilation). The mechanism of this effect is uncertain but it may involve effects on "whole body" or renal autoregulation, or direct vasodilator actions either through inhibition of carbonic anhydrase or by desensitizing the vascular smooth muscle cells to the rise in intracellular calcium induced by norepinephrine.

Other

Thiazides also lower urinary calcium excretion, making them useful in preventing calcium-containing kidney stones. This effect is associated with positive calcium balance and is associated with an increase in bone mineral density and reductions in fracture rates attributable to osteoporosis. By a lesser understood mechanism, thiazides directly stimulate osteoblast differentiation and bone mineral formation, further slowing the course of osteoporosis.

Because of their promotion of calcium retention, thiazides are used in the the following treatments are:

- Dent's Disease;
- Hypocalcemia;
- Nephrolithiasis (idiopathic hypercalciuria);
- Bromide intoxication and
- Nephrogenic diabetes insipidus.

Mechanisms of Action

The members of this class of diuretics are derived from benzothiadiazine. They control hypertension in part by inhibiting reabsorption of sodium (Na^+) and chloride(Cl^-) ions from the distal convoluted tubules in the kidneys by blocking the thiazide-sensitive Na^+-Cl^- symporter. The term "thiazide" is also often used for drugs with a similar action that do not have the thiazide chemical structure, such as chlorthalidone and metolazone. These agents are more properly termed thiazide-like diuretics.

Thiazide diuretics also increase calcium reabsorption at the distal tubule. By lowering the sodium concentration in the tubule epithelial cells, thiazides indirectly increase the activity of the basolateral Na^+/Ca^{2+} antiporter. This facilitates the transport of Ca^{2+} from the epithelial cells into the renal interstitium. This movement of Ca^{2+}, in turn, decreases the intracellular Ca^{2+} concentration, which allows more Ca^{2+} to diffuse from the lumen of the tubules into epithelial cells via apical Ca^{2+}-selective channels (TRPV5). In other words, less Ca^{2+} in the cell increases the driving force for reabsorption from the lumen.

Thiazides are also thought to increase the reabsorption of Ca^{2+} by a mechanism involving the reabsorption of sodium and calcium in the proximal tubule in response to sodium depletion. Some of this response is due to augmentation of the action of parathyroid hormone.

Denomination

That thiazide refers to both the type of molecule and the medication can sometimes lead to confusion, because some molecules (thiazide-like diuretics) are often considered as thiazide diuretics, although they are not thiazides from a chemical perspective. In this context, "thiazide" is taken to refer to a drug which acts at a "thiazide receptor", which is believed to be a sodium-chloride symporter.

Breast milk

Thiazides pass into breast milk, and can decrease the flow of breast milk. Thiazides are classed as "Drugs That Have Been Associated with Significant Effects on Some Nursing Infants and Should be Given to Nursing Mother's With Caution" by the American Academy of Pediatrics Committee on Drugs.

Contraindications

Contraindications include:

- Hypotension
- Allergy to sulphur-containing medications
- Gout
- Renal failure
- Lithium therapy
- Hypokalemia

- May worsen diabetes

Thiazides reduce the clearance of uric acid since they compete for the same transporter, and therefore raise the levels of uric acid in the blood. Hence they are prescribed with caution in patients with gout or hyperuricemia.

Chronic administration is associated with hyperglycemia.

Thiazides cause loss of blood potassium, while conserving blood calcium.

Thiazides can decrease placental perfusion and adversely affect the fetus so should be avoided in pregnancy.

Mechanisms of Hypokalemia

There are several mechanisms by which thiazide diuretics cause hypokalemia (decreased plasma potassium concentration):

- Increased delivery of sodium to the collecting ducts causes increased cellular uptake of Na from the lumen by apical Epithelial Na Channels (ENaCs). This then causes the basolateral Na/K exchanger to more actively exchange Na for K, which is then passively secreted into the lumen through apical channels, resulting in K loss. (Moreover, the increased delivery of K to the collecting ducts facilitates the exchange of K for H by the H/K exchangers on the intercalated alpha cells, resulting in loss of H [metabolic alkalosis].)
- Activation of the renin-angiotensin-aldosterone system by the diuretic hypovolemia: the body responds to hypovolemia by opposing diuresis, one effect of which is to produce aldosterone which stimulates the Na/K exchanger, resulting in further loss of potassium. For this reason, ACE inhibitors, which inhibit angiotensin IIproduction and therefore aldosterone activation, are frequently used in combination with thiazides to combat hypokalemia. There are fixed-dose ACE inhibitor and thiazide combinations.
- Flow rate in the nephron is increased under diuresis, reducing potassium concentration in the lumen, thus increasing the potassium gradient. Potassium is lost through the many potassium channels, such as ROMK. These are not exchangers; they allow facilitated diffusion, so the increased gradient is directly responsible for increased diffusion.

Mechanism of Action

Drug classes that share a common molecular mechanism of action by modulating the activity of a specific biological target. The definition of a mechanism of action also includes the type of activity at that biological target. For receptors, these activities include agonist, antagonist, inverse agonist, or modulator. Enzyme target mechanisms include activator or inhibitor. Ion channel modulators include opener or blocker. The following are specific examples of drug classes whose definition is based on a specific mechanism of action:

- 5-Alpha-reductase inhibitor
- Angiotensin II receptor antagonist

- ACE inhibitor
- Alpha-adrenergic agonist
- Beta blocker
- Dopamine agonist
- Dopamine antagonist
- Incretin mimetic
- Nonsteroidal anti-inflammatory drug – cyclooxygenase inhibitor
- Proton-pump inhibitor
- Renin inhibitor
- Selective glucocorticoid receptor modulator
- Selective serotonin reuptake inhibitor
- Statin – HMG-CoA reductase inhibitor

Mode of Action

Drug classes that are defined by common cellular mode of action include:

- Diuretic
- Cholinergic
- Dopaminergic
- GABAergic
- Serotonergic

THERAPEUTIC CLASS

Drug classes that are defined by their therapeutic use include:

- Analgesic
- Antibiotic
- Anticoagulant
- Antidepressant
- Anticancer
- Antiepileptic
- Antipsychotic
- Antiviral
- Sedative

Analgesic

An analgesic or painkiller is any member of the group of drugs used to achieve analgesia, relief from pain.

Analgesic drugs act in various ways on the peripheral and central nervous systems. They are distinct from anesthetics, which temporarily affect, and in some instances completely eliminate, sensation. Analgesics include paracetamol (known in North America as acetaminophen or simply APAP), the non-steroidal anti-inflammatory drugs (NSAIDs) such as the salicylates, and opioid drugs such as morphine and oxycodone.

In choosing analgesics, the severity and response to other medication determines the choice of agent; the World Health Organization (WHO) pain ladder specifies mild analgesics as its first step.

Analgesic choice is also determined by the type of pain: For neuropathic pain, traditional analgesics are less effective, and there is often benefit from classes of drugs that are not normally considered analgesics, such as tricyclic antidepressants and anticonvulsants.

Uses

Topical Nonsteroidal anti-inflammatory drugs provided pain relief in common conditions such as muscle sprains and overuse injuries. Since the side effects are also lesser, topical preparations could be preferred over oral medications in these conditions.

Contraindications

There are several classes of analgesic drugs. Each class has a different history of use for treating different sorts of pain and in different sorts of people. It is difficult to make a statement about when such drugs should be avoided.

In general, pain medication should not be used when there is another, less risky alternative. At the same time, people in pain should not experience undertreatment of pain. When a treatment is available to address the pain, a health care provider should recommend that correct treatment and not a lessor treatment which leaves too much pain.

Classification

Drugs for pain are typically classified by chemical structure.

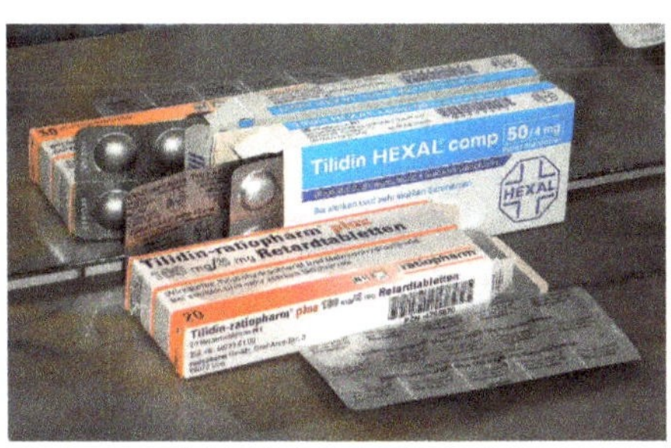

Tilidine, a type of painkiller

They may also be classified in other ways. Sometimes they are classified by use for various classes of medical condition. Other times they are sorted by the needs of special populations who would use them.They might be listed by availability in a geographical area, perhaps to prevent recommending a drug which is illegal in one place even if it is easily available elsewhere.

Paracetamol/Acetaminophen

Paracetamol, also known as acetaminophen or APAP, is a medication used to treat pain and fever. It is typically used for mild to moderate pain. In combination with opioid pain medication, paracetamol is used for more severe pain such as cancer pain and after surgery. It is typically used either by mouth or rectally but is also available intravenously. Effects last between two and four hours. Paracetamol is classified as a mild analgesic. Paracetamol is generally safe at recommended doses.

NSAIDs

Nonsteroidal anti-inflammatory drugs (usually abbreviated to NSAIDs), are a drug class that groups together drugs that provide analgesic (pain-killing) and antipyretic (fever-reducing) effects, and, in higher doses, anti-inflammatory effects. The most prominent members of this group of drugs, aspirin, ibuprofen and naproxen, are all available over the counter in most countries. As analgesics, NSAIDs are unusual in that they are non-narcotic and thus are used as a non-addictive alternative to narcotics.

COX-2 Inhibitors

These drugs have been derived from NSAIDs. The cyclooxygenase enzyme inhibited by NSAIDs was discovered to have at least 2 different versions: COX1 and COX2. Research suggested most of the adverse effects of NSAIDs to be mediated by blocking the COX1 (constitutive) enzyme, with the analgesic effects being mediated by the COX2 (inducible) enzyme. Thus, the COX2 inhibitors were developed to inhibit only the COX2 enzyme (traditional NSAIDs block both versions in general). These drugs (such as rofecoxib, celecoxib, and etoricoxib) are equally effective analgesics when compared with NSAIDs, but cause less gastrointestinal hemorrhage in particular.

After widespread adoption of the COX-2 inhibitors, it was discovered that most of the drugs in this class increase the risk of cardiovascular events by 40% on average. This led to the withdrawal of rofecoxib and valdecoxib, and warnings on others. Etoricoxib seems relatively safe, with the risk of thrombotic events similar to that of non-coxib NSAID diclofenac.

Opioids

Morphine, the archetypal opioid, and other opioids (e.g., codeine, oxycodone, hydrocodone, dihydromorphine, pethidine) all exert a similar influence on the cerebralopioid receptor system. Buprenorphine is a partial agonist of the μ-opioid receptor, and tramadol is a serotonin norepinephrine reuptake inhibitor (SNRI) with weak μ-opioid receptor agonist properties. Tramadol is structurally closer to venlafaxine than to codeine and delivers analgesia by not only delivering "opioid-like" effects (through mild agonism of the mu receptor) but also by acting as a weak but fast-acting serotonin releasing agent and norepinephrine reuptake inhibitor. Tapentadol, with some structural similarities to tramadol, presents what is believed to be a novel drug working through two (and possibly three) different modes of action in the fashion of both a traditional opioid and as a SNRI. The effects of serotonin and norepinephrine on pain, while not completely understood, have had causal links established and drugs in the SNRI class are commonly used in conjunction with opioids (especially tapentadol and tramadol) with greater success in pain relief. Dosing of all opioids may be limited by opioid toxicity (confusion, respiratory depression, myoclonic jerks and pinpoint pupils), seizures (tramadol), but opioid-tolerant individuals usually have higher dose ceilings than patients without tolerance.

Opioids, while very effective analgesics, may have some unpleasant side-effects. Patients starting morphine may experience nausea and vomiting (generally relieved by a short course of antiemetics such as phenergan). Pruritus (itching) may require switching to a different opioid. Constipation occurs in almost all patients on opioids, and laxatives (lactulose, macrogol-containing or co-danthramer) are typically co-prescribed.

When used appropriately, opioids and other central analgesics are otherwise safe and effective, however risks such as addiction and the body's becoming used to the drug (tolerance) can occur. The effect of tolerance means that frequent use of the drug may result in its diminished effect so, when safe to do so, the dosage may need to be increased to maintain effectiveness. This may be of particular concern regarding patients suffering with chronic pain. Opioid tolerance is often addressed with "opioid rotation therapy" in which a patient is routinely switched between two or more non-cross-tolerant opioid medications in order to prevent exceeding safe dosages in the attempt to achieve an adequate analgesic effect.

Alcohol

Describing the effects of using alcohol to treat pain is difficult. Alcohol has biological, mental, and social effects which influence the consequences of using alcohol for pain. Moderate use of alcohol can lessen certain types of pain in certain circumstances. Attempting to use alcohol to treat pain has also been observed to lead to negative outcomes including excessive drinking and alcohol use disorder.

Medical Cannabis

Medical cannabis or medical marijuana, can refer to the use of cannabis and its cannabinoids to treat disease or improve symptoms. There is evidence suggesting that cannabis can be used to treat chronic pain and muscle spasms with some trials indicating improved relief of neuropathic pain over opioids.

Combinations

Analgesics are frequently used in combination, such as the paracetamol and codeine preparations found in many non-prescription pain relievers. They can also be found in combination with vasoconstrictor drugs such as pseudoephedrine for sinus-related preparations, or with antihistamine drugs for allergy sufferers.

While the use of paracetamol, aspirin, ibuprofen, naproxen, and other NSAIDS concurrently with weak to mid-range opiates (up to about the hydrocodone level) has been said to show beneficial synergistic effects by combatting pain at multiple sites of action, several combination analgesic products have been shown to have few efficacy benefits when compared to similar doses of their individual components. Moreover, these combination analgesics can often result in significant adverse events, including accidental overdoses, most often due to confusion that arises from the multiple (and often non-acting) components of these combinations.

Alternative Medicine

Many people use alternative medicine treatments including drugs for pain relief. There is some evidence that some treatments using alternative medicine can relieve some types of pain more effectively than placebo. The available research concludes that more research would be necessary to better understand the use of alternative medicine.

Psychotropic Agents

Other psychotropic analgesic agents include ketamine (an NMDA receptor antagonist), clonidine and other α_2-adrenoreceptor agonists, and mexiletine and other local anaesthetic analogues.

Other Drugs

Drugs that have been introduced for uses other than analgesics are also used in pain management. Both first-generation (such as amitriptyline) and newer anti-depressants (such as duloxetine) are used alongside NSAIDs and opioids for pain involving nerve damage and similar problems. Other agents directly potentiate the effects of analgesics, such as using hydroxyzine, promethazine, carisoprodol, or tripelennamine to increase the pain-killing ability of a given dose of opioid analgesic.

Adjuvant analgesics, also called atypical analgesics, include nefopam, orphenadrine, pregabalin, gabapentin, cyclobenzaprine, scopolamine, and other drugs possessing anticonvulsant, anticholinergic, and/or antispasmodic properties, as well as many other drugs with CNS actions. These drugs are used along with analgesics to modulate and/or modify the action of opioids when used against pain, especially of neuropathic origin.

Dextromethorphan has been noted to slow the development of tolerance to opioids and exert additional analgesia by acting upon the NMDA receptors some analgesics such as methadone and ketobemidone and perhaps piritramide have intrinsic NMDA action.

High-alcohol liquor, two forms of which were found in the US Pharmacopoeia up until 1916 and in common use by physicians well into the 1930's has been used in the past as an agent for dulling pain, due to the CNS depressant effects of ethyl alcohol, a notable example being the American Civil War. However, the ability of alcohol to relieve severe pain is likely inferior to many analgesics used today (e.g., morphine, codeine). As such, in general, the idea of alcohol for analgesia is considered a primitive practice in virtually all industrialized countries today.

The use of adjuvant analgesics is an important and growing part of the pain-control field and new discoveries are made practically every year. Many of these drugs combat the side-effects of opioid analgesics, an added bonus. For example, antihistamines including orphenadrine combat the release of histamine caused by many opioids. Stimulants such as methylphenidate, caffeine, ephedrine, dextroamphetamine, methamphetamine, and cocaine work against heavy sedation and may elevate mood in distressed patients as do the antidepressants. The use of medicinal cannabis remains a debated issue.

In patients with chronic or neuropathic pain, various other substances may have analgesic properties. Tricyclic antidepressants, especially clomipramine and amitriptyline, have been shown to improve pain in what appears to be a central manner. Nefopam is used in Europe for pain relief with concurrent opioids. The exact mechanism of carbamazepine, gabapentin, and pregabalin is similarly unclear, but these anticonvulsants are used to treat neuropathic pain with differing degrees of success. Anticonvulsants are most commonly used for neuropathic pain as their mechanism of action tends to inhibit pain sensation.

Flupirtine is a centrally acting K+ channel opener with weak NMDA antagonist properties. It is used in Europe for moderate to strong pain and migraine and its muscle-relaxant properties. It has no anticholinergic properties and is believed to be devoid of any activity on dopamine, serotonin, or histamine receptors. It is not addictive, and tolerance usually does not develop. However, tolerance may develop in single cases.

Antibiotics

Antibiotics, also called antibacterials, are a type of antimicrobial drug used in the treatment and prevention of bacterial infections. They may either kill or inhibit the growth of bacteria. A limited number of antibiotics also possess antiprotozoal activity. Antibiotics are not effective against viruses such as the common cold or influenza, and their inappropriate use allows the emergence of resistant organisms. In 1928, Alexander Fleming identified penicillin, the first chemical compound with antibiotic properties. Fleming was working on a culture of disease-causing bacteria when he noticed the spores of a little green mold (*Penicillium chrysogenum*), in one of his culture plates. He observed that the presence of the mold killed or prevented the growth of the bacteria.

Antibiotics revolutionized medicine in the 20th century, and have together with vaccination led to the near eradication of diseases such as tuberculosis in the developed world. Their effectiveness and easy access led to overuse, especially in livestock raising, prompting bacteria to develop resistance. This has led to widespread problems with antimicrobial and antibiotic resistance, so much as to prompt the World Health Organization to classify antimicrobial resistance as a "serious threat that is no longer a prediction for the future, it is happening right now in every region of the world and has the potential to affect anyone, of any age, in any country".

The era of antibacterial treatment began with the discovery of arsphenamine, first synthesized by Alfred Bertheim and Paul Ehrlich in 1907, and used to treat syphilis. The first systemically active antibacterial drug, prontosil was discovered in 1933 by Gerhard Domagk, for which he was awarded the 1939 Nobel Prize. All classes of antibiotics in use today were first discovered prior to the mid 1980s.

Sometimes the term antibiotic is used to refer to any substance used against microbes, synonymous with antimicrobial, leading to the widespread but incorrect belief that antibiotics can be used against viruses. Some sources distinguish between antibacterial and antibiotic; antibacterials are used in soaps and cleaners generally and antibiotics are used as medicine.

Medical Uses

Antibiotics are used to treat or prevent bacterial infections, and sometimes protozoan infections. (Metronidazole is effective against a number of parasitic diseases). When an infection is suspected of being responsible for an illness but the responsible pathogen has not been identified, an empiric therapy is adopted. This involves the administration of a broad-spectrum antibiotic based on the signs and symptoms presented and is initiated pending laboratory results that can take several days.

When the responsible pathogenic microorganism is already known or has been identified, definitive therapy can be started. This will usually involve the use of a narrow-spectrum antibiotic. The choice of antibiotic given will also be based on its cost. Identification is critically important as it can reduce the cost and toxicity of the antibiotic therapy and also reduce the possibility of the emergence of antimicrobial resistance. To avoid surgery antibiotics may be given for non-complicated acute appendicitis. Effective treatment has been evidenced.

Antibiotics may be given as a preventive measure (prophylactic) and this is usually limited to at-risk populations such as those with a weakened immune system(particularly in HIV cases to prevent pneumonia), those taking immunosuppressive drugs, cancer patients and those having surgery. Their use in surgical procedures is to help prevent infection of incisions made. They have an important role in dental antibiotic prophylaxis where their use may prevent bacteremia and consequent infective endocarditis. Antibiotics are also used to prevent infection in cases of neutropenia particularly cancer-related.

Administration

There are different routes of administration for antibiotic treatment. Antibiotics are usually taken by mouth. In more severe cases, particularly deep-seated systemic infections, antibiotics can be given intravenously or by injection. Where the site of infection is easily accessed antibiotics may be given topically in the form of eye drops onto the conjunctiva for conjunctivitis or ear drops for ear infections and acute cases of swimmer's ear. Topical use is also one of the treatment options for some skin conditions including acne and cellulitis. Advantages of topical application include achieving high and sustained concentration of antibiotic at the site of infection; reducing the potential for systemic absorption and toxicity, and total volumes of antibiotic required are reduced, thereby also reducing the risk of antibiotic misuse. Topical antibiotics applied over certain types of surgical wounds have been reported to reduce the risk of surgical site infections. However, there are certain general causes for concern with topical administration of antibiotics. Some systemic absorption of the antibiotic may occur; the quantity of antibiotic applied is difficult to accurately dose, and there is also the possibility of local hypersensitivity reactions or contact dermatitis occurring.

Side-Effects

Antibiotics are screened for any negative effects before their approval for clinical use, and are usually considered safe and well tolerated. However, some antibiotics have been associated with a wide extent of adverse side effects ranging from mild to very severe depending on the type of antibiotic used, the microbes targeted, and the individual patient. Side effects may reflect the pharmacological or toxicological properties of the antibiotic or may involve hypersensitivity or allergic reactions. Adverse effects range from fever and nausea to major allergic reactions, including photodermatitis and anaphylaxis. Safety profiles of newer drugs are often not as well established as for those that have a long history of use.

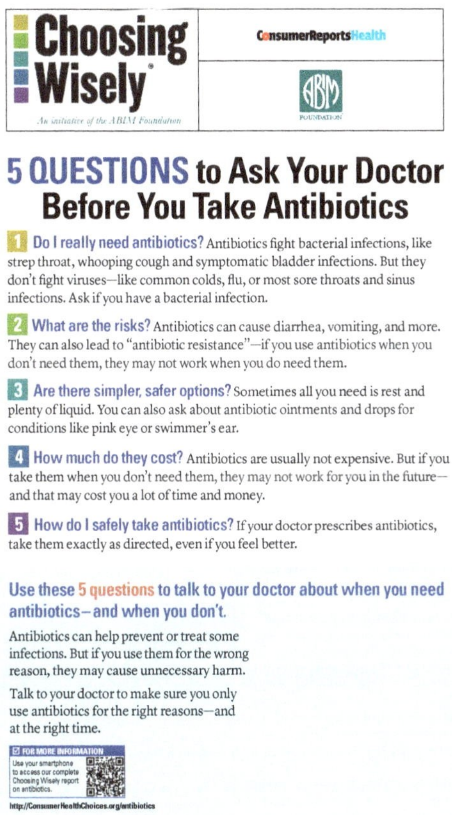

Health advocacy messages such as this one encourage patients to talk with their doctor about safety in using antibiotics.

Common side-effects include diarrhea, resulting from disruption of the species composition in the intestinal flora, resulting, for example, in overgrowth of pathogenic bacteria, such as *Clostridium difficile*. Antibacterials can also affect the vaginal flora, and may lead to overgrowth of yeast species of the genus *Candida* in the vulvo-vaginal area. Additional side-effects can result from interaction with other drugs, such as the possibility of tendon damage from the administration of a quinoloneantibiotic with a systemic corticosteroid.

Obesity

Exposure to antibiotics early in life is associated with increased body mass in humans and mouse models. Early life is a critical period for the establishment of the intestinal microbiota and for metabolic development. Mice exposed to subtherapeutic antibiotic treatment (STAT)– with either penicillin, vancomycin, or chlortetracycline had altered composition of the gut microbiota as well as its metabolic capabilities. One study has reported that mice given low-dose penicillin (1 μg/g body weight) around birth and throughout the weaning process had an increased body mass and fat mass, accelerated growth, and increased hepatic expression of genes involved in adipogenesis, compared to control mice. In addition, penicillin in combination with a high-fat diet increased fasting insulin levels in mice. However, it is unclear whether or not antibiotics cause obesity in humans. Studies have found a correlation between early exposure of antibiotics (<6 months) and increased body mass (at 10 and 20 months). Another study found that the type of antibiotic exposure was also significant with the highest risk of being overweight in those given macrolides compared to penicillin and cephalosporin. Therefore, there is correlation between antibiotic exposure in early life and obesity in humans, but whether or not there is a causal relationship remains unclear. Although there is a correlation between antibiotic use in early life and obesity, the effect of antibiotics on obesity in humans needs to be weighed against the beneficial effects of clinically indicated treatment with antibiotics in infancy.

Interactions

Birth Control Pills

The majority of studies indicate antibiotics do interfere with birth control pills, such as clinical studies that suggest the failure rate of contraceptive pills caused by antibiotics is very low (about 1%). In cases where antibiotics have been suggested to affect the efficiency of birth control pills, such as for the broad-spectrum antibiotic rifampicin, these cases may be due to an increase in the activities of hepatic liver enzyme's causing increased breakdown of the pill's active ingredients. Effects on the intestinal flora, which might result in reduced absorption of estrogens in the colon, have also been suggested, but such suggestions have been inconclusive and controversial. Clinicians have recommended that extra contraceptive measures be applied during therapies using antibiotics that are suspected to interact with oral contraceptives.

Alcohol

Interactions between alcohol and certain antibiotics may occur and may cause side-effects and decreased effectiveness of antibiotic therapy. While moderate alcohol consumption is unlikely to interfere with many common antibiotics, there are specific types of antibiotics with which alcohol consumption may cause serious side-effects. Therefore, potential risks of side-effects and effectiveness depend on the type of antibiotic administered.

Antibiotics such as metronidazole, tinidazole, cephamandole, latamoxef, cefoperazone, cefmenoxime, and furazolidone, cause a disulfiram-like chemical reaction with alcohol by inhibiting its breakdown by acetaldehyde dehydrogenase, which may result in vomiting, nausea, and shortness of breath. In addition, the efficacy of doxycycline and erythromycin succinate may be reduced by alcohol consumption. Other effects of alcohol on antibiotic activity include altered activity of the liver enzymes that break down the antibiotic compound.

Combination Therapy

In important infectious diseases, including tuberculosis, combination therapy (i.e., the concurrent application of two or more antibiotics) has been used to delay or prevent the emergence of resistance. In acute bacterial infections, antibiotics as part of combination therapy are prescribed for their synergistic effects to improve treatment outcome as the combined effect of both antibiotics is better than their individual effect. Methicillin-resistant Staphylococcus aureus infections may be treated with a combination therapy of fusidic acid and rifampin. Antibiotics used in combination may also be antagonistic and the combined effects of the two antibiotics may be less than if the individual antibiotic was given as part of a monotherapy. For example, Chloramphenicol and tetracyclines are antagonists to penicillins and aminoglycosides. However, this can vary depending on the species of bacteria. In general, combinations of a bacteriostatic antibiotic and bactericidal antibiotic are antagonistic.

Classes

Antibiotics are commonly classified based on their mechanism of action, chemical structure, or spectrum of activity.

Most target bacterial functions or growth processes. Those that target the bacterial cell wall (penicillins and cephalosporins) or the cell membrane (polymyxins), or interfere with essential bacterial enzymes (rifamycins, lipiarmycins, quinolones, and sulfonamides) have bactericidal activities. Those that target protein synthesis (macrolides, lincosamides and tetracyclines) are usually bacteriostatic (with the exception of bactericidal aminoglycosides). Further categorization is based on their target specificity. "Narrow-spectrum" antibiotics target specific types of bacteria, such as gram-negative or gram-positive, whereas broad-spectrum antibiotics affect a wide range of bacteria. Following a 40-year break in discovering new classes of antibacterial compounds, four new classes of antibiotics have been brought into clinical use in the late 2000's and early 2010's: cyclic lipopeptides (such as daptomycin), glycylcyclines (such as tigecycline), oxazolidinones (such as linezolid), and lipiarmycins (such as fidaxomicin).

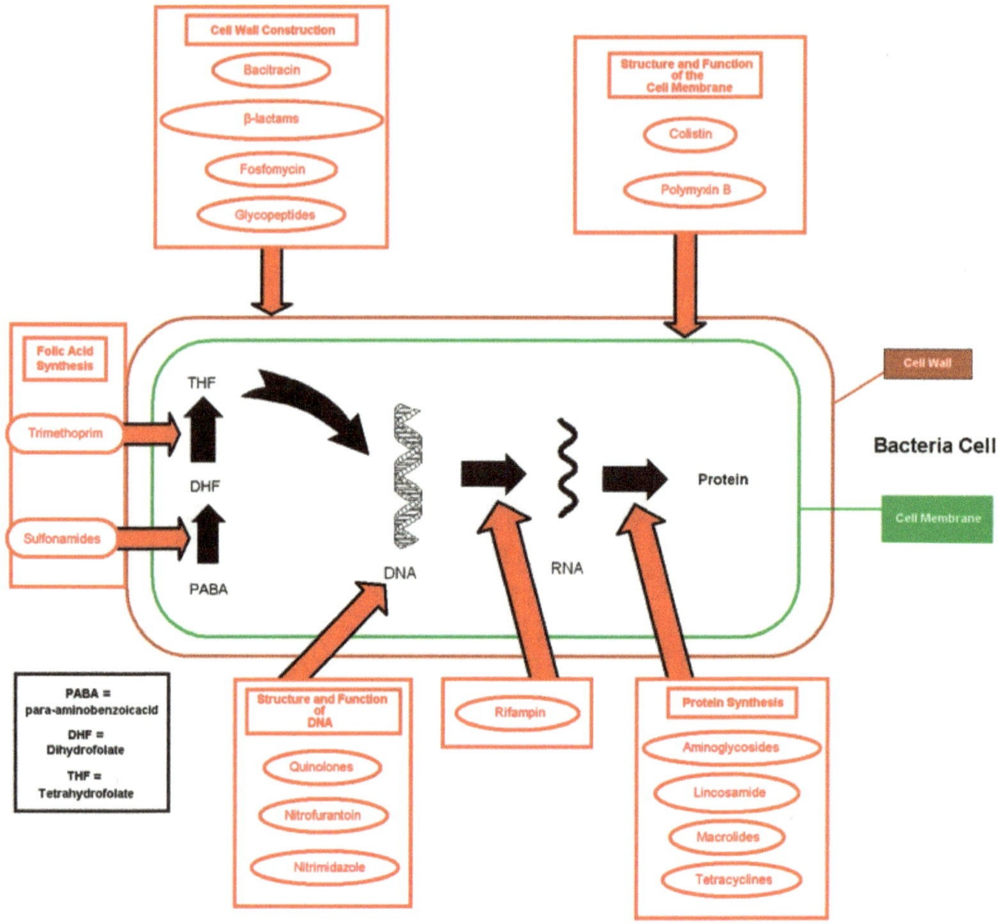

Molecular targets of antibiotics on the bacteria cell

Production

With advances in medicinal chemistry, most modern antibacterials are semisynthetic modifications of various natural compounds. These include, for example, the beta-lactam antibiotics, which include the penicillins (produced by fungi in the genus *Penicillium*), the cephalosporins, and the carbapenems. Compounds that are still isolated from living organisms are the aminoglycosides, whereas other antibacterials—for example, the sulfonamides, the quinolones, and the oxazolidinones—are produced solely by chemical synthesis. Many antibacterial compounds are relatively small molecules with a molecular weight of less than 1000 daltons.

Since the first pioneering efforts of Florey and Chain in 1939, the importance of antibiotics, including antibacterials, to medicine has led to intense research into producing antibacterials at large scales. Following screening of antibacterials against a wide range of bacteria, production of the active compounds is carried out using fermentation, usually in strongly aerobic conditions.

Anticoagulant

Anticoagulants are a class of drugs that work to prevent blood coagulation or which prolong the clotting time. Such substances occur naturally in leeches and blood-sucking insects. A group of pharmaceuticals called anticoagulants can be used as an injection as a medication for thrombotic disorders. Oral anticoagulants are also available. Some anticoagulants are used in medical equipment, such as test tubes, blood transfusion bags, and renal dialysisequipment.

Anticoagulants are closely related to antiplatelet drugs and thrombolytic drugs by manipulating the various pathways of blood coagulation. Specifically, anticoagulants manipulate the coagulation cascade that builds upon the initial platelet thrombus.

Medical Uses

The use of anticoagulants is a decision based upon the risks and benefits of anticoagulation. The biggest risk of anticoagulation therapy is the increased risk of bleeding. In otherwise healthy people, the increased risk of bleeding is minimal, but those who have had recent surgery, cerebral aneurysms, and other conditions may have too great of risk of bleeding. Generally, the benefit of anticoagulation is prevention of or reduction of progression of a disease. Some indications for anticoagulant therapy that are known to have benefit from therapy include:

- Atrial fibrillation — commonly forms an atrial appendage clot
- Coronary artery disease
- Deep vein thrombosis — can lead to pulmonary embolism
- Ischemic stroke
- Hypercoagulable states (e.g., Factor V Leiden) — can lead to deep vein thrombosis
- Myocardial infarction
- Pulmonary embolism
- Restenosis from stents

In these cases, anticoagulation therapy can prevent formation of dangerous clots or prevent growth of clots.

The decision to begin therapeutic anticoagulation often involves the use of multiple bleeding risk predictable outcome tools as non-invasive pre-test stratifications due to the potential for bleeds while on blood thinning agents. Among these tools are HAS-BLED, ATRIA, and CHA2DS2-VASc.

Adverse Effects

Patients aged 80 years or more may be especially susceptible to bleeding complications, with a rate of 13 bleeds per 100 person-years. Depletion of vitamin K by coumarin therapy increases risk of arterial calcification and heart valve calcification, especially if too much vitamin D is present.

Interactions

Foods and food supplements with blood-thinning effects include nattokinase, lumbrokinase, beer, bilberry, celery, cranberries, fish oil, garlic, ginger, ginkgo, ginseng, green tea, horse chestnut, licorice, niacin, onion, papaya, pomegranate, red clover, soybean, St. John's wort, turmeric, wheatgrass, and willow bark. Many herbal supplements have blood-thinning properties, such as danshen and feverfew. Multivitamins that do not interact with clotting are available for patients on anticoagulants.

However, some foods and supplements encourage clotting. These include alfalfa, avocado, cat's claw, coenzyme Q10, and dark leafy greens such as spinach. Their intake should be avoided whilst taking anticoagulants or, if coagulability is being monitored, their intake should be kept approximately constant so that anticoagulant dosage can be maintained at a level high enough to counteract this effect without fluctuations in coagulability.

Grapefruit interferes with some anticoagulant drugs, increasing the amount of time it takes for them to be metabolized out of the body, and so should be eaten only with caution when on anticoagulant drugs.

Anticoagulants are often used to treat acute deep vein thrombosis. People using anticoagulants to treat this condition should avoid using bed rest as a complementary treatment because there are clinical benefits to continuing to walk and remaining mobile while using anticoagulants in this way. Bed rest while using anticoagulants can harm patients in circumstances in which it is not medically necessary.

Types

A number of anticoagulants are available. The traditional ones (warfarin, other coumarins and heparins) are in widespread use. Since the 2000's a number of new agents have been introduced that are collectively referred to as the novel oral anticoagulants (NOACs) or directly acting oral anticoagulants (DOACs). These agents include inhibitors of factor IIa (dabigatran) and factor Xa (rivaroxaban, apixaban and edoxaban) and they have been shown to be as good or possibly better than the coumarins with less serious side effects. The newer anticoagulants (NOACs/DOACs), are more expensive than the traditional ones and should be used with care in patients with kidney problems. Additionally, there is no antidote for the factor Xa inhibitors, so it is difficult to stop their effects in the body in cases of emergency (accidents, urgent surgery). Idarucizumab was FDA approved for the reversal of dabigatran in 2015.

Novel Oral Anticoagulants

Novel oral anticoagulants (NOACs) are a new class of anticoagulant drugs that, like warfarin, can help inhibit clot formation. The most commonly prescribed NOACs are dabigatran, rivaroxaban, and apixaban.

Compared to warfarin, NOACs have a rapid onset action and relatively short half-lives, hence they carry out their function more rapidly and effectively, and allow for drugs to quickly reduce their anticoagulation effects. Routine monitoring and dose adjustments of

NOACs is less important than for warfarin, as they have better predictable anticoagulation activity. Both NOACs and warfarin are equivalently effect, but NOACs are less influenced by diet and medications compared to warfarin. However, there is presently no counter measure for most NOACs unlike in warfarin; nonetheless, the short half-lives of NOACs will result in its effects to swiftly recede. A reversal agent for dabigatran, idarucizumab, is currently the only NOAC reversal agent approved for use by the FDA.

NOACs are a lot costlier compared to warfarin, after having taken into consideration the cost of frequent blood testing associated with warfarin.

Relevance to Dental Treatments

With regards to NOAC medication and invasive dental treatments, there has not been enough clinical evidence and experience to prove any reliable side-effects, relevance or interaction between these two. Further clinical prospective studies on NOACs are required to investigate the bleeding risk and haemostasis associated to surgical dental procedures.

Recommendations of modifications to use/dosage of NOACs prior to dental treatments are made based on the balance of likely effects of each option of each procedure, and also the individual's bleeding risks and renal functionality. With low bleeding risk of dental procedures, it is recommended that NOAC medicine is still taken by patient as per normal, so as to avoid increase in the risk of thromboembolic event. For dental procedures with a higher risk of bleeding complications, the recommended practice is for patient to miss or delay a dose of their NOAC before such procedures so as to minimize the effect on thromboembolic risk.

Coumarins (vitamin K antagonists)

These oral anticoagulants are derived from coumarin, which is found in many plants. A prominent member of this class is warfarin (Coumadin). It takes at least 48 to 72 hours for the anticoagulant effect to develop. Where an immediate effect is required, heparin must be given concomitantly. These anticoagulants are used to treat patients with deep-vein thrombosis (DVT), pulmonary embolism (PE) and to prevent emboli in patients with atrial fibrillation (AF), and mechanical prosthetic heart valves. Other examples are acenocoumarol, phenprocoumon, atromentin, and phenindione.

The coumarins brodifacoum and difenacoum are used as rodenticides, but are not used medically.

Heparin and Derivative Substances

Heparin is a biological substance, usually made from pig intestines. It works by activating antithrombin III, which blocks thrombin from clotting blood. Heparin can be used *in vivo* (by injection), and also *in vitro* to prevent blood or plasma clotting in or on medical devices. In venipuncture, Vacutainer brand blood collecting tubes containing heparin usually have a green cap.

Low Molecular Weight Heparin

Low molecular weight heparin, a more highly processed product, is useful as it does not require monitoring of the APTT coagulation parameter (it has more predictable plasma levels) and has fewer side effects.

Synthetic Pentasaccharide Inhibitors of Factor Xa

- Fondaparinux is a synthetic sugar composed of the five sugars (pentasaccharide) in heparin that bind to antithrombin. It is a smaller molecule than low molecular weight heparin.
- Idraparinux

Direct Factor Xa Inhibitors

Drugs such as rivaroxaban, apixaban and edoxaban work by inhibiting factor Xa directly (unlike the heparins and fondaparinux, which work via antithrombin activation). Also betrixaban from Portola Pharmaceuticals, darexaban (YM150) from Astellas, and more recently letaxaban (TAK-442) from Takeda and eribaxaban(PD0348292) from Pfizer. The development of darexaban was discontinued in September 2011: in a trial for prevention of recurrences of myocardial infarction in top of dual antiplatelet therapy, the drug did not demonstrate effectiveness and the risk of bleeding was increased by approximately 300%. The development of letaxaban was discontinued for acute coronary syndrome in May 2011 following negative results from a Phase II study.

Direct Thrombin Inhibitors

Another type of anticoagulant is the direct thrombin inhibitor. Current members of this class include the bivalent drugs hirudin, lepirudin, and bivalirudin; and the monovalent drugs argatroban and dabigatran. An oral direct thrombin inhibitor, ximelagatran (Exanta) was denied approval by the Food and Drug Administration(FDA) in September 2004 and was pulled from the market entirely in February 2006 after reports of severe liver damage and heart attacks. In November 2010, dabigatran was approved by the FDA to treat atrial fibrillation.

Antithrombin Protein Therapeutics

The antithrombin protein itself is used as a protein therapeutic that can be purified from human plasma or produced recombinantly (for example, Atryn, which is produced in the milk of genetically modified goats.) Antithrombin is approved by the FDA as an anticoagulant for the prevention of clots before, during, or after surgery or birthing in patients with hereditary antithrombin deficiency.

Other Types of Anticoagulants

Many other anticoagulants exist, for use in research and development, diagnostics, or as drug candidates.

- Batroxobin, a toxin from a snake venom, clots platelet-rich plasma without affecting platelet functions (lyses fibrinogen).
- Hementin is an anticoagulant protease from the salivary glands of the giant Amazon leech, *Haementeria ghilianii*.
- Vitamin E

Antidepressant

Antidepressants are drugs used for the treatment of major depressive disorder and other conditions, including dysthymia, anxiety disorders, obsessive compulsive disorder, eating disorders, chronic pain, neuropathic pain and, in some cases, dysmenorrhoea, snoring, migraine, attention-deficit hyperactivity disorder (ADHD), addiction, dependence, and sleep disorders. They may be prescribed alone or in combination with other medications.

The most important classes of antidepressants are the selective serotonin reuptake inhibitors (SSRIs), serotonin–norepinephrine reuptake inhibitors (SNRIs), tricyclic antidepressants (TCAs), monoamine oxidase inhibitors (MAOIs), reversible monoamine oxidase A inhibitors (rMAO-A inhibitors), tetracyclic antidepressants (TeCAs), and noradrenergic and specific serotonergic antidepressant (NaSSAs). St John's wort is also used in the treatment of depression.

Medical Uses

For depression, the Hamilton Depression Rating Scale (HAM-D) is often used to measure the severity of depression. The maximum score for the 17-item HAM-D questionnaire is 52; the higher the score, the more severe the depression.

Anticarcinogen

An anticarcinogen (also known as a carcinopreventive agent) is a substance that counteracts the effects of a carcinogen or inhibits the development of cancer. Anticarcinogens are different from anticarcinoma agents (also known as anticancer or anti-neoplastic agents) in that anticarcinoma agents are used to selectively destroy or inhibit cancer cells *after* cancer has developed. Interest in anticarcinogens is motivated primarily by the principle that it is preferable to prevent disease (preventive medicine) than to have to treat it (rescue medicine).

In theory, anticarcinogens may act via different mechanisms including enhancement of natural defences against cancer, deactivation of carcinogens, and blocking the mechanisms by which carcinogens act (such as free radical damage to DNA). Confirmation that a substance possesses anticarcinogenic activity requires extensive *in vitro*, *in vivo*, and clinical investigation. Health claims for anticarcinogens are regulated by various national and international organizations like the US Food and Drug Administration (FDA) and European Food Safety Authority (EFSA).

Substances for which an anticarcinogenic health claim is approved

When consumed as part of a low fat diet, fiber-containing grain products, fruits, and vegetables may reduce the risk of some types of cancer. Cancer is, however, a disease associated with many factors, and the nature of the relationship between fiber, fruit, and vegetable intake and decreased cancer risk is not clear.

Anticonvulsant

Anticonvulsants (also commonly known as antiepileptic drugs or as antiseizure drugs) are a diverse group of pharmacological agents used in the treatment of epileptic seizures. Anticonvulsants are also increasingly being used in the treatment of bipolar disorder and borderline personality disorder, since many seem to act as mood stabilizers, and for the treatment of neuropathic pain. Anticonvulsants suppress the rapid and excessive firing of neurons during seizures. Anticonvulsants also prevent the spread of the seizure within the brain. Some investigators have observed that anticonvulsants themselves may cause reduced IQin children. However these adverse effects must be balanced against the significant risk epileptic seizures pose to children and the distinct possibility of death and devastating neurological sequelae secondary to seizures. Anticonvulsants are more accurately called antiepileptic drugs (abbreviated "AEDs"), and are often referred to as antiseizure drugs because they provide symptomatic treatment only and have not been demonstrated to alter the course of epilepsy.

Conventional antiepileptic drugs may block sodium channels or enhance γ-aminobutyric acid (GABA) function. Several antiepileptic drugs have multiple or uncertain mechanisms of action. Next to the voltage-gated sodium channels and components of the GABA system, their targets include $GABA_A$ receptors, the GAT-1 GABA transporter, and GABA transaminase. Additional targets include voltage-gated calcium channels, SV2A, and α2δ. By blocking sodium or calcium channels, antiepileptic drugs reduce the release of excitatory glutamate, whose release is considered to be elevated in epilepsy, but also that of GABA. This is probably a side effect or even the actual mechanism of action for some antiepileptic drugs, since GABA can itself, directly or indirectly, act proconvulsively. Another potential target of antiepileptic drugs is the peroxisome proliferator-activated receptor alpha. The drug class was the 5th-best-selling in the US in 2007.

Some anticonvulsants have shown antiepileptogenic effects in animal models of epilepsy. That is, they either prevent the development of epilepsy or can halt or reverse the progression of epilepsy. However, no drug has been shown in human trials to prevent epileptogenesis (the development of epilepsy in an individual at risk, such as after a head injury).

Antipsychotic

Antipsychotics also known as neuroleptics or major tranquilizers, are a class of medication primarily used to manage psychosis (including delusions, hallucinations, paranoia or disordered thought), principally in schizophreniaand bipolar disorder. They are increasingly being used in the management of non-psychotic disorders. Antipsychotics are usually effective in relieving symptoms of psychosis in the short term.

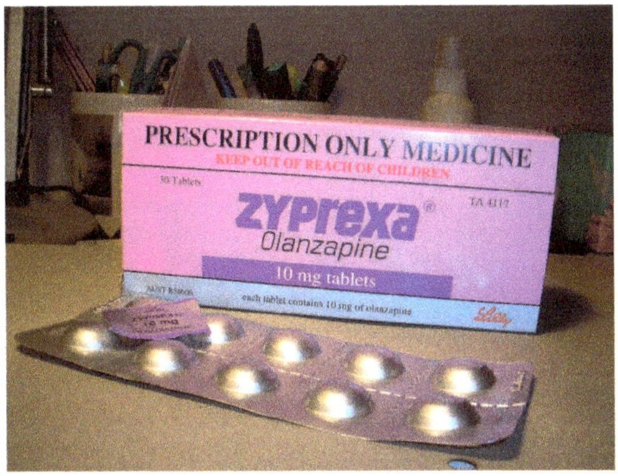

Olanzapine, an example of a second-generation antipsychotic

The long-term use of antipsychotics is associated with side effects such as involuntary movement disorders and metabolic syndrome. They are also associated with increased mortality in elderly people with dementia.

First-generation antipsychotics, known as typical antipsychotics, were discovered in the 1950's. Most second-generation drugs, known as atypical antipsychotics, have been developed more recently, although the first atypical antipsychotic, clozapine, was discovered in the 1960's and introduced clinically in the 1970's. Both generations of medication tend to block receptors in the brain's dopamine pathways, but atypicals tend to act on serotoninreceptors as well. Neuroleptic, which originates from the Greek word νεῦρον *neuron* ("nerve") and λῆψις *lepsis*("seizure" or "fit"), is a reference to neurological side effects.

MEDICAL uses

Antipsychotics are most frequently used for the following conditions:

- Schizophrenia
- Schizoaffective disorder most commonly in conjunction with either an antidepressant (in the case of the depressive subtype) or a mood stabiliser (in the case of the bipolar subtype).
- Bipolar disorder (acute mania and mixed episodes) may be treated with either typical or atypical antipsychotics, although atypical antipsychotics are usually preferred because they tend to have more favourable adverse effect profiles and, according to a recent meta-analysis, they tend to have a lower liability for causing conversion from mania to depression.
- Psychotic depression. In this indication it is a common practice for the psychiatrist to prescribe a combination of an atypical antipsychotic and an antidepressant as this practice is best supported by the evidence.

- Treatment-resistant (and not necessarily psychotic) major depression as an adjunct to standard antidepressant therapy.

They are not recommended for dementia or insomnia unless other treatments have not worked. They are not recommended in children unless other treatments are not effective or unless the child has psychosis.

Schizophrenia

Antipsychotic drug treatment is a key component of schizophrenia treatment algorithms recommended by the National Institute of Health and Clinical Excellence (NICE), the American Psychiatric Association, and the British Society for Psychopharmacology. The main effect of treatment with antipsychotics is to reduce the so-called "positive" symptoms, including delusions and hallucinations. There is mixed evidence to support a significant impact of antipsychotic use on negative symptoms (such as apathy, lack of emotional affect, and lack of interest in social interactions) or on the cognitive symptoms (disordered thinking, reduced ability to plan and execute tasks) of schizophrenia. In general, the efficacy of antipsychotic treatment in reducing both positive and negative symptoms appears to increase with increasing severity of baseline symptoms.

Applications of antipsychotic drugs in the treatment of schizophrenia include prophylaxis in those showing symptoms that suggest that they are at high risk of developing psychosis, treatment of first episode psychosis, maintenance therapy, and treatment of recurrent episodes of acute psychosis.

Prevention of Psychosis and Symptom Improvement

Test batteries such as the PACE (Personal Assessment and Crisis Evaluation Clinic) and COPS (Criteria of Prodromal Syndromes), which measure low level psychotic symptoms, and others focused on cognitive disturbances (Basic symptoms"), are used to evaluate people with early, low level symptoms of psychosis. Used in combination with family history information, these tests can identify a "high risk" group having a 20–40% risk of progression to frank psychosis within 2 years. These patients are often treated with low doses of antipsychotic drugs with the goal of reducing their symptoms and preventing progression to frank psychosis. While generally useful for reducing symptoms, the clinical trials performed to date provide little evidence that early use of antipsychotics, alone or in combination with cognitive-behavioral therapy, provides improved long term outcomes in those with prodromal symptoms.

First Episode Psychosis

NICE recommends that all persons presenting with a first episode of frank psychosis be treated with both an antipsychotic drug and cognitive-behavioral therapy (CBT). NICE further recommends that those expressing a preference for CBT alone be informed that combination treatment is more efficacious. A diagnosis of schizophrenia is not normally made at this time, as up to 25% of those presenting with first episode psychosis are eventually found to suffer from bipolar disorder instead. The goals of treatment of these patients include reducing symptoms and potentially improving long-term treatment outcomes.

Randomized clinical trials have provided evidence for the efficacy of antipsychotic drugs in achieving the former goal, with first-generation and second generation antipsychotics showing about equal efficacy. Evidence that early treatment has a favorable effect on long term outcomes is equivocal.

Recurrent Psychotic Episodes

Placebo-controlled trials of both first and second generation antipsychotic drugs consistently demonstrate the superiority of active drug to placebo in suppressing psychotic symptoms. A large meta-analysis of 38 trials of antipsychotic drugs in schizophrenia acute psychotic episodes showed an effect size of about 0.5. There is little or no difference in efficacy among approved antipsychotic drugs, including both first- and second-generation agents. The efficacy of such drugs is suboptimal. Few patients achieve complete resolution of symptoms. Response rates, calculated using various cutoff values for symptom reduction, are low and their interpretation is complicated by high placebo response rates and selective publication of clinical trial results.

Maintenance Therapy

The majority of patients treated with an antipsychotic drug will experience a response within 4 weeks. The goals of continuing treatment are to maintain suppression of symptoms, prevent relapse, improve quality of life, and support engagement in psychosocial therapy.

Maintenance therapy with antipsychotic drugs is clearly superior to placebo in preventing relapse, but is associated with weight gain, movement disorders, and high dropout rates. A 3-year trial following persons receiving maintenance therapy after an acute psychotic episode found that 33% obtained long-lasting symptom reduction, 13% achieved remission, and only 27% experienced satisfactory quality of life. The effect of relapse prevention on long term outcomes is uncertain, as historical studies show little difference in long term outcomes before and after the introduction of antipsychotic drugs.

A significant challenge in the use of antipsychotic drugs for the prevention of relapse is the poor rate of compliance. In spite of the relatively high rates of adverse effects associated with these drugs, some evidence, including higher dropout rates in placebo arms compared to treatment arms in randomized clinical trials, suggest that most patients who discontinue treatment do so because of suboptimal efficacy.

Bipolar Disorder

Antipsychotics are routinely used, often in conjunction with mood stabilisers such as lithium/valproate, as a first-line treatment for manic and mixed episodes associated with bipolar disorder. The reason for this combination is the therapeutic delay of the aforementioned mood stabilisers (for valproate therapeutic effects are usually seen around five days after treatment is commenced whereas lithium usually takes at least a week before the full therapeutic effects are seen) and the comparatively rapid antimanic effects of antipsychotic drugs. The antipsychotics have a documented efficacy when used alone in acute mania/mixed episodes.

Three atypical antipsychotics (lurasidone, olanzapine and quetiapine) have also been found to possess efficacy in the treatment of bipolar depression as a monotherapy. Whereas only olanzapine and quetiapine have been proven to be effective broad-spectrum (i.e. against all three types of relapse— manic, mixed and depressive) prophylactic (or *maintenance*) treatments in patients with bipolar disorder. A recent Cochrane review also found that olanzapine had a less favourable risk/benefit ratio than lithium as a maintenance treatment for bipolar disorder.

The American Psychiatric Association and the UK National Institute for Health and Care Excellence recommend antipsychotics for managing acute psychotic episodes in schizophrenia or bipolar disorder, and as a longer-term maintenance treatment for reducing the likelihood of further episodes. They state that response to any given antipsychotic can be variable so that trials may be necessary, and that lower doses are to be preferred where possible. A number of studies have looked at levels of "compliance" or "adherence" with antipsychotic regimes and found that discontinuation (stopping taking them) by patients is associated with higher rates of relapse, including hospitalization.

Dementia

An assessment for an underlying cause of behavior is needed before prescribing antipsychotic medication for symptoms of dementia. Antipsychotics in old age dementia showed a modest benefit compared to placebo in managing aggression or psychosis, but this is combined with a fairly large increase in serious adverse events. Thus, antipsychotics should not be used routinely to treat dementia with aggression or psychosis, but may be an option in a few cases where there is severe distress or risk of physical harm to others. Psychosocial interventions may reduce the need for antipsychotics.

Unipolar Depression

A number of atypical antipsychotics have some benefits when used in addition to other treatments in major depressive disorder. Aripiprazole, quetiapine, and olanzapine (when used in conjunction with fluoxetine) have received the Food and Drug Administration (FDA) labelling for this indication. There is, however, a greater risk of side effects with their use.

Other

Besides the above uses antipsychotics may be used for obsessive-compulsive disorder, posttraumatic stress disorder, personality disorders, Tourette syndrome, autism and agitation in those with dementia. Evidence however does not support the use of atypical antipsychotics in eating disorders or personality disorder. Risperidone may be useful for obsessive compulsive disorder. The use of low doses of antipsychotics for insomnia, while common, is not recommended as there is little evidence of benefit and concerns regarding adverse effects. Low dose antipsychotics may also be used in treatment of impulse-behavioral and cognitive-perceptual symptoms of borderline personality disorder.

In children they may be used in those with disruptive behavior disorders, mood disorders and pervasive developmental disorders or intellectual disability. Antipsychotics are only weakly recommended for Tourette syndrome, because although they are effective, side effects are common. The situation is similar for those on the autism spectrum. Much of the evidence for the off-label use of antipsychotics (for example, for dementia, OCD, PTSD, Personality Disorders, Tourette's) was of insufficient scientific quality to support such use, especially as there was strong evidence of increased risks of stroke, tremors, significant weight gain, sedation, and gastrointestinal problems. A UK review of unlicensed usage in children and adolescents reported a similar mixture of findings and concerns. A survey of children with pervasive developmental disorder found that 16.5% were taking an antipsychotic drug, most commonly for irritability, aggression, and agitation. Risperidone has been approved by the US FDA for the treatment of irritability in autistic children and adolescents.

Aggressive challenging behavior in adults with intellectual disability is often treated with antipsychotic drugs despite lack of an evidence base. A recent randomized controlled trial, however, found no benefit over placebo and recommended that the use of antipsychotics in this way should no longer be regarded as an acceptable routine treatment.

Typicals versus Atypicals

It is unclear whether the atypical (second-generation) antipsychotics offer advantages over older, first generation antipsychotics. Amisulpride, olanzapine, risperidone and clozapine may be more effective but are associated with greater side effects. Typical antipsychotics have equal drop-out and symptom relapse rates to atypicals when used at low to moderate dosages.

Clozapine is an effective treatment for those who respond poorly to other drugs ("treatment-resistant" or "refractory" schizophrenia), but it has the potentially serious side effect of agranulocytosis (lowered white blood cell count) in less than 4% of people.

Due to bias in the research the accuracy of comparisons of atypical antipsychotics is a concern.

In 2005, a US government body, the National Institute of Mental Health published the results of a major independent study (the CATIE project). No other atypical studied (risperidone, quetiapine, and ziprasidone) did better than the typical perphenazine on the measures used, nor did they produce fewer adverse effects than the typical antipsychotic perphenazine, although more patients discontinued perphenazine owing to extrapyramidal effects compared to the atypical agents (8% vs. 2% to 4%).

Compliance has not been shown to be different between the two types.

Many researchers question the first-line prescribing of atypicals over typicals, and some even question the distinction between the two classes. In contrast, other researchers point to the significantly higher risk of tardive dyskinesia and other extrapyramidal symptoms with the typicals and for this reason alone recommend first-line treatment with the atypicals, notwithstanding a greater propensity for metabolic adverse effects in the latter. The UK government organization NICE recently revised its recommendation favoring atypicals, to advise that the choice should be an individual one based on the particular profiles of the individual drug and on the patient's preferences.

The re-evaluation of the evidence has not necessarily slowed the bias toward prescribing the atypicals.

Antiviral Drug

Antiviral drugs are a class of medication used specifically for treating viral infections rather than bacterial ones. Most antivirals are used for specific viral infections, while a broad-spectrum antiviral is effective against a wide range of viruses. Unlike most antibiotics, antiviral drugs do not destroy their target pathogen; instead they inhibit their development.

Antiviral drugs are one class of antimicrobials, a larger group which also includes antibiotic (also termed antibacterial), antifungal and antiparasitic drugs, or antiviral drugs based on monoclonal antibodies. Most antivirals are considered relatively harmless to the host, and therefore can be used to treat infections. They should be distinguished from viricides, which are not medication but deactivate or destroy virus particles, either inside or outside the body. Natural antivirals are produced by some plants such as eucalyptus.

Medical Uses

Most of the antiviral drugs now available are designed to help deal with HIV, herpes viruses, the hepatitis B and C viruses, and influenza A and B viruses. Researchers are working to extend the range of antivirals to other families of pathogens.

Designing safe and effective antiviral drugs is difficult, because viruses use the host's cells to replicate. This makes it difficult to find targets for the drug that would interfere with the virus without also harming the host organism's cells. Moreover, the major difficulty in developing vaccines and anti-viral drugs is due to viral variation.

The emergence of antivirals is the product of a greatly expanded knowledge of the genetic and molecular function of organisms, allowing biomedical researchers to understand the structure and function of viruses, major advances in the techniques for finding new drugs, and the intense pressure placed on the medical profession to deal with the human immunodeficiency virus (HIV), the cause of the deadly acquired immunodeficiency syndrome (AIDS) pandemic.

The first experimental antivirals were developed in the 1960's, mostly to deal with herpes viruses, and were found using traditional trial-and-error drug discovery methods. Researchers grew cultures of cells and infected them with the target virus. They then introduced into the cultures chemicals which they thought might inhibit viral activity, and observed whether the level of virus in the cultures rose or fell. Chemicals that seemed to have an effect were selected for closer study.

This was a very time-consuming, hit-or-miss procedure, and in the absence of a good knowledge of how the target virus worked, it was not efficient in discovering effective antivirals which had few side effects. Only in the 1980's when the full genetic sequences of viruses began to be unraveled, did researchers begin to learn how viruses worked in detail, and exactly what chemicals were needed to thwart their reproductive cycle.

Sedative

A sedative or tranquillizer is a substance that induces sedation by reducing irritability or excitement.

At higher doses it may result in slurred speech, staggering gait, poor judgment, and slow, uncertain reflexes. Doses of sedatives such as benzodiazepines, when used as a hypnotic to induce sleep, tend to be higher than amounts used to relieve anxiety, whereas only low doses are needed to provide a peaceful effect.

Sedatives can be misused to produce an overly-calming effect (alcohol being the classic and most common sedating drug). In the event of an overdose or if combined with another sedative, many of these drugs can cause unconsciousness and even death.

Therapeutic Use

Doctors often administer sedatives to patients in order to dull the patient's anxiety related to painful or anxiety-provoking procedures. Although sedatives do not relieve pain in themselves, they can be a useful adjunct to analgesics in preparing patients for surgery, and are commonly given to patients before they are anaesthetized, or before other highly uncomfortable and invasive procedures like cardiac catheterization, colonoscopy or MRI. They increase tractability and compliance of children or troublesome or demanding patients.

AMALGAMATED CLASSES

Some drug classes have been amalgamated from these three principles to meet practical needs. The class of non-steroidal anti-inflammatory drugs (NSAIDs) is one such example. Strictly speaking, and also historically, the wider class of anti-inflammatory drugs also comprises *steroidal* anti-inflammatory drugs. These drugs were in fact the predominant anti-inflammatories during the decade leading up to the introduction of the term "non-steroidal anti-inflammatory drugs". Because of the disastrous reputation that the corticosteroids had got in the 1950s, the new term, which offered to signal that an anti-inflammatory drug was not a steroid, rapidly gained currency. The drug class of "non-steroidal anti-inflammatory drugs" (NSAIDs) is thus composed by one element ("anti-inflammatory") that designates the mechanism of action, and one element ("non-steroidal") that separates it from other drugs with that same mechanism of action. Similarly, one might argue that the class of disease-modifying anti-rheumatic drugs (DMARD) is composed by one element ("disease-modifying") that albeit vaguely designates a mechanism of action, and one element ("anti-rheumatic drug") that indicates its therapeutic use.

- Nonsteroidal anti-inflammatory drug (NSAID)
- Disease-modifying antirheumatic drug (DMARD)

REFERENCES

1. Mahoney A, Evans J (2008). "Comparing drug classification systems". AMIA Annual Symposium Proceedings: 1039. PMID 18999016.

2. World Health Organization (2003). Introduction to drug utilization research (PDF). Geneva: World Health Organization. p. 33. ISBN 924156234X.
3. Imming P, Sinning C, Meyer A (Oct 2006). "Drugs, their targets and the nature and number of drug targets". Nature Reviews. Drug Discovery. 5 (10): 821–34. doi:10.1038/nrd2132. PMID 17016423.
4. Buer JK (Oct 2014). "Origins and impact of the term 'NSAID'". Inflammopharmacology. 22 (5): 263–7. doi:10.1007/s10787-014-0211-2. PMID 25064056.
5. Buer JK (Aug 2015). "A history of the term "DMARD"". Inflammopharmacology. 23 (4): 163–71. doi:10.1007/s10787-015-0232-5. PMC 4508364Freely accessible. PMID 26002695.
6. Holten KB, Onusko EM (August 2000). "Appropriate prescribing of oral beta-lactam antibiotics". American Family Physician. 62 (3): 611–20. PMID 10950216.
7. Elander, R. P. (2003). "Industrial production of beta-lactam antibiotics". Applied microbiology and biotechnology. 61 (5–6): 385–392. doi:10.1007/s00253-003-1274-y. PMID 12679848.
8. Rossi S (Ed.) (2004). Australian Medicines Handbook 2004. Adelaide: Australian Medicines Handbook. ISBN 0-9578521-4-2.
9. Pichichero ME (April 2005). "A review of evidence supporting the American Academy of Pediatrics recommendation for prescribing cephalosporin antibiotics for penicillin-allergic patients". Pediatrics. 115 (4): 1048–57. doi:10.1542/peds.2004-1276. PMID 15805383.
10. Fisher, J. F.; Meroueh, S. O.; Mobashery, S. (2005). "Bacterial Resistance to β-Lactam Antibiotics: Compelling Opportunism, Compelling Opportunity†». Chemical Reviews. 105 (2): 395–424. doi:10.1021/cr030102i. PMID 15700950.
11. Kasten, B.; Reski, R. (1997-01-01). «β-Lactam antibiotics inhibit chloroplast division in a moss (Physcomitrella patens) but not in tomato (Lycopersicon esculentum)». Journal of Plant Physiology. 150 (1): 137–140. doi:10.1016/S0176-1617(97)80193-9.
12. Nangia, Ashwini; Biradha, Kumar; Desiraju, Gautam R. (1996-01-01). «Correlation of biological activity in β-lactam antibiotics with Woodward and Cohen structural parameters—a Cambridge database study». J. Chem. Soc., Perkin Trans. 2 (5): 943–953. doi:10.1039/p29960000943. ISSN 1364-5471.
13. Woodward, R. B. (1980-05-16). «Penems and Related Substances». Philosophical Transactions of the Royal Society of London B: Biological Sciences. 289 (1036): 239–250. doi:10.1098/rstb.1980.0042. ISSN 0962-8436. PMID 6109320.
14. Cohen, N. Claude (1983-02-01). «.beta.-Lactam antibiotics: geometrical requirements for antibacterial activities». Journal of Medicinal Chemistry. 26 (2): 259–264. doi:10.1021/jm00356a027. ISSN 0022-2623.
15. Drawz, S. M.; Bonomo, R. A. (2010). «Three Decades of β-Lactamase Inhibitors». Clinical Microbiology Reviews. 23 (1): 160–201. doi:10.1128/CMR.00037-09. PMC 2806661Freely accessible. PMID 20065329.

16. Leonard, David A.; Bonomo, Robert A.; Powers, Rachel A. (2013-11-19). «Class D β-Lactamases: A Reappraisal after Five Decades». Accounts of Chemical Research. 46 (11): 2407–2415. doi:10.1021/ar300327a. ISSN 0001-4842. PMC 4018812Freely accessible. PMID 23902256.
17. Macdougall C (2011). «Beyond Susceptible and Resistant Part I: Treatment of Infections Due to Gram-Negative Organisms with Inducible B-lactamases». Journal of Pediatric Pharmacology and Therapeutics. 16 (1): 23–30. PMC 3136230Freely accessible. PMID 22477821.
18. Dalhoff, A.; Janjic, N.; Echols, R. (2006). «Redefining penems». Biochemical Pharmacology. 71 (7): 1085–1095. doi:10.1016/j.bcp.2005.12.003. PMID 16413506.
19. Lundberg, M.; Siegbahn, P. E. M.; Morokuma, K. (2008). «The Mechanism for Isopenicillin N Synthase from Density-Functional Modeling Highlights the Similarities with Other Enzymes in the 2-His-1-carboxylate Family†». Biochemistry. 47 (3): 1031–1042. doi:10.1021/bi701577q. PMID 18163649.
20. Bachmann, B. O.; Li, R.; Townsend, C. A. (1998). «B-Lactam synthetase: A new biosynthetic enzyme». Proceedings of the National Academy of Sciences of the United States of America. 95 (16): 9082–9086. doi:10.1073/pnas.95.16.9082. PMC 21295Freely accessible. PMID 9689037.
21. Townsend, CA; Brown, AM; Nguyen, LT (1983). «Nocardicin A: Stereochemical and biomimetic studies of monocyclic β-lactam formation». Journal of the American Society. 105 (4): 919–927. doi:10.1021/ja00342a047.

CHAPTER 9

Pharmacodynamics and Pharmacokinetics

Chapter Contents

Pharmacodynamics (sometimes described as what a drug does to the body) is the study of the biochemical, physiologic, and molecular effects of drugs on the body and involves receptor binding (including receptor sensitivity), postreceptor effects, and chemical interactions. Pharmacodynamics, with pharmacokinetics (what the body does to a drug, or the fate of a drug within the body), helps explain the relationship between the dose and response, i.e., the drug's effects. The pharmacologic response depends on the drug binding to its target. The concentration of the drug at the receptor site influences the drug's effect.

INTRODUCTION

Pharmacodynamics is the study of the biochemical and physiologic effects of drugs (especially pharmaceutical drugs). The effects can include those manifested within animals (including humans), microorganisms, or combinations of organisms (for example, infection). Pharmacodynamics is the study of how a drug affects an organism, whereas pharmacokinetics is the study of how the organism affects the drug. Both together influence dosing, benefit, and adverse effects. Pharmacodynamics is sometimes abbreviated as **PD** and pharmacokinetics as PK, especially in combined reference (for example, when speaking of PK/PD models).

Pharmacodynamics places particular emphasis on dose–response relationships, that is, the relationships between drug concentration and effect. One dominant example is drug-receptor interactions as modeled by

$$L + R \rightleftharpoons L{\cdot}R$$

where *L*, *R*, and *LR* represent ligand (drug), receptor, and ligand-receptor complex concentrations, respectively. This equation represents a simplified model of reaction dynamics that can be studied mathematically through tools such as free energy maps.

EFFECTS ON THE BODY

The majority of drugs either

(a) mimic or inhibit normal physiological/biochemical processes or inhibit pathological processes in animals or

(b) inhibit vital processes of endo- or ectoparasites and microbial organisms. There are 7 main drug actions:

- stimulating action through direct receptor agonism and downstream effects;
- depressing action through direct receptor agonism and downstream effects (ex.: inverse agonist);
- blocking/antagonizing action (as with silent antagonists), the drug binds the receptor but does not activate it;
- stabilizing action, the drug seems to act neither as a stimulant or as a depressant (ex.: some drugs possess receptor activity that allows them to stabilize general receptor activation, like buprenorphine in opioid dependent individuals or aripiprazole in schizophrenia, all depending on the dose and the recipient);
- exchanging/replacing substances or accumulating them to form a reserve (ex.: glycogen storage);
- direct beneficial chemical reaction as in free radical scavenging and
- direct harmful chemical reaction which might result in damage or destruction of the cells, through induced toxic or lethal damage (cytotoxicity or irritation).

DESIRED ACTIVITY

The desired activity of a drug is mainly due to successful targeting of one of the following:

- Cellular membrane disruption;
- Chemical reaction with downstream effects;
- Interaction with enzyme proteins;
- Interaction with structural proteins;
- Interaction with carrier proteins;
- Interaction with ion channels and

- Ligand binding to receptors:
  - Hormone receptors
  - Neuromodulator receptors
  - Neurotransmitter receptors.

General anesthetics were once thought to work by disordering the neural membranes, thereby altering the Na^+ influx. Antacids and chelating agents combine chemically in the body. Enzyme-substrate binding is a way to alter the production or metabolism of key endogenous chemicals, for example aspirin irreversibly inhibits the enzyme prostaglandin synthetase (cyclooxygenase) thereby preventing inflammatory response. Colchicine, a drug for gout, interferes with the function of the structural protein tubulin, while Digitalis, a drug still used in heart failure, inhibits the activity of the carrier molecule, Na-K-ATPase pump. The widest class of drugs act as ligands which bind to receptors which determine cellular effects. Upon drug binding, receptors can elicit their normal action (agonist), blocked action (antagonist), or even action opposite to normal (inverse agonist).

In principle, a pharmacologist would aim for a target plasma concentration of the drug for a desired level of response. In reality, there are many factors affecting this goal. Pharmacokinetic factors determine peak concentrations, and concentrations cannot be maintained with absolute consistency because of metabolic breakdown and excretory clearance. Genetic factors may exist which would alter metabolism or drug action itself, and a patient's immediate status may also affect indicated dosage.

Undesirable Effects

Undesirable effects of a drug include:

- Increased probability of cell mutation (carcinogenic activity);
- A multitude of simultaneous assorted actions which may be deleterious;
- Interaction (additive, multiplicative, or metabolic) and
- Induced physiological damage, or abnormal chronic conditions.

Therapeutic Window

The therapeutic window is the amount of a medication between the amount that gives an effect (effective dose) and the amount that gives more adverse effects than desired effects. For instance, medication with a small pharmaceutical window must be administered with care and control, e.g. by frequently measuring blood concentration of the drug, since it easily loses effects or gives adverse effects.

Duration of Action

The *duration of action* of a drug is the length of time that particular drug is effective. Duration of action is a function of several parameters including plasma half-life, the time to equilibrate between plasma and target compartments, and the off rate of the drug from its biological target.

Receptor binding and effect

The binding of ligands (drug) to receptors is governed by the *law of mass action* which relates the large-scale status to the rate of numerous molecular processes. The rates of formation and un-formation can be used to determine the equilibrium concentration of bound receptors. The *equilibrium dissociation constant* is defined by:

$$L + R \leftrightarrow L{\cdot}R \qquad\qquad K_d = \frac{[L][R]}{[L{\cdot}R]}$$

where L=ligand, R=receptor, square brackets denote concentration. The fraction of bound receptors is

$$Fraction\ Bound = \frac{[L{\cdot}R]}{[R]+[L{\cdot}R]} = \frac{1}{1+\frac{K_d}{[L]}}$$

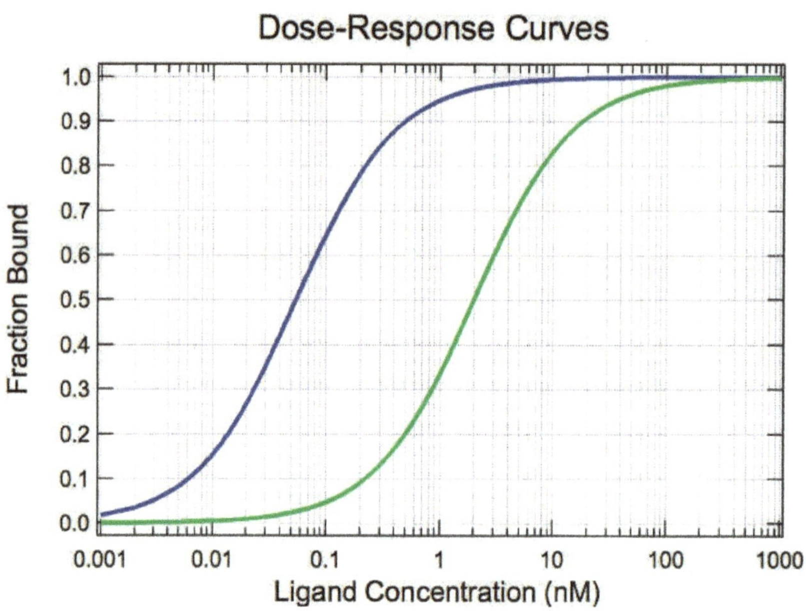

Semi-log plots of two agonists with different K_d. The blue curve represents the ligand with greater potency.

This expression is one way to consider the effect of a drug, in which the response is related to the fraction of bound receptors. The fraction of bound receptors is known as occupancy. The relationship between occupancy and pharmacological response is usually non-linear. This explains the so-called *receptor reserve* phenomenon i.e. the concentration producing 50% occupancy is typically higher than the concentration producing 50% of maximum response. More precisely, receptor reserve refers to a phenomenon whereby stimulation of only a fraction of the whole receptor population apparently elicits the maximal effect achievable in a particular tissue.

The simplest interpretation of receptor reserve is that it is a model that states there are excess receptors on the cell surface than what is necessary for full effect. Taking a more sophisticated approach, receptor reserve is an integrative measure of the response-inducing capacity of an agonist (in some receptor models it is termed intrinsic efficacy or intrinsic activity) and of the signal amplification capacity of the corresponding receptor (and its downstream signaling pathways). Thus, the existence (and magnitude) of receptor reserve depends on the agonist (efficacy), tissue (signal amplification ability) and measured effect (pathways activated to cause signal amplification). As receptor reserve is very sensitive to agonist's intrinsic efficacy, it is usually defined only for full (high-efficacy) agonists.

Often the response is determined as a function of $log[L]$ to consider many orders of magnitude of concentration. However, there is no biological or physical theory which relates effects to the log of concentration. It is just convenient for graphing purposes. It is useful to note that 50% of the receptors are bound when $[L]=K_d$.

The graph shown represents the conc-response for two hypothetical receptor agonists, plotted in a semi-log fashion. The curve toward the left represents a higher potency (potency arrow does not indicate direction of increase) since lower concentrations are needed for a given response. The effect increases as a function of concentration.

MULTICELLULAR PHARMACODYNAMICS

The concept of pharmacodynamics has been expanded to include Multicellular Pharmacodynamics (MCPD). MCPD is the study of the static and dynamic properties and relationships between a set of drugs and a dynamic and diverse multicellular four-dimensional organization. It is the study of the workings of a drug on a minimal multicellular system (mMCS), both *in vivo* and *in silico*. Networked Multicellular Pharmacodynamics (Net-MCPD) further extends the concept of MCPD to model regulatory genomic networks together with signal transduction pathways, as part of a complex of interacting components in the cell.

Toxicodynamics

Pharmacokinetics and pharmacodynamics are termed toxicokinetics and toxicodynamics in the field of ecotoxicology. Here, the focus is on toxic effects on a wide range of organisms. The corresponding models are called toxicokinetic-toxicodynamic models.

ANTIMICROBIAL PHARMACODYNAMICS

Antimicrobial pharmacodynamics is the relationship between concentration of antibiotic and its ability to inhibit vital processes of endo- or ectoparasites and microbial organisms. This branch of pharmacodynamics relates concentration of an anti-infective agent to effect, but specifically to its antimicrobial effect.

Concentration-dependent effects

The minimum inhibitory concentration and minimum bactericidal concentration are used to measure *in vitro* activity antimicrobial and is an excellent indicator of antimicrobial potency. They don't give any information relating to time-dependent antimicrobial killing the so-called post antibiotic effect.

Post Antibiotic Effect

The post antibiotic effect (PAE) is defined as persistent suppression of bacterial growth after a brief exposure (1 or 2 hours) of bacteria to an antibiotic even in the absence of host defense mechanisms. Factors that affect the duration of the post antibiotic effect include duration of antibiotic exposure, bacterial species, culture medium and class of antibiotic. It has been suggested that an alteration of DNA function is possibly responsible for post antibiotic effect following the observation that most inhibitors of protein and nucleic acid synthesis (aminoglycosides, fluoroquinolones, tetracyclines, clindamycin, certain newer macrolides/ketolides, and rifampicin and rifabutin) induce long-term PAE against susceptible bacteria. Theoretically, the ability of an antibiotic to induce a PAE is an attractive property of an antibiotic since antibiotic concentrations could fall below the MIC for the bacterium yet retain their effectiveness in their ability to suppress the growth. Therefore, an antibiotic with PAE would require less frequent administration and it could improve patient adherence with regard to pharmacotherapy. Proposed mechanisms include (1) slow recovery after reversible nonlethal damage to cell structures; (2) persistence of the drug at a binding site or within the periplasmic space; and (3) the need to synthesize new enzymes before growth can resume. Most antimicrobials possess significant in vitro PAEs ($\geq$ 1.5 hours) against susceptible gram-positive cocci . Antimicrobials with significant PAEs against susceptible gram-negative bacilli are limited to carbapenems and agents that inhibit protein or DNA synthesis.

PHARMACOKINETICS

Pharmacokinetics (from Ancient Greek *pharmakon* "drug" and *kinetikos* "moving, putting in motion"; see chemical kinetics), sometimes abbreviated as **PK**, is a branch of pharmacology dedicated to determining the fate of substances administered to a living organism. The substances of interest include any chemical xenobiotic such as: pharmaceutical drugs, pesticides, food additives, cosmetic ingredients, etc. It attempts to analyze chemical metabolism and to discover the fate of a chemical from the moment that it is administered up to the point at which it is completely eliminated from the body. Pharmacokinetics is the study of how an organism affects a drug, whereas pharmacodynamics is the study of how the drug affects the organism. Both together influence dosing, benefit, and adverse effects, as seen in PK/PD models.

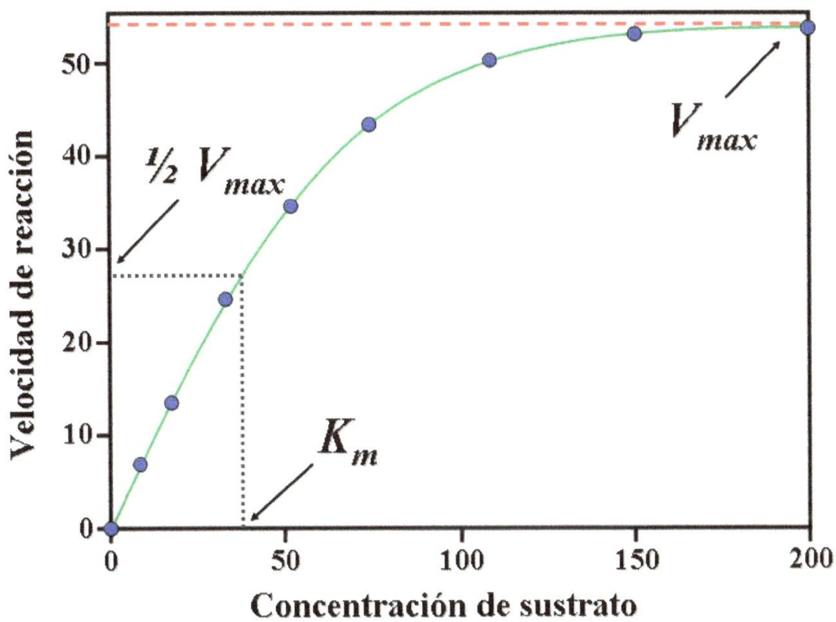

Graph that demonstrates the Michaelis-Menten kinetics model for the relationship between an enzyme and a substrate: one of the parameters studies in pharmacokinetics, where the substrate is a pharmaceutical drug.

Pharmacokinetics describes how the body affects a specific xenobiotic/chemical after administration through the mechanisms of absorption and distribution, as well as the metabolic changes of the substance in the body (e.g. by metabolic enzymes such as cytochrome P450 or glucuronosyltransferase enzymes), and the effects and routes of excretion of the metabolites of the drug. Pharmacokinetic properties of chemicals are affected by the route of administration and the dose of administered drug. These may affect the absorption rate.

Models have been developed to simplify conceptualization of the many processes that take place in the interaction between an organism and a chemical substance. One of these, the multi-compartmental model, gives the best approximation to reality; however, the complexity involved means that *monocompartmental models* and above all *two compartmental models* are the most-frequently used. The various compartments that the model is divided into are commonly referred to as the ADME scheme (also referred to as LADME if liberation is included as a separate step from absorption):

- **L**iberation - the process of release of a drug from the pharmaceutical formulation.
- **A**bsorption - the process of a substance entering the blood circulation.
- **D**istribution - the dispersion or dissemination of substances throughout the fluids and tissues of the body.

- **M**etabolism (or biotransformation, or inactivation) – the recognition by the organism that a foreign substance is present and the irreversible transformation of parent compounds into daughter metabolites.
- **E**xcretion - the removal of the substances from the body. In rare cases, some drugs irreversibly accumulate in body tissue.

The two phases of metabolism and excretion can also be grouped together under the title elimination. The study of these distinct phases involves the use and manipulation of basic concepts in order to understand the process dynamics. For this reason in order to fully comprehend the *kinetics* of a drug it is necessary to have detailed knowledge of a number of factors such as: the properties of the substances that act as excipients, the characteristics of the appropriate biological membranes and the way that substances can cross them, or the characteristics of the enzyme reactions that inactivate the drug.

All these concepts can be represented through mathematical formulas that have a corresponding graphical representation. The use of these models allows an understanding of the characteristics of a molecule, as well as how a particular drug will behave given information regarding some of its basic characteristics such as its acid dissociation constant (pKa), bioavailability and solubility, absorption capacity and distribution in the organism.

The model outputs for a drug can be used in industry (for example, in calculating bioequivalence when designing generic drugs) or in the clinical application of pharmacokinetic concepts. Clinical pharmacokinetics provides many performance guidelines for effective and efficient use of drugs for human-health professionals and in veterinary medicine.

Metrics

The following are the most commonly measured pharmacokinetic metrics:

Characteristic	Description	Example value	Symbol	Formula
Dose	Amount of drug administered.	500 mg	D	Design parameter
Dosing interval	Time between drug dose administrations.	24 h	τ	Design parameter
C_{max}	The peak plasma concentration of a drug after administration.	60.9 mg/L	C_{max}	Direct measurement
t_{max}	Time to reach C_{max}.	3.9 h	t_{max}	Direct measurement
C_{min}	The lowest (trough) concentration that a drug reaches before the next dose is administered.	27.7 mg/L	$C_{min,ss}$	Direct measurement

Volume of distribution	The apparent volume in which a drug is distributed (i.e., the parameter relating drug concentration to drug amount in the body).	6.0 L	V_d	$= \frac{D}{C_0}$
Concentration	Amount of drug in a given volume of plasma.	83.3 mg/L	C_0, C_{ss}	$= \frac{D}{V_d}$
Elimination half-life	The time required for the concentration of the drug to reach half of its original value.	12 h	$t_{\frac{1}{2}}$	$= \frac{\ln(2)}{k_e}$
Elimination rate constant	The rate at which a drug is removed from the body.	0.0578 h^{-1}	k_e	$= \frac{\ln(2)}{t_{\frac{1}{2}}} = \frac{CL}{V_d}$
Infusion rate	Rate of infusion required to balance elimination.	50 mg/h	k_{in}	$= C_{ss} \cdot CL$
Area under the curve	The integral of the concentration-time curve (after a single dose or in steady state).	1,320 mg/L·h	$AUC_{0-\infty}$	$= \int_0^\infty C \, dt$
			$AUC_{\tau,ss}$	$= \int_t^{t+\tau} C \, dt$
Clearance	The volume of plasma cleared of the drug per unit time.	0.38 L/h	CL	$= V_d \cdot k_e = \frac{D}{AUC}$
Bioavailability	The systemically available fraction of a drug.	0.8	f	$= \frac{AUC_{po} \cdot D_{iv}}{AUC_{iv} \cdot D_{po}}$
Fluctuation	Peak trough fluctuation within one dosing interval at steady state	41.8 %	$\%PTF$	$= \frac{C_{max,ss} - C_{min,ss}}{C_{av,ss}} \cdot 100$ Where $C_{av,ss} = \frac{1}{\tau} AUC_{\tau,ss}$

In pharmacokinetics, *steady state* refers to the situation where the overall intake of a drug is fairly in dynamic equilibrium with its elimination. In practice, it is generally considered that steady state is reached when a time of 4 to 5 times the half-life for a drug after regular dosing is started.

The following graph depicts a typical time course of drug plasma concentration and illustrates main pharmacokinetic metrics:

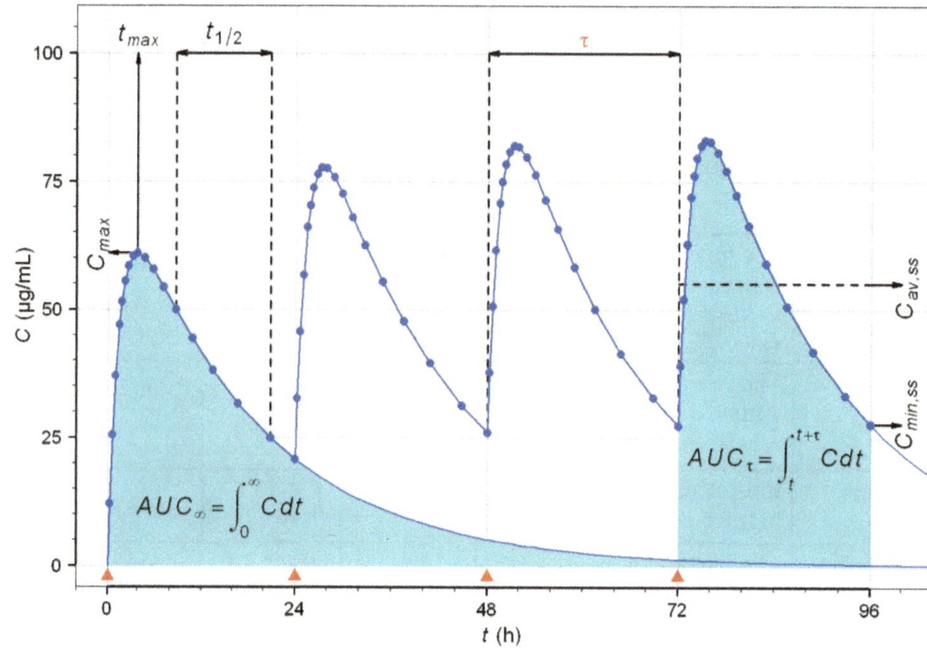

The time course of drug plasma concentrations over 96 hours following oral administrations every 24 hours. Note that the AUC in steady state equals AUC_∞ after the first dose.

Pharmacokinetic Models

Pharmacokinetic modelling is performed by noncompartmental or compartmental methods. Noncompartmental methods estimate the exposure to a drug by estimating the area under the curve of a concentration-time graph. Compartmental methods estimate the concentration-time graph using kinetic models. Noncompartmental methods are often more versatile in that they do not assume any specific compartmental model and produce accurate results also acceptable for bioequivalence studies. The final outcome of the transformations that a drug undergoes in an organism and the rules that determine this fate depend on a number of interrelated factors. A number of functional models have been developed in order to simplify the study of pharmacokinetics. These models are based on a consideration of an organism as a number of related compartments. The simplest idea is to think of an organism as only one homogenous compartment. This *monocompartimental model* presupposes that blood plasma concentrations of the drug are a true reflection of the drug's concentration in other fluids or tissues and that the elimination of the drug is directly proportional to the drug's concentration in the organism (first order kinetics).

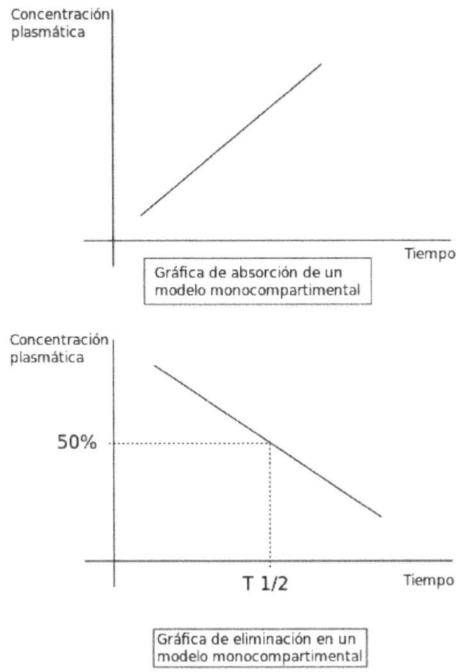

Graph representing the monocompartmental action model.

However, these models do not always truly reflect the real situation within an organism. For example, not all body tissues have the same blood supply, so the distribution of the drug will be slower in these tissues than in others with a better blood supply. In addition, there are some tissues (such as the brain tissue) that present a real barrier to the distribution of drugs, that can be breached with greater or lesser ease depending on the drug's characteristics. If these relative conditions for the different tissue types are considered along with the rate of elimination, the organism can be considered to be acting like two compartments: one that we can call the *central compartment* that has a more rapid distribution, comprising organs and systems with a well-developed blood supply; and a *peripheral compartment* made up of organs with a lower blood flow. Other tissues, such as the brain, can occupy a variable position depending on a drug's ability to cross the barrier that separates the organ from the blood supply.

This *two compartment model* will vary depending on which compartment elimination occurs in. The most common situation is that elimination occurs in the central compartment as the liver and kidneys are organs with a good blood supply. However, in some situations it may be that elimination occurs in the peripheral compartment or even in both. This can mean that there are three possible variations in the two compartment model, which still do not cover all possibilities.

This model may not be applicable in situations where some of the enzymes responsible for metabolizing the drug become saturated, or where an active elimination mechanism is present that is independent of the drug's plasma concentration. In the real world each tissue will have its own distribution characteristics and none of them will be strictly linear. If we label the drug's volume of distribution within the organism $\mathbf{Vd_F}$ and its volume of distribution in a tissue $\mathbf{Vd_T}$the former will be described by an equation that takes into account all the tissues that act in different ways, that is:

$$Vd_F = Vd_{T1} + Vd_{T2} + Vd_{T3} + \ldots + Vd_{Tn}$$

This represents the *multi-compartment model* with a number of curves that express complicated equations in order to obtain an overall curve. A number of computer programs have been developed to plot these equations. However complicated and precise this model may be, it still does not truly represent reality despite the effort involved in obtaining various distribution values for a drug. This is because the concept of distribution volume is a relative concept that is not a true reflection of reality. The choice of model therefore comes down to deciding which one offers the lowest margin of error for the drug involved.

Noncompartmental Analysis

Noncompartmental PK analysis is highly dependent on estimation of total drug exposure. Total drug exposure is most often estimated by area under the curve (AUC) methods, with the trapezoidal rule (numerical integration) the most common method. Due to the dependence on the length of 'x' in the trapezoidal rule, the area estimation is highly dependent on the blood/plasma sampling schedule. That is, the closer time points are, the closer the trapezoids reflect the actual shape of the concentration-time curve.

Compartmental Analysis

Compartmental PK analysis uses kinetic models to describe and predict the concentration-time curve. PK compartmental models are often similar to kinetic models used in other scientific disciplines such as chemical kinetics and thermodynamics. The advantage of compartmental over some noncompartmental analyses is the ability to predict the concentration at any time. The disadvantage is the difficulty in developing and validating the proper model. Compartment-free modelling based on curve stripping does not suffer this limitation. The simplest PK compartmental model is the one-compartmental PK model with IV bolus administration and first-order elimination. The most complex PK models (called PBPK models) rely on the use of physiological information to ease development and validation.

Single-Compartment Model

Linear pharmacokinetics is so-called because the graph of the relationship between the various factors involved (dose, blood plasma concentrations, elimination, etc.) gives a straight line or an approximation to one. For drugs to be effective they need to be able to move rapidly from blood plasma to other body fluids and tissues.

The change in concentration over time can be expressed as $C = C_{initial} * e^{-kelt}$

Multi-Compartmental Models

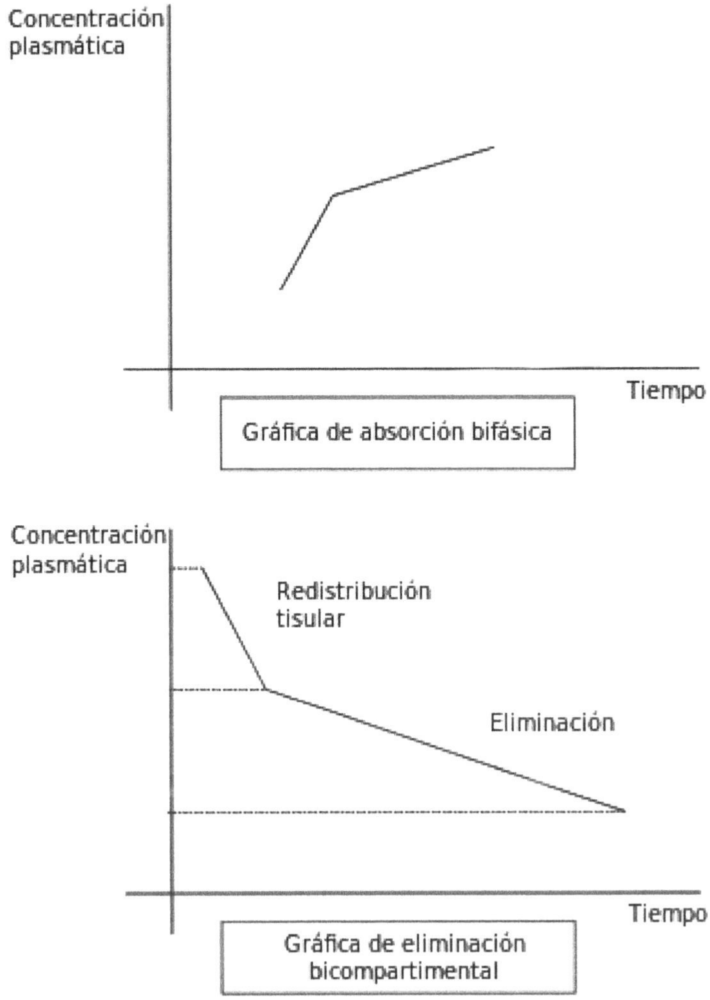

Graphs for absorption and elimination for a non-linear pharmacokinetic model.

The graph for the non-linear relationship between the various factors is represented by a curve, the relationships between the factors can then be found by calculating the dimensions of different areas under the curve. The models used in '*non linear pharmacokinetics* are largely based on Michaelis-Menten kinetics. A reaction's factors of non linearity include the following:

- Multiphasic absorption: Drugs injected intravenously are removed from the plasma through two primary mechanisms: (1) Distribution to body tissues and (2) metabolism + excretion of the drugs. The resulting decrease of the drug's plasma concentration follows a biphasic pattern (see figure).

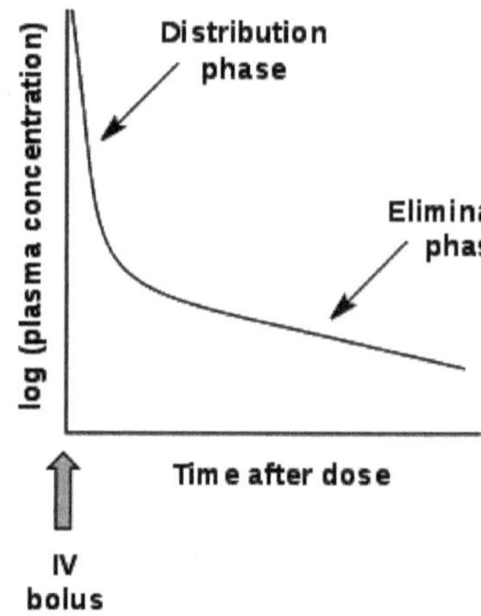

Plasma drug concentration vs time after an IV dose

- **Alpha phase**: An initial phase of rapid decrease in plasma concentration. The decrease is primarily attributed to drug distribution from the central compartment (circulation) into the peripheral compartments (body tissues). This phase ends when a pseudo-equilibrium of drug concentration is established between the central and peripheral compartments.
- **Beta phase**: A phase of gradual decrease in plasma concentration after the alpha phase. The decrease is primarily attributed to drug metabolism and excretion.
- Additional phases (gamma, delta, etc.) are sometimes seen.
- A drug's characteristics make a clear distinction between tissues with high and low blood flow.
- Enzymatic saturation: When the dose of a drug whose elimination depends on biotransformation is increased above a certain threshold the enzymes responsible for its metabolism become saturated. The drug's plasma concentration will then increase disproportionately and its elimination will no longer be constant.
- Induction or enzymatic inhibition: Some drugs have the capacity to inhibit or stimulate their own metabolism, in negative or positive feedback reactions. As occurs with fluvoxamine, fluoxetine and phenytoin. As larger doses of these pharmaceuticals are administered the plasma concentrations of the unmetabolized drug increases and the elimination half-life increases. It is therefore necessary to adjust the dose or other treatment parameters when a high dosage is required.
- The kidneys can also establish active elimination mechanisms for some drugs, independent of plasma concentrations.

It can therefore be seen that non-linearity can occur because of reasons that affect the entire pharmacokinetic sequence: absorption, distribution, metabolism and elimination.

Variable Volume in Time Models

Variable volume pharmacokinetic models can be a drug centered models that assign a volume of drug distribution to be where the drug is at that time. Another possibility occurs when the body volume is changing in time, which would occur, for example, during dialysis when the volume in which a drug can be distributed is itself changing in time.

At a practical level, a drug's bioavailability can be defined as the proportion of the drug that reaches its site of action. From this perspective the intravenousadministration of a drug provides the greatest possible bioavailability, and this method is considered to yield a bioavailability of 1 (or 100%). Bioavailability of other delivery methods is compared with that of intravenous injection («absolute bioavailability») or to a standard value related to other delivery methods in a particular study («relative bioavailability»).

$$B_A = \frac{[ABC]_P . D_{IV}}{[ABC]_{IV} . D_P}$$

$$B_R = \frac{[ABC]_A . dose_B}{[ABC]_B . dose_A}$$

Once a drug's bioavailability has been established it is possible to calculate the changes that need to be made to its dosage in order to reach the required blood plasma levels. Bioavailability is therefore a mathematical factor for each individual drug that influences the administered dose. It is possible to calculate the amount of a drug in the blood plasma that has a real potential to bring about its effect using the formula: $De = B. Da$; where *De* is the effective dose, *B* bioavailability and *Da* the administered dose.

Therefore, if a drug has a bioavailability of 0.8 (or 80%) and it is administered in a dose of 100 mg, the equation will demonstrate the following:

De = 0.8 x 100 mg = 80 mg

That is the 100 mg administered represents a blood plasma concentration of 80 mg that has the capacity to have a pharmaceutical effect.

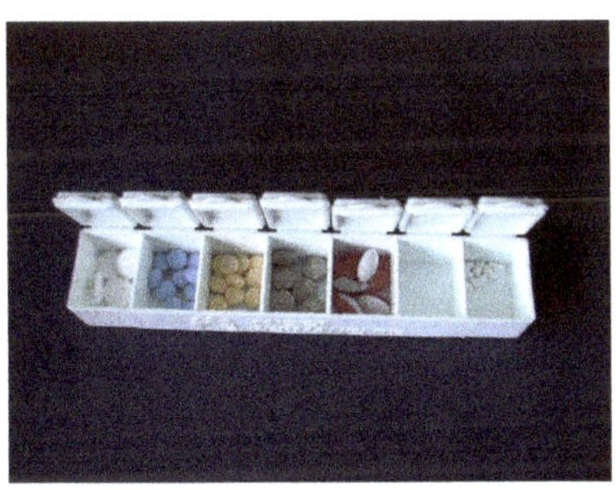

Different forms of tablets, which will have different pharmacokinetic behaviors after their administration.

This concept depends on a series of factors inherent to each drug, such as:

- Pharmaceutical form;

- Chemical form;
- Route of administration;
- Stability and
- Metabolism.

These concepts, which are discussed in detail in their respective titled articles, can be mathematically quantified and integrated to obtain an overall mathematical equation:

$$De = Q.Da.B$$

where **Q** is the drug's purity.

$$Va = \frac{Da.B.Q}{\tau}$$

where V_a is the drug's rate of administration and t is the rate at which the absorbed drug reaches the circulatory system.

Finally, using the Henderson-Hasselbalch equation, and knowing the drug's pKa (pH at which there is an equilibrium between its ionized and non ionized molecules), it is possible to calculate the non ionized concentration of the drug and therefore the concentration that will be subject to absorption:

$$pH = pKa + log\frac{B}{A}$$

When two drugs have the same bioavailability, they are said to be biological equivalents or bioequivalents. This concept of bioequivalence is important because it is currently used as a yardstick in the authorization of generic drugs in many countries .

LADME

A number of phases occur once the drug enters into contact with the organism, these are described using the acronym LADME:

- Liberation of the active substance from the delivery system,
- Absorption of the active substance by the organism,
- Distribution through the blood plasma and different body tissues,
- Metabolism that is, inactivation of the xenobiotic substance, and finally
- Excretion or elimination of the substance or the products of its metabolism.

Some textbooks combine the first two phases as the drug is often administered in an active form, which means that there is no liberation phase. Others include a phase that combines distribution, metabolism and excretion into a «disposition phase». Other authors include the drug's toxicological aspect in what is known as *ADME-Tox* or *ADMET*.

Each of the phases is subject to physico-chemical interactions between a drug and an organism, which can be expressed mathematically. Pharmacokinetics is therefore based on mathematical equations that allow the prediction of a drug's behavior and which place great emphasis on the relationships between drug plasma concentrations and the time elapsed since the drug's administration.

Analysis

Bioanalytical Methods

Bioanalytical methods are necessary to construct a concentration-time profile. Chemical techniques are employed to measure the concentration of drugs in biological matrix, most often plasma. Proper bioanalytical methods should be selective and sensitive. For example, microscale thermophoresis can be used to quantify how the biological matrix/ liquid affects the affinity of a drug to its target.

Mass Spectrometry

Pharmacokinetics is often studied using mass spectrometry because of the complex nature of the matrix (often plasma or urine) and the need for high sensitivity to observe concentrations after a low dose and a long time period. The most common instrumentation used in this application is LC-MS with a triple quadrupole mass spectrometer. Tandem mass spectrometry is usually employed for added specificity. Standard curves and internal standards are used for quantitation of usually a single pharmaceutical in the samples. The samples represent different time points as a pharmaceutical is administered and then metabolized or cleared from the body. Blank samples taken before administration are important in determining background and ensuring data integrity with such complex sample matrices. Much attention is paid to the linearity of the standard curve; however it is common to use curve fitting with more complex functions such as quadratics since the response of most mass spectrometers is less than linear across large concentration ranges.

There is currently considerable interest in the use of very high sensitivity mass spectrometry for microdosing studies, which are seen as a promising alternative to animal experimentation.

Population Pharmacokinetics

Population pharmacokinetics is the study of the sources and correlates of variability in drug concentrations among individuals who are the target patient population receiving clinically relevant doses of a drug of interest. Certain patient demographic, pathophysiological, and therapeutical features, such as body weight, excretory and metabolic functions, and the presence of other therapies, can regularly alter dose-concentration relationships. For example, steady-state concentrations of drugs eliminated mostly by the kidney are usually greater in patients suffering from renal failure than they are in patients with normal renal function receiving the same drug dosage. Population pharmacokinetics seeks to identify the measurable pathophysiologic factors that cause changes in the dose-concentration relationship and the extent of these changes so that, if such changes are associated with clinically significant shifts in the therapeutic index, dosage can be appropriately modified.

An advantage of population pharmacokinetic modelling is its ability to analyse sparse data sets (sometimes only one concentration measurement per patient is available).

Software packages used in population pharmacokinetics modelling include NONMEM, which was developed at the UCSF and newer packages which incorporate GUIs like Monolix as well as graphical model building tools; Phoenix NLME.

Clinical Pharmacokinetics

Clinical pharmacokinetics (arising from the clinical use of population pharmacokinetics) is the direct application to a therapeutic situation of knowledge regarding a drug's pharmacokinetics and the characteristics of a population that a patient belongs to (or can be ascribed to).

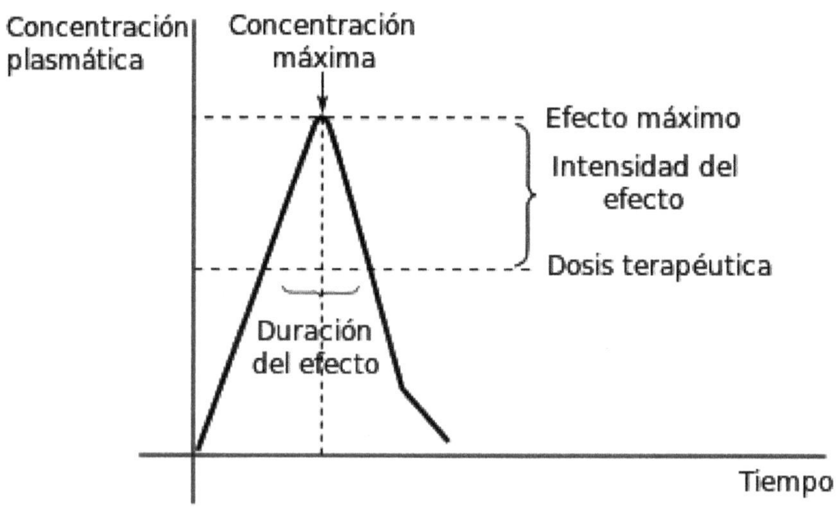

Basic graph for evaluating the therapeutic implications of pharmacokinetics.

An example is the relaunch of the use of ciclosporin as an immunosuppressor to facilitate organ transplant. The drug's therapeutic properties were initially demonstrated, but it was almost never used after it was found to cause nephrotoxicity in a number of patients. However, it was then realized that it was possible to individualize a patient's dose of ciclosporin by analyzing the patients plasmatic concentrations (pharmacokinetic monitoring). This practice has allowed this drug to be used again and has facilitated a great number of organ transplants.

Clinical monitoring is usually carried out by determination of plasma concentrations as this data is usually the easiest to obtain and the most reliable. The main reasons for determining a drug's plasma concentration include:

- Narrow therapeutic range (difference between toxic and therapeutic concentrations)
- High toxicity
- High risk to life.

Drugs where pharmacokinetic monitoring is recommended include:

Medication for which monitoring is recommended.			
• Antiepileptic medication + Phenytoin + Carbamazepine + Valproic acid + Lamotrigine + Ethosuximide + Phenobarbital + Primidone	• Cardioactive medication + Digoxin + Lidocaine	• Immunosuppressor medication + Ciclosporin + Tacrolimus + Sirolimus + Everolimus + Mycophenolate	• Antibiotic medication + Gentamicin + Tobramycin + Amikacin + Vancomycin
• Bronchodilator medication + Theophylline	• Cytostatic medication + Methotrexate + 5-Fluorouracil + Irinotecan	* Antiviral (HIV) medication + Efavirenz + Tenofovir + Ritonavir	• Coagulation factors + Factor VIII, + Factor IX, + Factor VIIa, + Factor XI

Ecotoxicology

Ecotoxicology is the branch of science that deals with the nature, effects, and interactions of substances that are harmful to the environment.

REFERENCES

1. Lees P, Cunningham FM, Elliott J (2004). "Principles of pharmacodynamics and their applications in veterinary pharmacology". J. Vet. Pharmacol. Ther. 27 (6): 397–414. doi:10.1111/j.1365-2885.2004.00620.x. PMID 15601436.
2. Carruthers SG (February 1980). "Duration of drug action". Am. Fam. Physician. 21 (2): 119–26. PMID 7352385.
3. Vauquelin G, Charlton SJ (October 2010). "Long-lasting target binding and rebinding as mechanisms to prolong in vivo drug action". Br. J. Pharmacol. 161 (3): 488–508. doi:10.1111/j.1476-5381.2010.00936.x. PMC 2990149Freely accessible. PMID 20880390.
4. Ruffolo RR Jr (December 1982). "Review important concepts of receptor theory". J. Auton. Pharmacol. 2 (4): 277–295. PMID 7161296.
5. Dhalla AK, Shryock JC, Shreeniwas R, Belardinelli L (2003). "Pharmacology and therapeutic applications of A1 adenosine receptor ligands". Curr. Top. Med. Chem. 3 (4): 369–385. PMID 12570756.

6. Gesztelyi R, Kiss Z, Wachal Z, Juhasz B, Bombicz M, Csepanyi E, Pak K, Zsuga J, Papp C, Galajda Z, Branzaniuc K, Porszasz R, Szentmiklosi AJ, Tosaki A (2013). "The surmountable effect of FSCPX, an irreversible A(1) adenosine receptor antagonist, on the negative inotropic action of A(1) adenosine receptor full agonists in isolated guinea pig left atria". Arch. Pharm. Res. 36 (3): 293–305. doi:10.1007/s12272-013-0056-z. PMID 23456693.
7. Li Q, Hickman M (2011). "Toxicokinetic and toxicodynamic (TK/TD) evaluation to determine and predict the neurotoxicity of artemisinins". Toxicology. 279 (1-3): 1–9. doi:10.1016/j.tox.2010.09.005. PMID 20863871.
8. C.H. Nightingale, T. Murakawa, P.G. Ambrose (2002) Antimicrobial Pharmacodynamics in Theory and Clinical Practice Informa Health Care ISBN 0-8247-0561-0
9. Drusano GL (2004). "Antimicrobial pharmacodynamics: critical interactions of 'bug and drug'". Nat. Rev. Microbiol. 2 (4): 289–300. doi:10.1038/nrmicro862. PMID 15031728.
10. "Archived copy" (PDF). Archived from the original (PDF) on 2015-07-13. Retrieved 2008-11-13.
11. Guan L, Blumenthal RM, Burnham JC (October 1992). "Analysis of macromolecular biosynthesis to define the quinolone-induced postantibiotic effect in Escherichia coli". Antimicrob. Agents Chemother. 36 (10): 2118–24. doi:10.1128/aac.36.10.2118. PMC 245465Freely accessible. PMID 1280055.
12. Zarrini G, Bahari-Delgosha Z, Mollazadeh-Moghaddam K, Shahverdi AR (2010). "Post-antibacterial effect of thymol". Pharmaceutical biology. 48 (6): 633–636. doi:10.3109/13880200903229098. PMID 20645735.
13. Katzung basic and clinical pharmacology 13th edition 2015
14. Pharmacokinetics. (2006). In Mosby's Dictionary of Medicine, Nursing & Health Professions. Philadelphia, PA: Elsevier Health Sciences. Retrieved December 11, 2008, from http://www.credoreference.com/entry/6686418
15. Kathleen Knights; Bronwen Bryant (2002). Pharmacology for Health Professionals. Amsterdam: Elsevier. ISBN 0-7295-3664-5.
16. Koch HP, Ritschel WA (1986). "Liberation". Synopsis der Biopharmazie und Pharmakokinetik (in German). Landsberg, München: Ecomed. pp. 99–131. ISBN 3-609-64970-4.
17. Ruiz-Garcia A, Bermejo M, Moss A, Casabo VG (February 2008). "Pharmacokinetics in drug discovery". J Pharm Sci. 97 (2): 654–90. doi:10.1002/jps.21009. PMID 17630642.
18. AGAH working group PHARMACOKINETICS (2004-02-16). "Collection of terms, symbols, equations, and explanations of common pharmacokinetic and pharmacodynamic parameters and some statistical functions" (PDF). Arbeitsgemeinschaft für Angewandte Humanpharmakologie (AGAH) (Association for Applied Human Pharmacology). Retrieved 2011-04-04.

19. Milo Gibaldi, Donald Perrier. FarmacocinéticaReverté 1982 pages 1-10. ISBN 84-291-5535-X, 9788429155358
20. Gill SC, Moon-Mcdermott L, Hunt TL, Deresinski S, Blaschke T, Sandhaus RA (Sep 1999). "Phase I Pharmacokinetics of Liposomal Amikacin (MiKasome) in Human Subjects: Dose Dependence and Urinary Clearance". Abstr Intersci Conf Antimicrob Agents Chemother. 39: 33 (abstract no. 1195).
21. Weiner, Daniel; Johan Gabrielsson (2000). "PK24 - Non-linear kinetics - flow II". Pharmacokinetic/pharmacodynamic data analysis: concepts and applications. Apotekarsocieteten. pp. 527–36. ISBN 91-86274-92-9.
22. Niazi, S. "Volume of distribution as a function of time". Journal of Pharmaceutical Sciences. 65: 452–454. PMID 1263103.
23. Wesolowski, Carl A. (12 July 2016). "Time Varying Apparent Volume of Distribution and Drug Half-Lives Following Intravenous Bolus Injections". PLOS ONE. Retrieved 9 September 2016.
24. Michael E. Winter, Mary Anne Koda-Kimple, Lloyd Y. Young, Emilio Pol Yanguas Farmacocinética clínica básica Ediciones Díaz de Santos, 1994 pgs. 8-14 ISBN 84-7978-147-5, 9788479781477 (in Spanish)
25. Baaske P, Wienken CJ, Reineck P, Duhr S, Braun D (Feb 2010). "Optical Thermophoresis quantifies Buffer dependence of Aptamer Binding". Angew. Chem. Int. Ed. 49 (12): 1–5. doi:10.1002/anie.200903998. PMID 20186894. Lay summary – Phsyorg.com.
26. Wienken CJ, Baaske P, Rothbauer U, Braun D, Duhr S (2010). "Protein-binding assays in biological liquids using microscale thermophoresis". Nature Communications. 1 (7): 100. Bibcode:2010NatCo...1E.100W. doi:10.1038/ncomms1093. PMID 20981028.
27. Hsieh Y, Korfmacher WA (June 2006). "Increasing speed and throughput when using HPLC-MS/MS systems for drug metabolism and pharmacokinetic screening". Current Drug Metabolism. 7 (5): 479–89. doi:10.2174/138920006777697963. PMID 16787157.
28. Covey TR, Lee ED, Henion JD (October 1986). "High-speed liquid chromatography/tandem mass spectrometry for the determination of drugs in biological samples". Anal. Chem. 58 (12): 2453–60. doi:10.1021/ac00125a022. PMID 3789400.
29. Covey TR, Crowther JB, Dewey EA, Henion JD (February 1985). "Thermospray liquid chromatography/mass spectrometry determination of drugs and their metabolites in biological fluids". Anal. Chem. 57 (2): 474–81. doi:10.1021/ac50001a036. PMID 3977076.
30. Committee for Medicinal Products for Human Use (CHMP) (December 2009). "ICH guideline M3(R2) on non-clinical safety studies for the conduct of human clinical trials and marketing authorisation for pharmaceuticals" (PDF). European Medicines Agency, Evaluation of Medicines for Human Use. EMA/CPMP/ICH/286/1995. Retrieved 4 May 2013.

31. Sheiner LB, Rosenberg B, Marathe VV (October 1977). "Estimation of population characteristics of pharmacokinetic parameters from routine clinical data". J Pharmacokinet Biopharm. 5 (5): 445–79. doi:10.1007/BF01061728. PMID 925881.
32. Sheiner LB, Beal S, Rosenberg B, Marathe VV (September 1979). "Forecasting individual pharmacokinetics". Clin. Pharmacol. Ther. 26 (3): 294–305. PMID 466923.
33. Bonate PL (2005). "Recommended reading in population pharmacokinetic pharmacodynamics". AAPS J. 7 (2): E363–73. doi:10.1208/aapsj070237. PMC 2750974Freely accessible. PMID 16353916.
34. R. García del Moral, M. Andújar y F. O'Valle Mecanismos de nefrotoxicidad por ciclosporina A a nivel celular (in Spanish). NEFROLOGIA. Vol. XV. Supplement 1, 1995. Consulted 23 February 2008.
35. Joaquín Herrera Carranza Manual de farmacia clínica y Atención Farmacéutica (in Spanish). Published by Elsevier España, 2003; page 159. ISBN 84-8174-658-4
36. Jager T, Albert C, Preuss TG, Ashauer R (April 2011). "General unified threshold model of survival--a toxicokinetic-toxicodynamic framework for ecotoxicology". Environ. Sci. Technol. 45 (7): 2529–40. Bibcode:2011EnST...45.2529J. doi:10.1021/es103092a. PMID 21366215.
37. Ashauer R. "Toxicokinetic-Toxicodynamic Models - Ecotoxicology and Models". Swiss Federal Institute of Aquatic Science and Technology. Retrieved 2011-12-03.

CHAPTER 10

Pharmacology

Chapter Contents

- **Introduction**
- **Divisions**
- **Scientific Background**
- **Medicine Development And Safety Testing**
- **Drug Legislation And Safety**
- **Pharmacophore**

In general terms, pharmacology is the science of drug action on biological systems. In it's entirety, it embraces knowledge of the sources, chemical properties, biological effects and therapeutic uses of drugs. It is a science that is basic not only to medicine, but also to pharmacy, nursing, dentistry and veterinary medicine. Pharmacological studies range from those that determine the effects of chemical agents upon subcellular mechanisms, to those that deal with the potential hazards of pesticides and herbicides, to those that focus on the treatment and prevention of major diseases by drug therapy. Pharmacologists are also involved in molecular modeling of drugs, and the use of drugs as tools to dissect aspects of cell function.

INTRODUCTION

Pharmacology is the branch of medicine and biology concerned with the study of drug action, where a drug can be broadly defined as any man-made, natural, or endogenous (from within body) molecule which exerts a biochemical and/or physiological effect on the cell, tissue, organ, or organism (sometimes the word pharmacon is used as a term to encompass these endogenous and exogenous bioactive species). More specifically, it is the study of the interactions that occur between a living organism and chemicals that affect normal or abnormal biochemical function. If substances have medicinal properties, they are considered pharmaceuticals.

The field encompasses drug composition and properties, synthesis and drug design, molecular and cellular mechanisms, organ/systems mechanisms, signal transduction/ cellular communication, molecular diagnostics, interactions, toxicology, chemical biology, therapy, and medical applications and antipathogenic capabilities. The two main areas of pharmacology are pharmacodynamics and pharmacokinetics. The former studies the effects of the drug on biological systems, and the latter the effects of biological systems on the drug. In broad terms, pharmacodynamics discusses the chemicals with biological receptors, and pharmacokinetics discusses the absorption, distribution, metabolism, and excretion (ADME) of chemicals from the biological systems. Pharmacology is not synonymous with pharmacy and the two terms are frequently confused. Pharmacology, a biomedical science, deals with the research, discovery, and characterization of chemicals which show biological effects and the elucidation of cellular and organismal function in relation to these chemicals. In contrast, pharmacy, a health services profession, is concerned with application of the principles learned from pharmacology in its clinical settings; whether it be in a dispensing or clinical care role. In either field, the primary contrast between the two are their distinctions between direct-patient care, for pharmacy practice, and the science-oriented research field, driven by pharmacology.

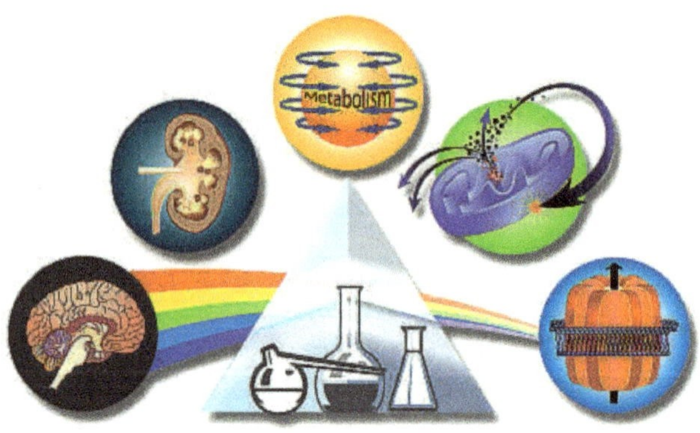

A variety of topics involved with pharmacology, including neuropharmacology, renal pharmacology, human metabolism, intracellular metabolism, and intracellular regulation

The origins of clinical pharmacology date back to the Middle Ages in Avicenna's *The Canon of Medicine*, Peter of Spain's *Commentary on Isaac*, and John of St Amand's *Commentary on the Antedotary of Nicholas*. Clinical pharmacology owes much of its foundation to the work of William Withering. Pharmacology as a scientific discipline did not further advance until the mid-19th century amid the great biomedical resurgence of that period. Before the second half of the nineteenth century, the remarkable potency and specificity of the actions of drugs such as morphine, quinine and digitalis were explained vaguely and with reference to extraordinary chemical powers and affinities to certain organs or tissues. The first pharmacology department was set up by Rudolf Buchheim in 1847, in recognition of the need to understand how therapeutic drugs and poisons produced their effects. Early pharmacologists focused on natural substances, mainly plant extracts. Pharmacology developed in the 19th century as a biomedical science that applied the principles of scientific experimentation to therapeutic contexts. Today pharmacologists use genetics, molecular biology, chemistry, and other advanced tools to transform information about molecular mechanisms and targets into therapies directed against disease, defects or pathogens, and create methods for preventative care, diagnostics, and ultimately personalized medicine.

DIVISIONS

The discipline of pharmacology can be divided into many sub disciplines each with a specific focus.

Clinical Pharmacology

Clinical pharmacology is the basic science of pharmacology with an added focus on the application of pharmacological principles and methods in the medical clinic and towards patient care and outcomes.

Neuropharmacology

Neuropharmacology is the study of the effects of medication on central and peripheral nervous system functioning.

Psychopharmacology

Psychopharmacology, also known as behavioral pharmacology, is the study of the effects of medication on the psyche (psychology), observing changed behaviors of the body and mind, and how molecular events are manifest in a measurable behavioral form. This is similar to the closely related ethnopharmacology. Psychopharmacology is an interdisciplinary field which studies behavioral effects of psychoactive drugs. It incorporates approaches and techniques from neuropharmacology, animal behavior and behavioral neuroscience, and is interested in the behavioral and neurobiological mechanisms of action of psychoactive drugs. Another goal of behavioral pharmacology is to develop animal behavioral models to screen chemical compounds with therapeutic potentials. People in this field (called behavioral pharmacologists) typically use small animals (e.g. rodents) to study psychotherapeutic drugs such as antipsychotics, antidepressants and anxiolytics, and drugs of abuse such as nicotine, cocaine, methamphetamine, etc. study of drugs which affect behavior. *Ethopharmacology* (not to be confused with ethnopharmacology) is a term which has been in use since the 1960's and derives from the Greek word "*ethos*" meaning character and "pharmacology" the study of drug actions and mechanism.

Cardiovascular Pharmacology

Cardiovascular pharmacology is the study of the effects of drugs on the entire cardiovascular system, including the heart and blood vessels.

Pharmacogenetics

Pharmacogenetics is clinical testing of genetic variation that gives rise to differing response to drugs.

Pharmacogenomics

Pharmacogenomics is the application of genomic technologies to drug discovery and further characterization of older drugs.

Pharmacoepidemiology

Pharmacoepidemiology is the study of the effects of drugs in large numbers of people.

Systems Pharmacology

Systems pharmacology is the application of systems biology principles to the field of pharmacology.

Toxicology

Toxicology is the study of the adverse effects, molecular targets, and characterization of drugs or any chemical substance in excess (including those beneficial in lower doses).

Theoretical Pharmacology

Theoretical pharmacology is a relatively new and rapidly expanding field of research activity in which many of the techniques of computational chemistry, in particular computational quantum chemistry and the method of molecular mechanics, are proving to be of great value. Theoretical pharmacologists aim at rationalizing the relation between the activity of a particular drug, as observed experimentally, and its structural features as derived from computer experiments. They aim to find structure—activity relations. Furthermore, on the basis of the structure of a given organic molecule, the theoretical pharmacologist aims at predicting the biological activity of new drugs that are of the same general type as existing drugs. More ambitiously, it aims to predict entirely new classes of drugs, tailor-made for specific purposes.

Posology

Posology is the study of how medicines are dosed. It also depends upon various factors including age, climate, weight, sex, and time of administration. It is derived from the Greek words posos meaning how much and logos meaning science.

Pharmacognosy

Pharmacognosy is a branch of pharmacology dealing especially with the composition, use, and development of medicinal substances of biological origin and especially medicinal substances obtained from plants.

Environmental Pharmacology

Environmental pharmacology is a new discipline. Focus is being given to understand gene–environment interaction, drug-environment interaction and toxin-environment interaction. There is a close collaboration between environmental science and medicine in addressing these issues, as healthcare itself can be a cause of environmental damage or remediation. Human health and ecology are intimately related. Demand for more pharmaceutical products may place the public at risk through the destruction of species. The entry of chemicals and drugs into the aquatic ecosystem is a more serious concern today. In addition, the production of some illegal drugs pollutes drinking water supply by releasing carcinogens. This field is intimately linked with Public Health fields.

Dental Pharmacology

Dental pharmacology relates to the study of drugs commonly used in the treatment of dental disease.

SCIENTIFIC BACKGROUND

The study of chemicals requires intimate knowledge of the biological system affected. With the knowledge of cell biology and biochemistry increasing, the field of pharmacology has also changed substantially. It has become possible, through molecular analysis of receptors, to design chemicals that act on specific cellular signaling or metabolic pathways by affecting sites directly on cell-surface receptors (which modulate and mediate cellular signaling pathways controlling cellular function).

A chemical has, from the pharmacological point-of-view, various properties. Pharmacokinetics describes the effect of the body on the chemical (e.g. half-life and volume of distribution), and pharmacodynamics describes the chemical's effect on the body (desired or toxic).

When describing the pharmacokinetic properties of the chemical that is the active ingredient or active pharmaceutical ingredient (API), pharmacologists are often interested in *L-ADME*:

- Liberation – How is the API disintegrated (for solid oral forms (breaking down into smaller particles)), dispersed, or dissolved from the medication?
- Absorption – How is the API absorbed (through the skin, the intestine, the oral mucosa)?
- Distribution – How does the API spread through the organism?
- Metabolism – Is the API converted chemically inside the body, and into which substances. Are these active (as well)? Could they be toxic?
- Excretion – How is the API excreted (through the bile, urine, breath, skin)?

Medication is said to have a narrow or wide *therapeutic index* or *therapeutic window*. This describes the ratio of desired effect to toxic effect. A compound with a narrow therapeutic index (close to one) exerts its desired effect at a dose close to its toxic dose. A compound with a wide therapeutic index (greater than five) exerts its desired effect at a dose substantially below its toxic dose. Those with a narrow margin are more difficult to dose and administer, and may require therapeutic drug monitoring (examples are warfarin, some antiepileptics, aminoglycoside antibiotics). Most anti-cancer drugs have a narrow therapeutic margin: toxic side-effects are almost always encountered at doses used to kill tumors.

MEDICINE DEVELOPMENT AND SAFETY TESTING

Development of medication is a vital concern to medicine, but also has strong economical and political implications. To protect the consumer and prevent abuse, many governments regulate the manufacture, sale, and administration of medication. In the United States, the main body that regulates pharmaceuticals is the Food and Drug Administration and they enforce standards set by the United States Pharmacopoeia. In the European Union, the main body that regulates pharmaceuticals is the EMA and they enforce standards set by the European Pharmacopoeia.

The metabolic stability and the reactivity of a library of candidate drug compounds have to be assessed for drug metabolism and toxicological studies. Many methods have been proposed for quantitative predictions in drug metabolism; one example of a recent computational method is SPORCalc. If the chemical structure of a medicinal compound is altered slightly, this could slightly or dramatically alter the medicinal properties of the compound depending on the level of alteration as it relates to the structural composition of the substrate or receptor site on which it exerts its medicinal effect, a concept referred to as the structural activity relationship (SAR). This means that when a useful activity has been identified, chemists will make many similar compounds called analogues, in an attempt to maximize the desired medicinal effect(s) of the compound. This development phase can take anywhere from a few years to a decade or more and is very expensive.

These new analogues need to be developed. It needs to be determined how safe the medicine is for human consumption, its stability in the human body and the best form for delivery to the desired organ system, like tablet or aerosol. After extensive testing, which can take up to 6 years, the new medicine is ready for marketing and selling.

As a result of the long time required to develop analogues and test a new medicine and the fact that of every 5000 potential new medicines typically only one will ever reach the open market, this is an expensive way of doing things, often costing over 1 billion dollars. To recoup this outlay pharmaceutical companies may do a number of things:

- Carefully research the demand for their potential new product before spending an outlay of company funds.
- Obtain a patent on the new medicine preventing other companies from producing that medicine for a certain allocation of time.

DRUG LEGISLATION AND SAFETY

In the United States, the Food and Drug Administration (FDA) is responsible for creating guidelines for the approval and use of drugs. The FDA requires that all approved drugs fulfill two requirements:

- The drug must be found to be effective against the disease for which it is seeking approval (where 'effective' means only that the drug performed better than placebo or competitors in at least two trials).
- The drug must meet safety criteria by being subject to animal and controlled human testing.

Gaining FDA approval usually takes several years to attain. Testing done on animals must be extensive and must include several species to help in the evaluation of both the effectiveness and toxicity of the drug. The dosage of any drug approved for use is intended to fall within a range in which the drug produces a therapeutic effect or desired outcome.

The safety and effectiveness of prescription drugs in the U.S. is regulated by the federal Prescription Drug Marketing Act of 1987.

The Medicines and Healthcare products Regulatory Agency (MHRA) has a similar role in the UK.

Education

Students of pharmacology are trained as biomedical scientists, studying the effects of drugs on living organisms. This can lead to new drug discoveries, as well as a better understanding of the way in which the human body works.

Students of pharmacology must have detailed working knowledge of aspects in physiology, pathology and chemistry. During a typical degree they will cover areas such as (but not limited to) biochemistry, cell biology, basic physiology, genetics & the Central Dogma, medical microbiology, neuroscience, and depending on the department's interests, bio-organic chemistry and/or chemical biology.

Modern Pharmacology is highly interdisciplinary. Graduate programs accept students from most biological and chemical backgrounds. With the increasing drive towards biophysical and computational research to describe systems, pharmacologists may even consider themselves mainly physical scientists. In many instances, Analytical Chemistry is closely related to the studies and needs of pharmacological research. Therefore, many institutions will include pharmacology under a Chemistry or Biochemistry Department, especially if a separate Pharmacology Dept. does not exist. What makes an institutional department independent of another, or exist in the first place, is usually an artifact of historical times.

Whereas a pharmacy student will eventually work in a pharmacy dispensing medications, a pharmacologist will typically work within a laboratory setting. Careers for a pharmacologist include academic positions (medical and non-medical), governmental positions, private industrial positions, science writing, scientific patents and law, consultation, biotech and pharmaceutical employment, the alcohol industry, food industry, forensics/law enforcement, public health, and environmental/ecological sciences.

PHARMACOPHORE

A pharmacophore is an abstract description of molecular features that are necessary for molecular recognition of a ligand by a biological macromolecule. The IUPAC defines a pharmacophore to be "an ensemble of steric and electronic features that is necessary to ensure the optimal supramolecular interactions with a specific biological target and to trigger (or block) its biological response". A pharmacophore model explains how structurally diverse ligands can bind to a common receptor site. Furthermore, pharmacophore models can be used to identify through de novo design or virtual screening novel ligands that will bind to the same receptor.

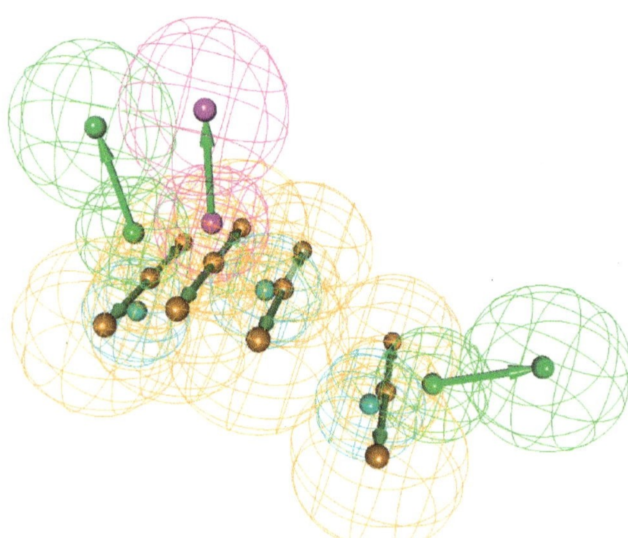

An example of a pharmacophore model.

Features

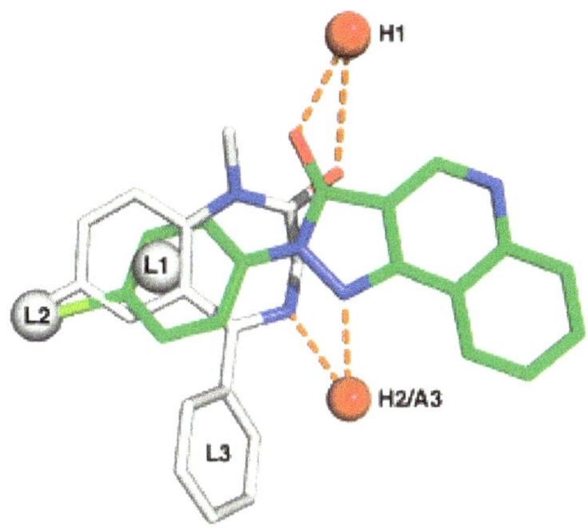

An example of a pharmacophore model of the benzodiazepine binding site on the $GABA_A$ receptor. White sticks represent the carbon atoms of the benzodiazepine diazepam, while green represents carbon atoms of the nonbenzodiazepine CGS-9896. Red and blue sticks are oxygen and nitrogen atoms that are present in both structures. The red spheres labeled H1 and H2/A3 are, respectively, hydrogen bond donating and accepting sites in the receptor, while L1, L2, and L3 denote lipophilic binding sites.

Typical pharmacophore features include hydrophobic centroids, aromatic rings, hydrogen bond acceptors or donors, cations, and anions. These pharmacophoric points may be located on the ligand itself or may be projected points presumed to be located in the receptor.

The features need to match different chemical groups with similar properties, in order to identify novel ligands. Ligand-receptor interactions are typically "polar positive", "polar negative" or "hydrophobic". A well-defined pharmacophore model includes both hydrophobic volumes and hydrogen bond vectors.

History

Historically, pharmacophores were established by Lemont Kier, who first mentions the concept in 1967 and uses the term in a publication in 1971.

The development of the concept is often erroneously accredited to Paul Ehrlich. However neither the alleged source nor any of his other works mention the term "pharmacophore" or make use of the concept.

Model Development

The process for developing a pharmacophore model generally involves the following steps:

- Select a training set of ligands – Choose a structurally diverse set of molecules that will be used for developing the pharmacophore model. As a pharmacophore model should be able to discriminate between molecules with and without bioactivity, the set of molecules should include both active and inactive compounds.

- Conformational analysis – Generate a set of low energy conformations that is likely to contain the bioactive conformation for each of the selected molecules.
- Molecular superimposition – Superimpose ("fit") all combinations of the low-energy conformations of the molecules. Similar (bioisosteric) functional groups common to all molecules in the set might be fitted (*e.g.*, phenyl rings or carboxylic acid groups). The set of conformations (one conformation from each active molecule) that results in the best fit is presumed to be the active conformation.
- Abstraction – Transform the superimposed molecules into an abstract representation. For example, superimposed phenyl rings might be referred to more conceptually as an 'aromatic ring' pharmacophore element. Likewise, hydroxy groups could be designated as a 'hydrogen-bond donor/acceptor' pharmacophore element.
- Validation – A pharmacophore model is a *hypothesis* accounting for the observed biological activities of a set of molecules that bind to a common biological target. The model is only valid insofar as it is able to account for differences in biological activity of a range of molecules.

As the biological activities of new molecules become available, the pharmacophore model can be updated to further refine it.

Applications

In modern computational chemistry, pharmacophores are used to define the essential features of one or more molecules with the same biological activity. A database of diverse chemical compounds can then be searched for more molecules which share the same features arranged in the same relative orientation. Pharmacophores are also used as the starting point for developing 3D-QSAR models. Such tools and a related concept of "privileged structures", which are "defined as molecular frameworks which are able of providing useful ligands for more than one type of receptor or enzyme target by judicious structural modifications", aid in drug discovery.

REFERENCES

1. Vallance P, Smart TG (January 2006). "The future of pharmacology". British Journal of Pharmacology. 147 Suppl 1 (S1): S304–7. doi:10.1038/sj.bjp.0706454. PMC 1760753Freely accessible. PMID 16402118.
2. Brater DC, Daly WJ (May 2000). "Clinical pharmacology in the Middle Ages: principles that presage the 21st century". Clin. Pharmacol. Ther. 67 (5): 447–50. doi:10.1067/mcp.2000.106465. PMID 10824622.
3. Mannfred A. Hollinger (2003)."Introduction to pharmacology". CRC Press. p.4. ISBN 0-415-28033-8

4. Rang HP (January 2006). "The receptor concept: pharmacology's big idea". Br. J. Pharmacol. 147 Suppl 1 (S1): S9–16. doi:10.1038/sj.bjp.0706457. PMC 1760743Freely accessible. PMID 16402126.
5. Maehle AH, Prüll CR, Halliwell RF (August 2002). "The emergence of the drug receptor theory". Nat Rev Drug Discov. 1 (8): 637–41. doi:10.1038/nrd875. PMID 12402503.
6. Rang, H.P.; M.M. Dale; J.M. Ritter; R.J. Flower (2007). Pharmacology. China: Elsevier. ISBN 0-443-06911-5.
7. Krsiak, M (1991). "Ethopharmacology: A historical perspective". Neuroscience and biobehavioral reviews. 15 (4): 439–45. doi:10.1016/s0149-7634(05)80124-1. PMID 1792005.
8. Rahman, SZ; Khan, RA (Dec 2006). "Environmental pharmacology: A new discipline". Indian J Pharmacol. 38 (4): 229–30. doi:10.4103/0253-7613.27017.
9. Sue Ruhoy Ilene; Daughton Christian G (2008). "Beyond the medicine cabinet: An analysis of where and why medications accumulate". Environment International. 34 (8): 1157–1169. doi:10.1016/j.envint.2008.05.002.
10. "Dental Pharmacology". nba.uth.tmc.edu. Texas Medical Center. Retrieved 22 May 2015.
11. James Smith; Viktor Stein (2009). "SPORCalc: A development of a database analysis that provides putative metabolic enzyme reactions for ligand-based drug design". Computational Biology and Chemistry. 33 (2): 149–159. doi:10.1016/j.compbiolchem.2008.11.002. PMID 19157988.
12. Newton, David; Alasdair Thorpe; Chris Otter (2004). Revise A2 Chemistry. Heinemann Educational Publishers. p. 1. ISBN 0-435-58347-6.
13. Nagle, Hinter; Barbara Nagle (2005). Pharmacology: An Introduction. Boston: McGraw Hill. ISBN 0-07-312275-0.
14. Wermuth CG, Ganellin CR, Lindberg P, Mitscher LA (1998). "Glossary of terms used in medicinal chemistry (IUPAC Recommendations 1998)". Pure and Applied Chemistry. 70 (5): 1129–1143. doi:10.1351/pac199870051129.
15. Madsen U, Bräuner-Osborne H, Greenwood JR, Johansen TN, Krogsgaard-Larsen P, Liljefors T, Nielsen M, Frølund B (2005). "GABA and Glutamate receptor ligands and their therapeutic potential in CNS disorders". In Gad SC. Drug Discovery Handbook. Hoboken, N.J: Wiley-Interscience/J. Wiley. pp. 797–907. ISBN 0-471-21384-5.
16. Duarte, CD; et al. (2007), "Privileged structures: a useful concept for the rational design of new lead drug candidates", Mini Rev Med Chem, 7 (11): 1108–1119, doi:10.2174/138955707782331722, PMID 18045214.
17. Kier LB (September 1967). "Molecular orbital calculation of preferred conformations of acetylcholine, muscarine, and muscarone". Mol. Pharmacol. 3 (5): 487–94. PMID 6052710.

18. Kier LB (1971). Molecular orbital theory in drug research. Boston: Academic Press. pp. 164–169. ISBN 0-12-406550-3.
19. Ehrlich P (1909). "Über den jetzigen Stand der Chemotherapie". Ber. Dtsch. Chem. Ges. 42: 17–47. doi:10.1002/cber.19090420105.
20. J.H. van Drie (2007). "Monty Kier and the Origin of the Pharmacophore Concept" (PDF). Internet Electronic Journal of Molecular Design. 6: 271–279.

CHAPTER 11

Enzyme inhibitor and Ligand Efficiency

Chapter Contents

- **Introduction**
- **Reversible Inhibitors**
- **Irreversible Inhibitors**
- **Discovery and Design of Inhibitors**
- **Ligand Efficiency**

Enzyme inhibitors are molecules that interact in some way with the enzyme to prevent it from working in the normal manner. There are a variety of types of inhibitors including: nonspecific, irreversible, reversible - competitive and noncompetitive. Poisons and drugs are examples of enzyme inhibitors.

Ligand efficiency (LE) is most commonly defined as the ratio of the affinity of a ligand divided by the number of heavy (nonhydrogen) atoms in the molecule (LE = ΔG/ [number of heavy atoms]). This ratio was first described in 1999 and gained widespread popularity in drug discovery circles shortly thereafter. The rapid uptake of LE in drug discovery was likely facilitated by the already widespread use of Lipinski's rules (another size restraining metric) and a burgeoning interest in fragment-based approaches to drug discovery. Ligand efficiency validated fragment-based design and offered a simple measure to keep molecular size in check while undertaking a lead optimization program.

INTRODUCTION

An enzyme inhibitor is a molecule that binds to an enzyme and decreases its activity. Since blocking an enzyme's activity can kill a pathogen or correct a metabolic imbalance, many drugs are enzyme inhibitors. They are also used in pesticides. Not all molecules that bind to enzymes are inhibitors; *enzyme activators* bind to enzymes and increase their enzymatic activity, while enzyme substrates bind and are converted to products in the normal catalytic cycle of the enzyme.

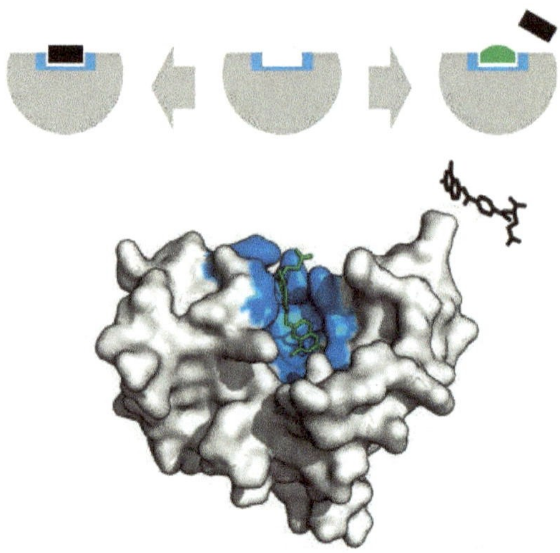

An enzyme binding site that would normally bind substrate can alternatively bind a competitive inhibitor, preventing substrate access. Dihydrofolate reductase is inhibited by methotrexate which prevents binding of its substrate, folic acid. Binding site in blue, inhibitor in green, and substrate in black.

The binding of an inhibitor can stop a substrate from entering the enzyme's active site and/or hinder the enzyme from catalyzing its reaction. Inhibitor binding is either reversible or irreversible. Irreversible inhibitors usually react with the enzyme and change it chemically (e.g. via covalent bond formation). These inhibitors modify key amino acid residues needed for enzymatic activity. In contrast, reversible inhibitors bind non-covalently and different types of inhibition are produced depending on whether these inhibitors bind to the enzyme, the enzyme-substrate complex, or both.

Many drug molecules are enzyme inhibitors, so their discovery and improvement is an active area of research in biochemistry and pharmacology. A medicinal enzyme inhibitor is often judged by its specificity (its lack of binding to other proteins) and its potency (its dissociation constant, which indicates the concentration needed to inhibit the enzyme). A high specificity and potency ensure that a drug will have few side effects and thus low toxicity.

Enzyme inhibitors also occur naturally and are involved in the regulation of metabolism. For example, enzymes in a metabolic pathway can be inhibited by downstream products. This type of negative feedback slows the production line when products begin to build up and is an important way to maintain homeostasis in a cell. Other cellular enzyme inhibitors are proteins that specifically bind to and inhibit an enzyme target. This can help control enzymes that may be damaging to a cell, like proteases or nucleases. A well-characterized example of this is the ribonuclease inhibitor, which binds to ribonucleases in one of the tightest known protein–protein interactions. Natural enzyme inhibitors can also be poisons and are used as defenses against predators or as ways of killing prey.

REVERSIBLE INHIBITORS

Types of Reversible Inhibitors

Reversible inhibitors attach to enzymes with non-covalent interactions such as hydrogen bonds, hydrophobic interactions and ionic bonds. Multiple weak bonds between the inhibitor and the active site combine to produce strong and specific binding. In contrast to substrates and irreversible inhibitors, reversible inhibitors generally do not undergo chemical reactions when bound to the enzyme and can be easily removed by dilution or dialysis.

There are four kinds of reversible enzyme inhibitors. They are classified according to the effect of varying the concentration of the enzyme's substrate on the inhibitor.

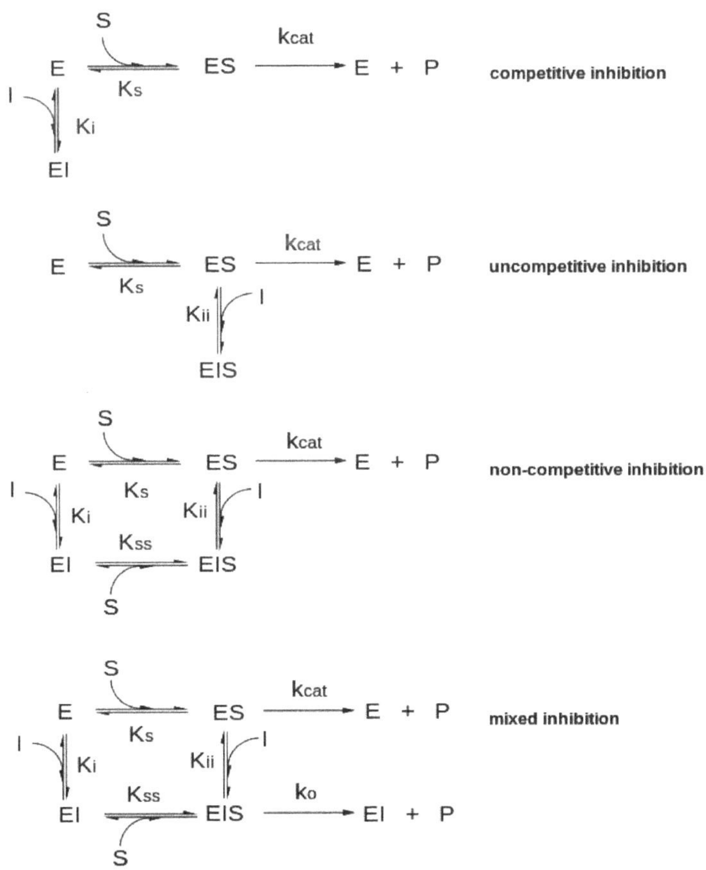

Types of inhibition. This classification was introduced by W.W. Cleland.

- In *competitive inhibition*, the substrate and inhibitor cannot bind to the enzyme at the same time, as shown in the figure on the right. This usually results from the inhibitor having an affinity for the active site of an enzyme where the substrate also binds; the substrate and inhibitor *compete* for access to the enzyme's active site. This type of inhibition can be overcome by sufficiently high concentrations of substrate (V_{max} remains constant), i.e., by out-competing the inhibitor. However, the apparent K_m will increase as it takes a higher concentration of the substrate to reach the K_m point, or half the V_{max}. Competitive inhibitors are often similar in structure to the real substrate (see examples below).
- In *uncompetitive inhibition*, the inhibitor binds only to the substrate-enzyme complex. This type of inhibition causes V_{max} to decrease (maximum velocity decreases as a result of removing activated complex) and K_m to decrease (due to better binding efficiency as a result of Le Chatelier's principle and the effective elimination of the ES complex thus decreasing the K_m which indicates a higher binding affinity).
- In *non-competitive inhibition*, the binding of the inhibitor to the enzyme reduces its activity but does not affect the binding of substrate. As a result, the extent of inhibition depends only on the concentration of the inhibitor. V_{max} will decrease due to the inability for the reaction to proceed as efficiently, but K_m will remain the same as the actual binding of the substrate, by definition, will still function properly.
- In *mixed inhibition*, the inhibitor can bind to the enzyme at the same time as the enzyme's substrate. However, the binding of the inhibitor affects the binding of the substrate, and vice versa. This type of inhibition can be reduced, but not overcome by increasing concentrations of substrate. Although it is possible for mixed-type inhibitors to bind in the active site, this type of inhibition generally results from an allosteric effect where the inhibitor binds to a different site on an enzyme. Inhibitor binding to this allosteric site changes the conformation(i.e., tertiary structure or three-dimensional shape) of the enzyme so that the affinity of the substrate for the active site is reduced.

Quantitative Description of Reversible Inhibition

Reversible inhibition can be described quantitatively in terms of the inhibitor's binding to the enzyme and to the enzyme-substrate complex, and its effects on the kinetic constants of the enzyme. In the classic Michaelis-Menten scheme below, an enzyme (E) binds to its substrate (S) to form the enzyme–substrate complex ES. Upon catalysis, this complex breaks down to release product P and free enzyme. The inhibitor (I) can bind to either E or ES with the dissociation constants K_i or K_i', respectively.

- Competitive inhibitors can bind to E, but not to ES. Competitive inhibition increases Km (i.e., the inhibitor interferes with substrate binding), but does not affect V_{max} (the inhibitor does not hamper catalysis in ES because it cannot bind to ES).

- Uncompetitive inhibitors bind to ES. Uncompetitive inhibition decreases both Km' and 'V_{max}. The inhibitor affects substrate binding by increasing the enzyme's affinity for the substrate (decreasing Km) as well as hampering catalysis (decreases V_{max}).
- Non-competitive inhibitors have identical affinities for E and ES (Ki = Ki'). Non-competitive inhibition does not change Km (i.e., it does not affect substrate binding) but decreases V_{max} (i.e., inhibitor binding hampers catalysis).

Mixed-type inhibitors bind to both E and ES, but their affinities for these two forms of the enzyme are different (Ki ≠ Ki'). Thus, mixed-type inhibitors interfere with substrate binding (increase K_m) and hamper catalysis in the ES complex (decrease V_{max}).

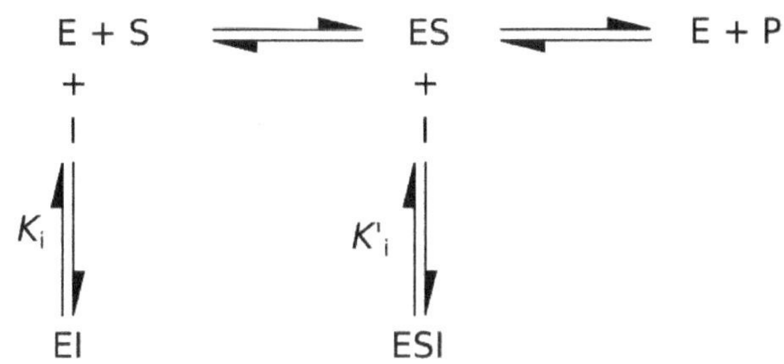

Kinetic scheme for reversible enzyme inhibitors

When an enzyme has multiple substrates, inhibitors can show different types of inhibition depending on which substrate is considered. This results from the active site containing two different binding sites within the active site, one for each substrate. For example, an inhibitor might compete with substrate A for the first binding site, but be a non-competitive inhibitor with respect to substrate B in the second binding site.

Measuring the Dissociation Constants of a Reversible Inhibitor

As noted above, an enzyme inhibitor is characterized by its two dissociation constants, K_i and K_i', to the enzyme and to the enzyme-substrate complex, respectively. The enzyme-inhibitor constant K_i can be measured directly by various methods; one extremely accurate method is isothermal titration calorimetry, in which the inhibitor is titrated into a solution of enzyme and the heat released or absorbed is measured. However, the other dissociation constant K_i' is difficult to measure directly, since the enzyme-substrate complex is short-lived and undergoing a chemical reaction to form the product. Hence, K_i' is usually measured indirectly, by observing the enzyme activity under various substrate and inhibitor concentrations, and fitting the data to a modified Michaelis–Menten equation

$$V = \frac{V_{max}[S]}{\alpha K_m + \alpha'[S]} = \frac{(1/\alpha')V_{max}[S]}{(\alpha/\alpha')K_m + [S]}$$

where the modifying factors α and α' are defined by the inhibitor concentration and its two dissociation constants

$$\alpha = 1 + \frac{[I]}{K_i}$$
$$\alpha' = 1 + \frac{[I]}{K_i'}.$$

Thus, in the presence of the inhibitor, the enzyme's effective K_m and V_{max} become $(\alpha/\alpha')K_m$ and $(1/\alpha')V_{max}$, respectively. However, the modified Michaelis-Menten equation assumes that binding of the inhibitor to the enzyme has reached equilibrium, which may be a very slow process for inhibitors with sub-nanomolar dissociation constants. In these cases, it is usually more practical to treat the tight-binding inhibitor as an irreversible inhibitor (see below); however, it can still be possible to estimate K_i' kinetically if K_i is measured independently.

The effects of different types of reversible enzyme inhibitors on enzymatic activity can be visualized using graphical representations of the Michaelis–Menten equation, such as Lineweaver–Burk and Eadie-Hofstee plots. For example, in the Lineweaver–Burk plots at the right, the competitive inhibition lines intersect on the *y*-axis, illustrating that such inhibitors do not affect V_{max}. Similarly, the non-competitive inhibition lines intersect on the *x*-axis, showing these inhibitors do not affect K_m. However, it can be difficult to estimate K_i and K_i' accurately from such plots, so it is advisable to estimate these constants using more reliable nonlinear regression methods, as described above.

Reversible Inhibitors

Traditionally reversible enzyme inhibitors have been classified as competitive, uncompetitive, or non-competitive, according to their effects on K_m and V_{max}. These different effects result from the inhibitor binding to the enzyme E, to the enzyme–substrate complex ES, or to both, respectively. The division of these classes arises from a problem in their derivation and results in the need to use two different binding constants for one binding event. The binding of an inhibitor and its effect on the enzymatic activity are two distinctly different things, another problem the traditional equations fail to acknowledge. In noncompetitive inhibition the binding of the inhibitor results in 100% inhibition of the enzyme only, and fails to consider the possibility of anything in between. The common form of the inhibitory term also obscures the relationship between the inhibitor binding to the enzyme and its relationship to any other binding term be it the Michaelis–Menten equation or a dose response curve associated with ligand receptor binding. To demonstrate the relationship the following rearrangement can be made:

$$\frac{V_{max}}{1 + \frac{[I]}{K_i}} = \frac{V_{max}}{\frac{[I] + K_i}{K_i}}$$

Adding zero to the bottom ([I]-[I])

$$\frac{V_{\max}}{\frac{[\mathrm{I}]+K_i}{[\mathrm{I}]+K_i-[\mathrm{I}]}}$$

Dividing by $[\mathrm{I}]+K_i$

$$\frac{V_{\max}}{\frac{1}{1-\frac{[\mathrm{I}]}{[\mathrm{I}]+K_i}}}=V_{\max}-V_{\max}\frac{[\mathrm{I}]}{[\mathrm{I}]+K_i}$$

This notation demonstrates that similar to the Michaelis–Menten equation,where the rate of reaction depends on the percent of the enzyme population interacting with substrate.

fraction of the enzyme population bound by substrate

$$\frac{[\mathrm{S}]}{[\mathrm{S}]+K_m}$$

fraction of the enzyme population bound by inhibitor

$$\frac{[\mathrm{I}]}{[\mathrm{I}]+K_i}$$

the effect of the inhibitor is a result of the percent of the enzyme population interacting with inhibitor. The only problem with this equation in its present form is that it assumes absolute inhibition of the enzyme with inhibitor binding, when in fact there can be a wide range of effects anywhere from 100% inhibition of substrate turn over to just >0%. To account for this the equation can be easily modified to allow for different degrees of inhibition by including a delta $V_{\max}$ term.

$$V_{\max}-\Delta V_{\max}\frac{[\mathrm{I}]}{[\mathrm{I}]+K_i}$$

or

$$V_{\max 1}-(V_{\max 1}-V_{\max 2})\frac{[\mathrm{I}]}{[\mathrm{I}]+K_i}$$

This term can then define the residual enzymatic activity present when the inhibitor is interacting with individual enzymes in the population. However the inclusion of this term has the added value of allowing for the possibility of activation if the secondary $V_{\max}$ term turns out to be higher than the initial term. To account for the possibly of activation as well the notation can then be rewritten replacing the inhibitor “I” with a modifier term denoted here as “X”.

$$V_{\max 1} - (V_{\max 1} - V_{\max 2})\frac{[\mathrm{X}]}{[\mathrm{X}] + K_x}$$

While this terminology results in a simplified way of dealing with kinetic effects relating to the maximum velocity of the Michaelis–Menten equation, it highlights potential problems with the term used to describe effects relating to the K_m. The K_m relating to the affinity of the enzyme for the substrate should in most cases relate to potential changes in the binding site of the enzyme which would directly result from enzyme inhibitor interactions. As such a term similar to the one proposed above to modulate V_{max} should be appropriate in most situations:

$$K_{m1} - (K_{m1} - K_{m2})\frac{[\mathrm{X}]}{[\mathrm{X}] + K_x}$$

Special Cases

- The mechanism of partially competitive inhibition is similar to that of non-competitive, except that the EIS complex has catalytic activity, which may be lower or even higher (partially competitive activation) than that of the enzyme–substrate (ES) complex. This inhibition typically displays a lower V_{max}, but an unaffected K_m value.
- Uncompetitive inhibition occurs when the inhibitor binds only to the enzyme–substrate complex, not to the free enzyme; the EIS complex is catalytically inactive. This mode of inhibition is rare and causes a decrease in both V_{max} and the K_m value.
- Substrate and product inhibition is where either the substrate or product of an enzyme reaction inhibit the enzyme's activity. This inhibition may follow the competitive, uncompetitive or mixed patterns. In substrate inhibition there is a progressive decrease in activity at high substrate concentrations. This may indicate the existence of two substrate-binding sites in the enzyme. At low substrate, the high-affinity site is occupied and normal kinetics are followed. However, at higher concentrations, the second inhibitory site becomes occupied, inhibiting the enzyme. Product inhibition is often a regulatory feature in metabolism and can be a form of negative feedback.
- Slow-tight inhibition occurs when the initial enzyme–inhibitor complex EI undergoes isomerisation to a second more tightly held complex, EI*, but the overall inhibition process is reversible. This manifests itself as slowly increasing enzyme inhibition. Under these conditions, traditional Michaelis–Menten kinetics give a false value for K_i, which is time–dependent. The true value of K_i can be obtained through more complex analysis of the on (k_{on}) and off (k_{off}) rate constants for inhibitor association.

Examples of Reversible Inhibitors

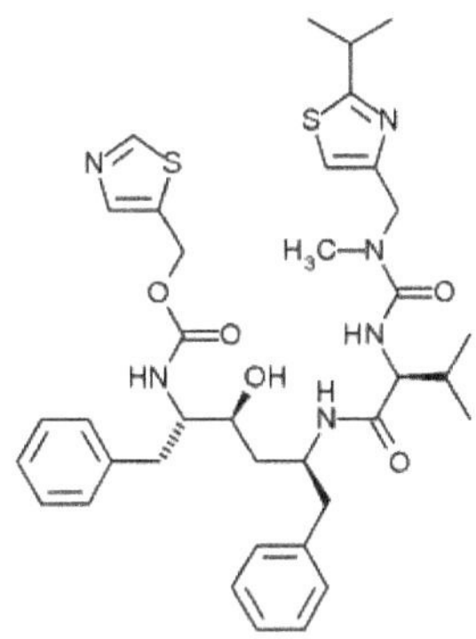

Peptide-based HIV-1 protease inhibitor ritonavir

As enzymes have evolved to bind their substrates tightly, and most reversible inhibitors bind in the active site of enzymes, it is unsurprising that some of these inhibitors are strikingly similar in structure to the substrates of their targets. An example of these substrate mimics are the protease inhibitors, a very successful class of antiretroviral drugs used to treat HIV. The structure of ritonavir, a protease inhibitor based on a peptide and containing three peptide bonds, is shown on the right. As this drug resembles the protein that is the substrate of the HIV protease, it competes with this substrate in the enzyme's active site.

Enzyme inhibitors are often designed to mimic the transition state or intermediate of an enzyme-catalyzed reaction. This ensures that the inhibitor exploits the transition state stabilizing effect of the enzyme, resulting in a better binding affinity (lower K_i) than substrate-based designs. An example of such a transition state inhibitor is the antiviral drug oseltamivir; this drug mimics the planar nature of the ring oxonium ion in the reaction of the viral enzyme neuraminidase.

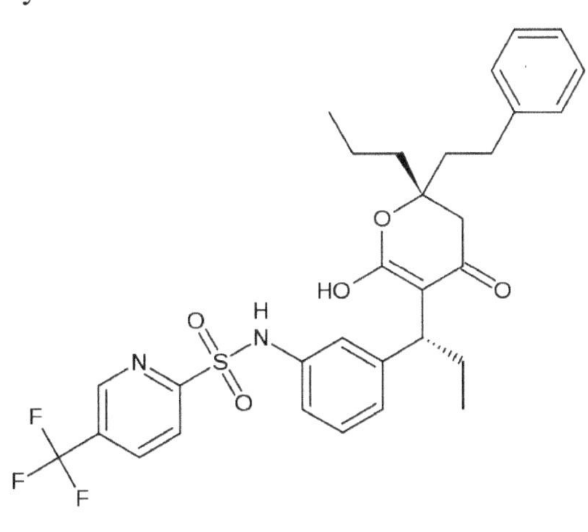

Nonpeptidic HIV-1 protease inhibitor tipranavir

However, not all inhibitors are based on the structures of substrates. For example, the structure of another HIV protease inhibitor tipranavir is shown on the left. This molecule is not based on a peptide and has no obvious structural similarity to a protein substrate. These non-peptide inhibitors can be more stable than inhibitors containing peptide bonds, because they will not be substrates for peptidases and are less likely to be degraded.

In drug design it is important to consider the concentrations of substrates to which the target enzymes are exposed. For example, some protein kinaseinhibitors have chemical structures that are similar to adenosine triphosphate, one of the substrates of these enzymes. However, drugs that are simple competitive inhibitors will have to compete with the high concentrations of ATP in the cell. Protein kinases can also be inhibited by competition at the binding sites where the kinases interact with their substrate proteins, and most proteins are present inside cells at concentrations much lower than the concentration of ATP. As a consequence, if two protein kinase inhibitors both bind in the active site with similar affinity, but only one has to compete with ATP, then the competitive inhibitor at the protein-binding site will inhibit the enzyme more effectively.

IRREVERSIBLE INHIBITORS

Types of Irreversible Inhibition

Irreversible inhibitors usually covalently modify an enzyme, and inhibition can therefore not be reversed. Irreversible inhibitors often contain reactive functional groups such as nitrogen mustards, aldehydes, haloalkanes, alkenes, Michael acceptors, phenyl sulfonates, or fluorophosphonates. These electrophilic groups react with amino acid side chains to form covalent adducts. The residues modified are those with side chains containing nucleophiles such as hydroxyl or sulfhydryl groups; these include the amino acids serine (as in DFP, right), cysteine, threonine, or tyrosine.

Irreversible inhibition is different from irreversible enzyme inactivation. Irreversible inhibitors are generally specific for one class of enzyme and do not inactivate all proteins; they do not function by destroying protein structure but by specifically altering the active site of their target. For example, extremes of pH or temperature usually cause denaturation of all protein structure, but this is a non-specific effect. Similarly, some non-specific chemical treatments destroy protein structure: for example, heating in concentrated hydrochloric acid will hydrolyze the peptide bonds holding proteins together, releasing free amino acids.

Irreversible inhibitors display time-dependent inhibition and their potency therefore cannot be characterized by an IC_{50} value. This is because the amount of active enzyme at a given concentration of irreversible inhibitor will be different depending on how long the inhibitor is pre-incubated with the enzyme. Instead, $k_{obs}/[I]$ values are used, wherek_{obs} is the observed pseudo-first order rate of inactivation (obtained by plotting the log of % activity vs. time) and $[I]$ is the concentration of inhibitor. The $k_{obs}/[I]$ parameter is valid as long as the inhibitor does not saturate binding with the enzyme (in which case $k_{obs} = k_{inact}$).

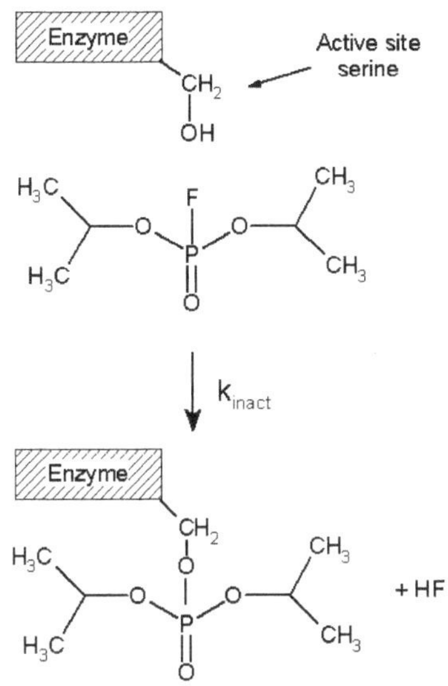

Reaction of the irreversible inhibitor diisopropylfluorophosphate (DFP) with a serine protease

Analysis of Irreversible Inhibition

As shown in the figure to the left, irreversible inhibitors form a reversible non-covalent complex with the enzyme (EI or ESI) and this then reacts to produce the covalently modified "dead-end complex" EI*. The rate at which EI* is formed is called the inactivation rate or k_{inact}. Since formation of EI may compete with ES, binding of irreversible inhibitors can be prevented by competition either with substrate or with a second, reversible inhibitor. This protection effect is good evidence of a specific reaction of the irreversible inhibitor with the active site.

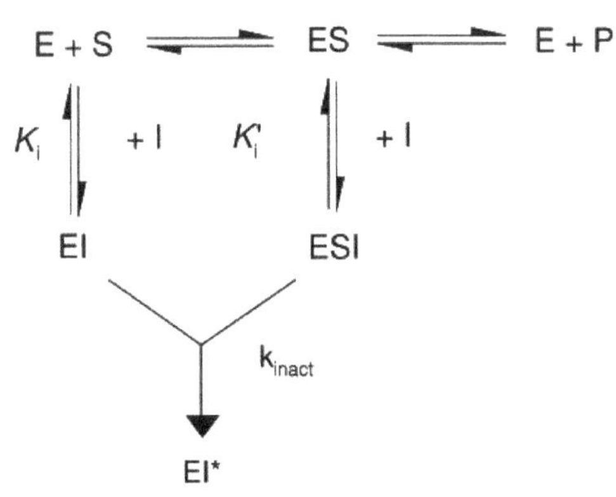

Kinetic scheme for irreversible inhibitors

The binding and inactivation steps of this reaction are investigated by incubating the enzyme with inhibitor and assaying the amount of activity remaining over time. The activity will be decreased in a time-dependent manner, usually following exponential decay. Fitting these data to a rate equation gives the rate of inactivation at this concentration of inhibitor. This is done at several different concentrations of inhibitor. If a reversible EI complex is involved the inactivation rate will be saturable and fitting this curve will give k_{inact} and K_i.

Another method that is widely used in these analyses is mass spectrometry. Here, accurate measurement of the mass of the unmodified native enzyme and the inactivated enzyme gives the increase in mass caused by reaction with the inhibitor and shows the stoichiometry of the reaction. This is usually done using a MALDI-TOF mass spectrometer. In a complementary technique, peptide mass fingerprinting involves digestion of the native and modified protein with a protease such as trypsin. This will produce a set of peptides that can be analyzed using a mass spectrometer. The peptide that changes in mass after reaction with the inhibitor will be the one that contains the site of modification.

Special Cases

Not all irreversible inhibitors form covalent adducts with their enzyme targets. Some reversible inhibitors bind so tightly to their target enzyme that they are essentially irreversible.

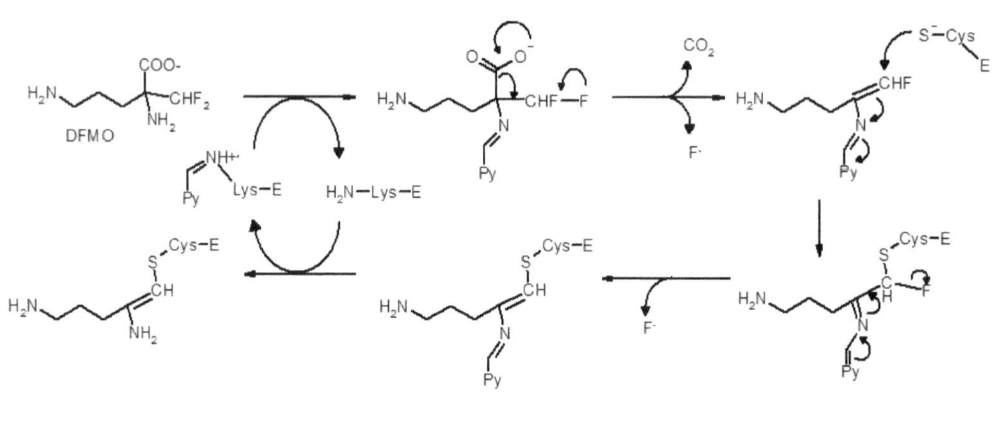

Chemical mechanism for irreversible inhibition of ornithine decarboxylase by DFMO. Pyridoxal 5'-phosphate (Py) and enzyme (E) are not shown. Adapted from

These tight-binding inhibitors may show kinetics similar to covalent irreversible inhibitors. In these cases, some of these inhibitors rapidly bind to the enzyme in a low-affinity EI complex and this then undergoes a slower rearrangement to a very tightly bound EI* complex (see figure above). This kinetic behaviour is called slow-binding. This slow rearrangement after binding often involves a conformational change as the enzyme "clamps down" around the inhibitor molecule. Examples of slow-binding inhibitors include some important drugs, such methotrexate, allopurinol, and the activated form of acyclovir.

Examples of Irreversible Inhibitors

Diisopropylfluorophosphate (DFP) is shown as an example of an irreversible protease inhibitor in the figure above right. The enzyme hydrolyses the phosphorus–fluorine bond, but the phosphate residue remains bound to the serine in the active site, deactivating it. Similarly, DFP also reacts with the active site of acetylcholine esterase in the synapses of neurons, and consequently is a potent neurotoxin, with a lethal dose of less than 100 mg.

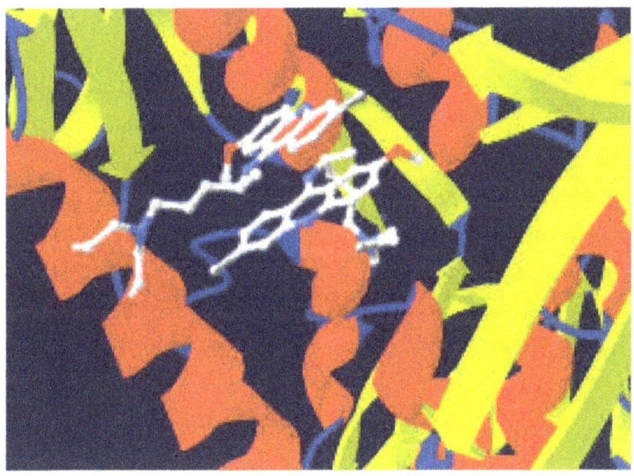

Trypanothione reductase with the lower molecule of an inhibitor bound irreversibly and the upper one reversibly. Created from PDB 1GXF.

Suicide inhibition is an unusual type of irreversible inhibition where the enzyme converts the inhibitor into a reactive form in its active site. An example is the inhibitor of polyamine biosynthesis, α-difluoromethylornithine or DFMO, which is an analogue of the amino acid ornithine, and is used to treat African trypanosomiasis (sleeping sickness). Ornithine decarboxylase can catalyse the decarboxylation of DFMO instead of ornithine, as shown above. However, this decarboxylation reaction is followed by the elimination of a fluorine atom, which converts this catalytic intermediate into a conjugated imine, a highly electrophilic species. This reactive form of DFMO then reacts with either a cysteine or lysine residue in the active site to irreversibly inactivate the enzyme.

Since irreversible inhibition often involves the initial formation of a non-covalent EI complex, it is sometimes possible for an inhibitor to bind to an enzyme in more than one way. For example, in the figure showing trypanothione reductase from the human protozoan parasite *Trypanosoma cruzi*, two molecules of an inhibitor called *quinacrine mustard* are bound in its active site. The top molecule is bound reversibly, but the lower one is bound covalently as it has reacted with an amino acid residue through its nitrogen mustard group.

DISCOVERY AND DESIGN OF INHIBITORS

New drugs are the products of a long drug development process, the first step of which is often the discovery of a new enzyme inhibitor. In the past the only way to discover these new inhibitors was by trial and error: screening huge libraries of compounds against a target enzyme and hoping that some useful leads would emerge. This brute force approach is still successful and has even been extended by combinatorial chemistry approaches that quickly produce large numbers of novel compounds and high-throughput screening technology to rapidly screen these huge chemical libraries for useful inhibitors.

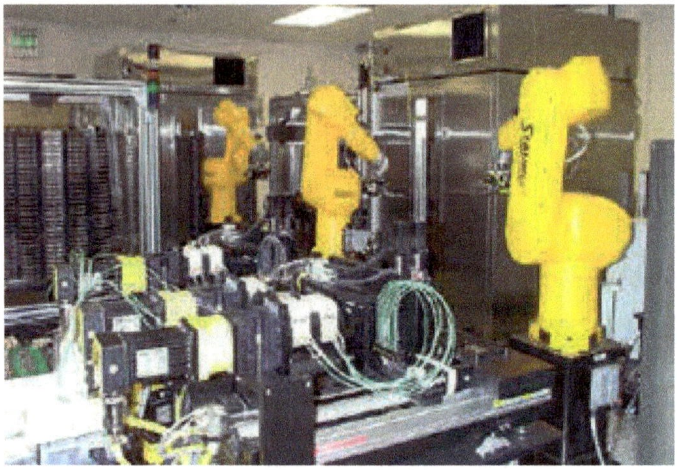

Robots used for the high-throughput screening of chemical libraries to discover new enzyme inhibitors

More recently, an alternative approach has been applied: rational drug design uses the three-dimensional structure of an enzyme's active site to predict which molecules might be inhibitors. These predictions are then tested and one of these tested compounds may be a novel inhibitor. This new inhibitor is then used to try to obtain a structure of the enzyme in an inhibitor/enzyme complex to show how the molecule is binding to the active site, allowing changes to be made to the inhibitor to try to optimize binding. This test and improve cycle is then repeated until a sufficiently potent inhibitor is produced. Computer-based methods of predicting the affinity of an inhibitor for an enzyme are also being developed, such as molecular docking and molecular mechanics.

Uses of Inhibitors

Enzyme inhibitors are found in nature and are also designed and produced as part of pharmacology and biochemistry. Natural poisons are often enzyme inhibitors that have evolved to defend a plant or animal against predators. These natural toxins include some of the most poisonous compounds known. Artificial inhibitors are often used as drugs, but can also be insecticides such as malathion, herbicides such as glyphosate, or disinfectants such as triclosan. Other artificial enzyme inhibitors block acetylcholinesterase, an enzyme which breaks down acetylcholine, and are used as nerve agents in chemical warfare.

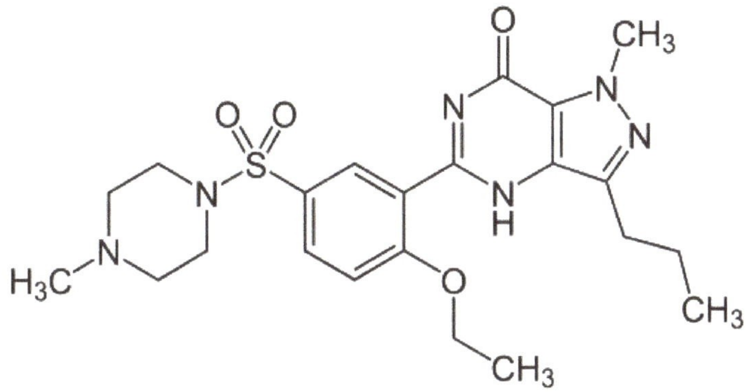

The structure of sildenafil (Viagra)

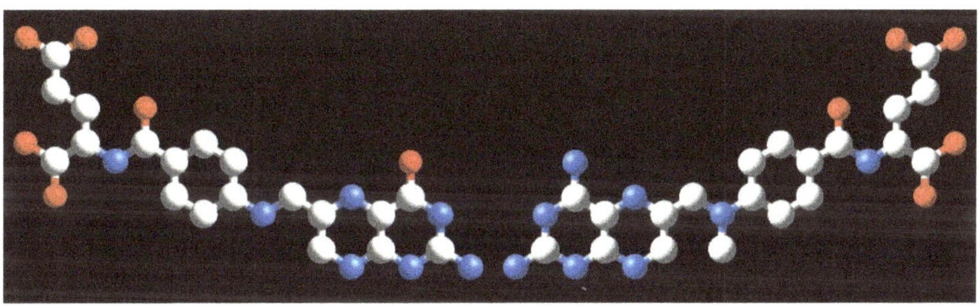

The coenzyme folic acid (left) compared to the anti-cancer drug methotrexate (right)

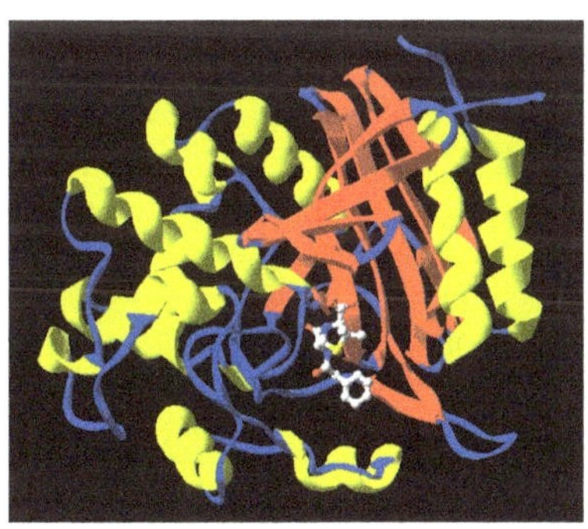

The structure of a complex between penicillin G and the Streptomyces transpeptidase. Generated from PDB 1PWC.

Chemotherapy

The most common uses for enzyme inhibitors are as drugs to treat disease. Many of these inhibitors target a human enzyme and aim to correct a pathological condition. However, not all drugs are enzyme inhibitors. Some, such as anti-epileptic drugs, alter enzyme activity by causing more or less of the enzyme to be produced. These effects are called enzyme induction and inhibition and are alterations in gene expression, which is unrelated to the type of enzyme inhibition discussed here. Other drugs interact with cellular targets that are not enzymes, such as ion channels or membrane receptors.

An example of a medicinal enzyme inhibitor is sildenafil (Viagra), a common treatment for male erectile dysfunction. This compound is a potent inhibitor of cGMP specific phosphodiesterase type 5, the enzyme that degrades the signalling molecule cyclic guanosine monophosphate. This signalling molecule triggers smooth muscle relaxation and allows blood flow into the corpus cavernosum, which causes an erection. Since the drug decreases the activity of the enzyme that halts the signal, it makes this signal last for a longer period of time.

Another example of the structural similarity of some inhibitors to the substrates of the enzymes they target is seen in the figure comparing the drug methotrexate to folic acid. Folic acid is a substrate of dihydrofolate reductase, an enzyme involved in making nucleotides that is potently inhibited by methotrexate. Methotrexate blocks the action of dihydrofolate reductase and thereby halts the production of nucleotides. This block of nucleotide biosynthesis is more toxic to rapidly growing cells than non-dividing cells, since a rapidly growing cell has to carry out DNA replication, therefore methotrexate is often used in cancer chemotherapy.

Antibiotics

Drugs also are used to inhibit enzymes needed for the survival of pathogens. For example, bacteria are surrounded by a thick cell wallmade of a net-like polymer called peptidoglycan. Many antibiotics such as penicillin and vancomycin inhibit the enzymes that produce and then cross-link the strands of this polymer together. This causes the cell wall to lose strength and the bacteria to burst. In the figure, a molecule of penicillin (shown in a ball-and-stick form) is shown bound to its target, the transpeptidase from the bacteria *Streptomyces* R61 (the protein is shown as a ribbon-diagram).

Antibiotic drug design is facilitated when an enzyme that is essential to the pathogen's survival is absent or very different in humans. In the example above, humans do not make peptidoglycan, therefore inhibitors of this process are selectively toxic to bacteria. Selective toxicity is also produced in antibiotics by exploiting differences in the structure of the ribosomes in bacteria, or how they make fatty acids.

Metabolic Control

Enzyme inhibitors are also important in metabolic control. Many metabolic pathways in the cell are inhibited by metabolites that control enzyme activity through allosteric regulation or substrate inhibition. A good example is the allosteric regulation of the glycolytic pathway. This catabolic pathway consumes glucose and produces ATP, NADH and pyruvate. A key step for the regulation of glycolysis is an early reaction in the pathway catalysed by phosphofructokinase-1 (PFK1). When ATP levels rise, ATP binds an allosteric site in PFK1 to decrease the rate of the enzyme reaction; glycolysis is inhibited and ATP production falls. This negative feedback control helps maintain a steady concentration of ATP in the cell. However, metabolic pathways are not just regulated through inhibition since enzyme activation is equally important. With respect to PFK1, fructose 2,6-bisphosphate and ADP are examples of metabolites that are allosteric activators.

Physiological enzyme inhibition can also be produced by specific protein inhibitors. This mechanism occurs in the pancreas, which synthesises many digestive precursor enzymes known as zymogens. Many of these are activated by the trypsin protease, so it is important to inhibit the activity of trypsin in the pancreas to prevent the organ from digesting itself. One way in which the activity of trypsin is controlled is the production of a specific and potent trypsin inhibitor protein in the pancreas. This inhibitor binds tightly to trypsin, preventing the trypsin activity that would otherwise be detrimental to the organ. Although the trypsin inhibitor is a protein, it avoids being hydrolysed as a substrate by the protease by excluding water from trypsin's active site and destabilising the transition state. Other examples of physiological enzyme inhibitor proteins include the barstar inhibitor of the bacterial ribonuclease barnaseand the inhibitors of protein phosphatases.

Pesticides

Many pesticides are enzyme inhibitors. Acetylcholinesterase (AChE) is an enzyme found in animals from insects to humans. It is essential to nerve cell function through its mechanism of breaking down the neurotransmitter acetylcholine into its constituents, acetate and choline. This is somewhat unique among neurotransmitters as most, including serotonin, dopamine, and norepinephrine, are absorbed from the synaptic cleft rather than cleaved. A large number of AChE inhibitors are used in both medicine and agriculture. Reversible competitive inhibitors, such as edrophonium, physostigmine, and neostigmine, are used in the treatment of myasthenia gravis and in anaesthesia. The carbamate pesticides are also examples of reversible AChE inhibitors. The organophosphate pesticides such as malathion, parathion, and chlorpyrifos irreversibly inhibit acetylcholinesterase.

The herbicide glyphosate is an inhibitor of 3-phosphoshikimate 1-carboxyvinyltransferase, other herbicides, such as the sulfonylureas inhibit the enzyme acetolactate synthase. Both these enzymes are needed for plants to make branched-chain amino acids. Many other enzymes are inhibited by herbicides, including enzymes needed for the biosynthesis of lipids and carotenoids and the processes of photosynthesis and oxidative phosphorylation.

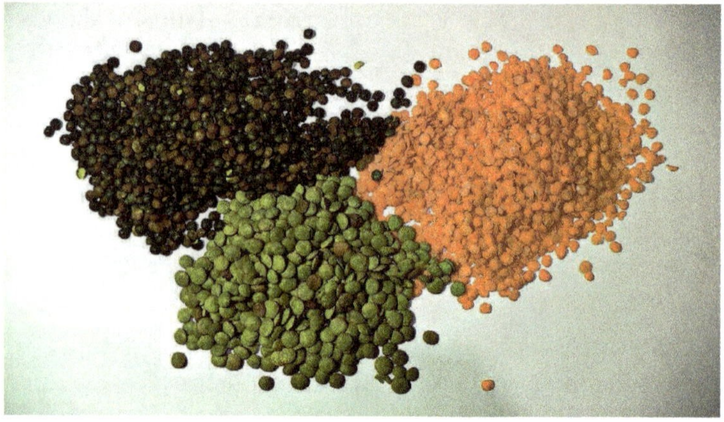

To discourage seed predators, pulses contain trypsin inhibitors that interfere with digestion.

Natural Poisons

Animals and plants have evolved to synthesize a vast array of poisonous products including secondary metabolites, peptides and proteins that can act as inhibitors. Natural toxins are usually small organic molecules and are so diverse that there are probably natural inhibitors for most metabolic processes. The metabolic processes targeted by natural poisons encompass more than enzymes in metabolic pathways and can also include the inhibition of receptor, channel and structural protein functions in a cell. For example, paclitaxel (taxol), an organic molecule found in the Pacific yew tree, binds tightly to tubulin dimers and inhibits their assembly into microtubules in the cytoskeleton.

Many natural poisons act as neurotoxins that can cause paralysis leading to death and have functions for defence against predators or in hunting and capturing prey. Some of these natural inhibitors, despite their toxic attributes, are valuable for therapeutic uses at lower doses. An example of a neurotoxin are the glycoalkaloids, from the plant species in the *Solanaceae* family (includes potato, tomato and eggplant), that are acetylcholinesterase inhibitors. Inhibition of this enzyme causes an uncontrolled increase in the acetylcholine neurotransmitter, muscular paralysis and then death. Neurotoxicity can also result from the inhibition of receptors; for example, atropine from deadly nightshade (*Atropa belladonna*) that functions as a competitive antagonist of the muscarinic acetylcholine receptors.

Although many natural toxins are secondary metabolites, these poisons also include peptides and proteins. An example of a toxic peptide is alpha-amanitin, which is found in relatives of the death cap mushroom. This is a potent enzyme inhibitor, in this case preventing the RNA polymerase II enzyme from transcribing DNA. The algal toxin microcystin is also a peptide and is an inhibitor of protein phosphatases. This toxin can contaminate water supplies after algal blooms and is a known carcinogen that can also cause acute liver hemorrhage and death at higher doses.

Proteins can also be natural poisons or antinutrients, such as the trypsin inhibitors (discussed above) that are found in some legumes, as shown in the figure above. A less common class of toxins are toxic enzymes: these act as irreversible inhibitors of their target enzymes and work by chemically modifying their substrate enzymes. An example is ricin, an extremely potent protein toxin found in castor oil beans. This enzyme is a glycosidase that inactivates ribosomes. Since ricin is a catalytic irreversible inhibitor, this allows just a single molecule of ricin to kill a cell.

LIGAND EFFICIENCY

Ligand efficiency is a measurement of the binding energy per atom of a ligand to its binding partner, such as a receptor or enzyme.

Ligand efficiency is used in drug discovery research programs to assist in narrowing focus to lead compounds with optimal combinations of physicochemical properties and pharmacological properties.

Mathematically, ligand efficiency (LE) can be defined as the ratio of Gibbs free energy (ΔG) to the number of non-hydrogen atoms of the compound:

$LE = (\Delta G)/N$

where $\Delta G = -RTlnK_i$ and N is the number of non-hydrogen atoms. It can be transformed to the equation:

$LE = 1.4(-log IC_{50})/N$

Other metrics

Some suggest that better metrics for ligand efficiency are percentage/potency efficiency index (PEI), binding efficiency index (BEI) and surface-binding efficiency index (SEI) because they are easier to calculate and take into account the differences between elements in different rows of the periodic table. It is important to note that PEI is a relative measure for comparing compounds tested in the same conditions (e.g. a single-point assay) and are not comparable at different inhibitor concentrations. Also for BEI and SEI, similar measurements must be used (e.g. always using pK_i).

PEI = (% inhibition at a given compound concentration as fraction: 0 – 1.0) / (molecular weight, kDa)

BEI = (pK_i, pK_d, or pIC_{50}) / (molecular weight, kDa)

SEI = (pK_i, pK_d, or pIC_{50}) / (PSA/100 Å)

where pK_i, pK_d and pIC_{50} is defined as $-log(K_i)$, $-log(K_d)$, or $-log(IC_{50})$, respectively. K_i and IC_{50} in mol/L.

The authors suggest plotting compounds SEI and BEI on a plane and optimizing compounds towards the diagonal and so optimizing both SEI and BEI which incorporate potency, molecular weight and PSA.

There are other metrics which can be useful during hit to lead optimization: group efficiency (GE), lipophilic efficiency/lipophilic ligand efficiency (LipE/LLE), ligand lipophilicity index (LLE_{AT}) ligand efficiency dependent lipophilicity (LELP), fit quality scaled ligand efficiency (LE_scale), size independent ligand efficiency (SILE).

REFERENCES

1. Shapiro, R; Vallee, BL (1991). "Interaction of human placental ribonuclease with placental ribonuclease inhibitor". Biochemistry. 30 (8): 2246–55. doi:10.1021/bi00222a030. PMID 1998683.
2. Berg J., Tymoczko J. and Stryer L. (2002) Biochemistry. W. H. Freeman and Company, ISBN 0-7167-4955-6.
3. Cleland WW (1963). "The kinetics of enzyme-catalyzed reactions with two or more substrates or products. II. Inhibition: nomenclature and theory". Biochim. Biophys. Acta. 67: 173–87. doi:10.1016/0926-6569(63)90226-8. PMID 14021668.
4. *Irwin H. Segel, Enzyme Kinetics : Behavior and Analysis of Rapid Equilibrium and Steady-State Enzyme Systems. Wiley–Interscience; New edition (1993), ISBN 0-471-30309-7
5. Holdgate, GA (2001). "Making cool drugs hot: isothermal titration calorimetry as a tool to study binding energetics". BioTechniques. 31 (1): 164–6, 168, 170 passim. PMID 11464510.
6. Leatherbarrow, RJ (1990). "Using linear and non-linear regression to fit biochemical data". Trends in Biochemical Sciences. 15 (12): 455–8. doi:10.1016/0968-0004(90)90295-M. PMID 2077683.
7. Tseng, SJ; Hsu, JP (1990). "A comparison of the parameter estimating procedures for the Michaelis-Menten model". Journal of Theoretical Biology. 145 (4): 457–64. doi:10.1016/S0022-5193(05)80481-3. PMID 2246896.
8. Walsh, R.; Martin, E.; Darvesh, S. (2011). "Limitations of conventional inhibitor classifications". Integrative Biology. Royal Society of Chemistry. 3 (12): 1197–1201. doi:10.1039/c1ib00053e. PMID 22038120.
9. Walsh, R.; Martin, E.; Darvesh, S. (2007). "A versatile equation to describe reversible enzyme inhibition and activation kinetics: Modeling β-galactosidase and butyrylcholinesterase. Biochimica et Biophysica Acta (BBA) - General Subjects. 1770 (5): 733–746. doi:10.1016/j.bbagen.2007.01.001. PMID 17307293.
10. Walsh, Ryan (2012). Ch. 17. Alternative Perspectives of Enzyme Kinetic Modeling. In Ekinci, Deniz. Medicinal Chemistry and Drug Design (PDF). InTech. pp. 357–371. ISBN 978-953-51-0513-8.
11. Segel, Irwin H. (1993) Enzyme Kinetics : Behavior and Analysis of Rapid Equilibrium and Steady-State Enzyme Systems. Wiley-Interscience; New edition , ISBN 0-471-30309-7.
12. Dixon, M. Webb, E.C., Thorne, C.J.R. and Tipton K.F., Enzymes (3rd edition) Longman, London (1979) p. 126
13. Hsu, JT; Wang, HC; Chen, GW; Shih, SR (2006). Antiviral drug discovery targeting to viral proteases. Current pharmaceutical design. 12 (11): 1301–14. doi:10.2174/138161206776361110. PMID 16611117.
14. Lew W, Chen X, Kim CU; Chen; Kim (2000). Discovery and development of GS 4104 (oseltamivir): an orally active influenza neuraminidase inhibitor. Curr. Med. Chem. 7 (6): 663–72. doi:10.2174/0929867003374886. PMID 10702632.

15. Fischer PM (2003). The design, synthesis and application of stereochemical and directional peptide isomers: a critical review. Curr. Protein Pept. Sci. 4 (5): 339–56. doi:10.2174/1389203033487054. PMID 14529528.

16. Bogoyevitch, MA; Barr, RK; Ketterman, AJ (2005). Peptide inhibitors of protein kinases-discovery, characterisation and use. Biochimica et Biophysica Acta. 1754 (1–2): 79–99. doi:10.1016/j.bbapap.2005.07.025. PMID 16182621.

17. Lundblad R. L. Chemical Reagents for Protein Modification CRC Press Inc (2004) ISBN 0-8493-1983-8

18. Price, N.; Hames, B. and Rickwood, D. (eds.) (1996) Proteins LabFax Academic Press, ISBN 0-12-564710-7.

19. Adam, GC; Cravatt, BF; Sorensen, EJ (2001). Profiling the specific reactivity of the proteome with non-directed activity-based probes. Chemistry & Biology. 8 (1): 81–95. doi:10.1016/S1074-5521(00)90060-7. PMID 11182321.

20. Maurer, T; Fung, HL (2000). Comparison of methods for analyzing kinetic data from mechanism-based enzyme inactivation: application to nitric oxide synthase. AAPS PharmSci. 2 (1): 68–77. doi:10.1208/ps020108. PMC 2751003Freely accessible. PMID 11741224.

21. Loo JA, DeJohn DE, Du P, Stevenson TI, Ogorzalek Loo RR; Dejohn; Du; Stevenson; Ogorzalek Loo (1999). Application of mass spectrometry for target identification and characterization. Med Res Rev. 19 (4): 307–19. doi:10.1002/(SICI)1098-1128(199907)19:4<307::AID-MED4>3.0.CO;2-2. PMID 10398927.

22. Poulin, R; Lu, L; Ackermann, B; Bey, P; Pegg, AE (1992). Mechanism of the irreversible inactivation of mouse ornithine decarboxylase by alpha-difluoromethylornithine. Characterization of sequences at the inhibitor and coenzyme binding sites. The Journal of Biological Chemistry. 267 (1): 150–8. PMID 1730582.

23. Szedlacsek, SE; Duggleby, RG (1995). Kinetics of slow and tight-binding inhibitors. Enzyme Kinetics and Mechanism Part D: Developments in Enzyme Dynamics. Methods in Enzymology. 249. pp. 144–80. doi:10.1016/0076-6879(95)49034-5. ISBN 978-0-12-182150-0. PMID 7791610.

24. Stone, SR; Morrison, JF (1986). Mechanism of inhibition of dihydrofolate reductases from bacterial and vertebrate sources by various classes of folate analogues. Biochimica et Biophysica Acta. 869 (3): 275–85. doi:10.1016/0167-4838(86)90067-1. PMID 3511964.

25. Pick, FM; McGartoll, MA; Bray, RC (1971). Reaction of formaldehyde and of methanol with xanthine oxidase. European Journal of Biochemistry / FEBS. 18 (1): 65–72. doi:10.1111/j.1432-1033.1971.tb01215.x. PMID 4322209.

26. Reardon, JE (1989). Herpes simplex virus type 1 and human DNA polymerase interactions with 2›-deoxyguanosine 5›-triphosphate analogues. Kinetics of incorporation into DNA and induction of inhibition. The Journal of Biological Chemistry. 264 (32): 19039–44. PMID 2553730.

27. Cohen, J.A.; Oosterbaan, R.A.; Berends, F. (1967). Organophosphorus compounds. Enzyme Structure. Methods in Enzymology. 11. p. 686. doi:10.1016/S0076-

6879(67)11085-9. ISBN 978-0-12-181860-9.

28. Brenner, G. M. (2000): Pharmacology. Philadelphia, PA: W.B. Saunders Company. ISBN 0-7216-7757-6

29. Saravanamuthu, A; Vickers, TJ; Bond, CS; Peterson, MR; Hunter, WN; Fairlamb, AH (2004). Two interacting binding sites for quinacrine derivatives in the active site of trypanothione reductase: a template for drug design. The Journal of Biological Chemistry. 279 (28): 29493–500. doi:10.1074/jbc.M403187200. PMC 3491871Freely accessible. PMID 15102853.

30. Koppitz M, Eis K; Eis (2006). Automated medicinal chemistry. Drug Discov. Today. 11 (11–12): 561–8. doi:10.1016/j.drudis.2006.04.005. PMID 16713909.

31. Scapin G (2006). Structural biology and drug discovery. Curr. Pharm. Des. 12 (17): 2087–97. doi:10.2174/138161206777585201. PMID 16796557.

32. Gohlke H, Klebe G; Klebe (August 2002). Approaches to the description and prediction of the binding affinity of small-molecule ligands to macromolecular receptors. Angew. Chem. Int. Ed. Engl. 41 (15): 2644–76. doi:10.1002/1521-3773(20020802)41:15<2644::AID-ANIE2644>3.0.CO;2-O. PMID 12203463.

33. Glen RC, Allen SC; Allen (May 2003). Ligand-protein docking: cancer research at the interface between biology and chemistry. Curr. Med. Chem. 10 (9): 763–7. doi:10.2174/0929867033457809. PMID 12678780.

34. Maggi, M; Filippi, S; Ledda, F; Magini, A; Forti, G (2000). Erectile dysfunction: from biochemical pharmacology to advances in medical therapy. European Journal of Endocrinology. Bioscientifica. 143 (2): 143–54. doi:10.1530/eje.0.1430143. PMID 10913932.

35. McGuire, JJ (2003). Anticancer antifolates: current status and future directions. Current pharmaceutical design. 9 (31): 2593–613. doi:10.2174/1381612033453712. PMID 14529544.

36. Katz, AH; Caufield, CE (2003). Structure-based design approaches to cell wall biosynthesis inhibitors. Current pharmaceutical design. 9 (11): 857–66. doi:10.2174/1381612033455305. PMID 12678870.

37. Okar, DA; Lange, AJ (1999). Fructose-2,6-bisphosphate and control of carbohydrate metabolism in eukaryotes. BioFactors (Oxford, England). 10 (1): 1–14. doi:10.1002/biof.5520100101. PMID 10475585.

38. Price, Nicholas and Stevens, Lewis (1999) Fundamentals of Enzymology, Oxford University Press, ISBN 0-19-850229-X.

39. Smyth, TP (2004). Substrate variants versus transition state analogues as noncovalent reversible enzyme inhibitors. Bioorganic & Medicinal Chemistry. 12 (15): 4081–8. doi:10.1016/j.bmc.2004.05.041. PMID 15246086.

40. Hartley, RW (1989). Barnase and barstar: two small proteins to fold and fit together. Trends in Biochemical Sciences. 14 (11): 450–4. doi:10.1016/0968-0004(89)90104-7. PMID 2696173.

41. Oliver, CJ; Shenolikar, S (1998). Physiologic importance of protein phosphatase inhibitors. Frontiers in Bioscience. 3: D961–72. PMID 9727084.

42. Tan S, Evans R, Singh B; Evans; Singh (March 2006). Herbicidal inhibitors of amino acid biosynthesis and herbicide-tolerant crops. Amino Acids. 30 (2): 195–204. doi:10.1007/s00726-005-0254-1. PMID 16547651.

43. Duke SO (1990). Overview of herbicide mechanisms of action. Environ. Health Perspect. Brogan &#38. 87: 263–71. doi:10.2307/3431034. JSTOR 3431034. PMC 1567841Freely accessible. PMID 1980104.

44. Tan, G; Gyllenhaal, C; Soejarto, DD (2006). Biodiversity as a source of anticancer drugs. Current drug targets. 7 (3): 265–77. doi:10.2174/138945006776054942. PMID 16515527.

45. Abal, M; Andreu, JM; Barasoain, I (2003). Taxanes: microtubule and centrosome targets, and cell cycle dependent mechanisms of action. Current cancer drug targets. 3 (3): 193–203. doi:10.2174/1568009033481967. PMID 12769688.

46. Hostettmann, K.; Borloz, A.; Urbain, A.; Marston, A. (2006). Natural Product Inhibitors of Acetylcholinesterase. Current Organic Chemistry. 10 (8): 825–847. doi:10.2174/138527206776894410.

47. Defrates, LJ; Hoehns, JD; Sakornbut, EL; Glascock, DG; Tew, AR (2005). Antimuscarinic intoxication resulting from the ingestion of moonflower seeds. The Annals of pharmacotherapy. 39 (1): 173–6. doi:10.1345/aph.1D536. PMID 15572604.

48. Vetter, J (1998). Toxins of Amanita phalloides. Toxicon. 36 (1): 13–24. doi:10.1016/S0041-0101(97)00074-3. PMID 9604278.

49. Holmes, CF; Maynes, JT; Perreault, KR; Dawson, JF; James, MN (2002). Molecular enzymology underlying regulation of protein phosphatase-1 by natural toxins. Current medicinal chemistry. 9 (22): 1981–9. doi:10.2174/0929867023368827. PMID 12369866.

50. Bischoff, K (2001). The toxicology of microcystin-LR: occurrence, toxicokinetics, toxicodynamics, diagnosis and treatment. Veterinary and human toxicology. 43 (5): 294–7. PMID 11577938.

51. Hartley, MR; Lord, JM (2004). Cytotoxic ribosome-inactivating lectins from plants. Biochimica et Biophysica Acta. 1701 (1–2): 1–14. doi:10.1016/j.bbapap.2004.06.004. PMID 15450171.

52. I. D. Kuntz; K. Chen; K. A. Sharp; P. A. Kollman (1999). The maximal affinity of ligands. Proc Natl Acad Sci U S A. 96 (18): 9997–10002. Bibcode:1999PNAS...96.9997K. doi:10.1073/pnas.96.18.9997. PMC 17830Freely accessible. PMID 10468550.

53. Abadzapatero, C; Metz, J (2005). Ligand efficiency indices as guideposts for drug discovery. Drug Discovery Today. 10 (7): 464–469. doi:10.1016/S1359-6446(05)03386-6. PMID 15809192.

54. Hopkins, Andrew L.; Groom, Colin R.; Alex, Alexander (2004). Ligand efficiency: A useful metric for lead selection. Drug Discovery Today. 9 (10): 430–431. doi:10.1016/S1359-6446(04)03069-7. PMID 15109945.

55. Shultz, Michael D. (2013). Setting expectations in molecular optimizations: strengths and limitations of commonly used composite parameters. Bioorganic & Medicinal Chemistry Letters. 23 (21): 5980–91. doi:10.1016/j.bmcl.2013.08.029. PMID 24018190.

Index